# Caregiving
Research • Practice • Policy

Ronda C. Talley, Series Editor

An official publication of
The Rosalynn Carter Institute for Caregiving

For further volumes:
http://www.springer.com/series/8274

# Editorial Board

**Peter S. Arno, Ph.D.**
School of Health Sciences and Practice, New York Medical College, Valhalla, NY, USA

**Brenda Yvonne Cartwright, Ph.D.**
University of Hawaii at Manoa, Honolulu, HI, USA

**Gilbert Cleeton, Ph.D.**
Walden University, Baltimore, MD, USA

**Michael D'Andrea, EdD**
University of Hawaii at Manoa, Honolulu, HI, USA

**Pam Doty, Ph.D.**
U.S. Department of Health and Human Services, Washington, USA

**Dothel W. Edwards, Jr., Rh.D., CRC, CLCP**
Alabama State University, Montgomery, AL, USA

**Clayton W. Faubion, Ph.D., CRC**
University of Maryland Eastern Shore, Princess Anne, MD, USA

**Alan Goldberg, PsyD, JD, ABPP**
Private Practice Psychology & Disability Law, Tuscon, AZ, USA

**Martin H. Greenberg, MD**
American Academy of Pediatrics, Savannah, GA, USA

**Andy Imperato**
American Association of People with Disabilities, Washington, DC, USA

**Kathryn Pekala Service, MSN, RNC, NP, CDDN**
Massachusetts Office of Health and Human Services, Northampton, MA, USA

**Henry Kautz, Ph.D.**
University of Rochester, Rochester, NY, USA

**Madan M. Kundu, Ph.D., FNRCA, CRC, NCC, LRC**
Southern University, Baton Rouge, LA, USA

**Donald Lollar, EdD**
Oregon Health & Science University, Portland, OR, USA

**James F. Malec, Ph.D., LP, ABPP-Cn, Rp**
Indiana University School of Medicine, Indianapolis, IN, USA

**Susan Palmer Mazrui, MA**
Federal Regulatory Affairs, AT&T, Washington, DC, USA

**Nancy A. Miller, Ph.D.**
University of Maryland Baltimore County, Baltimore, MD, USA

**Jan C. Orleck, LCSW, CCM**
Private Practice, Humana Military Health Services, Louisville, KY, USA

**Randolph B. Pipes, Ph.D.**
Auburn University, Auburn, AL, USA

**Lilliam Rangel-Diaz, CLA**
Center for Education Advocacy, Inc., Former Clinton Presidential Appointee, Board of Directors National Council on Disability, Miami, FL, USA

**Marcia J. Scherer, Ph.D., MPH, FACRM**
University of Rochester Medical Center, Webster, NY, USA

**Deborah M. Spitalnik, Ph.D.**
Elizabeth M. Boggs Center on Developmental Disabilities, New Brunswick, NJ, USA

**William B. Talley, Rh.D., CRC**
University of Maryland Eastern Shore, Princess Anne, MD, USA

**Patricia Walker-Hinton, Ph.D., RN, FAAN**
Uniformed Services University of the Health Sciences, Bethesda, MD, USA

**Peggy Wittman, EdD, OTR, FAOTA**
Eastern Kentucky University, Richmond, KY, USA

**Theda Zawaiza, Ph.D.**
Office of Elementary and Secondary Education, Organizational Structure and Offices, Washington, DC, USA

Ronda C. Talley • John E. Crews
Editors

# Multiple Dimensions of Caregiving and Disability

Research, Practice, Policy

Springer

*Editors*
Ronda C. Talley, PhD, MPH
Western Kentucky University
Bowling Green, KY, USA

John E. Crews, DPA
Div. Diabetes Translation
Vision Health Initiative (VHI)
Centers for Disease Control & Prevention
Atlanta, GA, USA

ISSN 2192-340X
ISSN 2192-3418 (Electronic)
ISBN 978-1-4614-3383-5
ISBN 978-1-4614-3384-2 (eBook)
DOI 10.1007/978-1-4614-3384-2
Springer New York Dordrecht Heidelberg London

Library of Congress Control Number: 2012940532

© Springer Science+Business Media New York 2012
This work is subject to copyright. All rights are reserved by the Publisher, whether the whole or part of the material is concerned, specifically the rights of translation, reprinting, reuse of illustrations, recitation, broadcasting, reproduction on microfilms or in any other physical way, and transmission or information storage and retrieval, electronic adaptation, computer software, or by similar or dissimilar methodology now known or hereafter developed. Exempted from this legal reservation are brief excerpts in connection with reviews or scholarly analysis or material supplied specifically for the purpose of being entered and executed on a computer system, for exclusive use by the purchaser of the work. Duplication of this publication or parts thereof is permitted only under the provisions of the Copyright Law of the Publisher's location, in its current version, and permission for use must always be obtained from Springer. Permissions for use may be obtained through RightsLink at the Copyright Clearance Center. Violations are liable to prosecution under the respective Copyright Law.
The use of general descriptive names, registered names, trademarks, service marks, etc. in this publication does not imply, even in the absence of a specific statement, that such names are exempt from the relevant protective laws and regulations and therefore free for general use.
While the advice and information in this book are believed to be true and accurate at the date of publication, neither the authors nor the editors nor the publisher can accept any legal responsibility for any errors or omissions that may be made. The publisher makes no warranty, express or implied, with respect to the material contained herein.

Printed on acid-free paper

Springer is part of Springer Science+Business Media (www.springer.com)

*To my mother, Ronda McCoy Talley, who educated hundreds of children with special needs. Using her intuition of children's needs and her skills as a master teacher, she taught children who others said could not learn. With her gentle and generous spirit, she showed compassion while bringing forth the best in each student who walked through her classroom door.*
Ronda C. Talley

*To Nancy, Kate, and Ripsi*
John E. Crews

# Foreword

From its inception in 1987, the Rosalynn Carter Institute for Caregiving (RCI) has sought to bring attention to the extraordinary contributions made by caregivers to their loved ones. I grew up in a home that was regularly transformed into a caregiving household when members of my family became seriously ill, disabled or frail with age, so my interest in the issue is personal. In my hometown of Plains, Georgia, as in most communities across our country, it was expected that family members and neighbors would take on the responsibility of providing care whenever illness struck close to home. Delivering such care with the love, respect, and attention it deserves is both labor intensive and personally demanding. Those who do so represent one of this nation's most significant yet underappreciated assets in our health delivery system.

When the RCI began, "caregiving" was found nowhere in the nation's health lexicon. Its existence was not a secret but rather simply accepted as a fact of life. In deciding on the direction and priorities of the new institute, we convened groups of family and professional caregivers from around the region to tell their personal stories. As I listened to neighbors describe caring for aged and/or chronically ill or disabled family members, I recognized that their experiences reflected mine. They testified that, while caregiving for them was full of personal meaning and significance and could be extremely rewarding, it could also be fraught with anxiety, stress, and feelings of isolation. Many felt unprepared and most were overwhelmed at times. A critical issue in the "field" of caregiving, I realized, was the need to better understand the kinds of policies and programs necessary to support those who quietly and consistently care for loved ones.

With the aging of America's Baby Boomers expecting to double the elderly population in the next 20 years, deinstitutionalization of individuals with chronic mental illnesses and developmental disabilities, a rising percentage of women in the workforce, smaller and more dispersed families, changes in the role of hospitals, and a range of other factors, caregiving has become one of the most significant issues of our time. Caregiving as an area of research, as a focus and concern of policy-making, and as an area of professional training and practice has reached a new and unparalleled level of importance in our society and indeed globally.

As we survey the field of caregiving today, we now recognize that it is an essential component of long-term care in the community, yet also a potential health risk for those who provide care. The basic features of a public health approach have emerged: a focus on populations of caregivers and recipients, tracking and surveillance of health risks, understanding the factors associated with risk status, and the development and testing of the effectiveness of various interventions to maximize benefits for both the recipients of care and their providers.

The accumulated wisdom from this work is represented in the volumes that make up the Springer Caregiving Series. This series presents a broad portrait of the nature of caregiving in the United States in the twenty-first century. Most Americans have been, are now, or will be caregivers. With our society's increasing demands for care, we cannot expect a high quality of life for our seniors and others living with limitations due to illness or disability unless we understand and support the work of caregivers. Without thoughtful planning, intelligent policies, and sensitive interventions, there is the risk that the work of family, paraprofessional, and professional caregivers will become intolerably difficult and burdensome. We cannot let this happen.

This volume examines the breadth and depth of caregiving. Readers will gain an appreciation of the fact that caregiving represents a process that occurs across the life span of those who need care and, in many respects, across the life span of those who provide it. Caregiving is received as well as provided by the young and the old; those involved represent all races, genders, and economic groups. Its complexity is reflected across four broad areas: (1) the characteristics, demands, and trends pertaining to caregivers and care recipients; (2) the practice of professionals who serve caregivers; (3) the public policies that support caregivers; and (4) the relationship between the quality of life of the caregiver and the care recipient. The structure of this volume provides readers with insights into each of these issues.

Readers of this series will find hope and evidence that improved support for family and professional caregivers lies within our reach. The field of caregiving has matured and, as evidenced in these volumes, has generated rigorous and practical research findings to guide effective and enlightened policy and program options. My hope is that these volumes will play an important role in documenting the research base, guiding practice, and moving our nation toward effective polices to support all of America's caregivers.

Rosalynn Carter

# Contents

1 Introduction: Multiple Dimensions of Caregiving and Disability ..... 1
John E. Crews and Ronda C. Talley

2 Family Dynamics and Caregiving for People with Disabilities ....... 11
Susan H. McDaniel and Anthony R. Pisani

3 Feelings of Family Caregivers ..................................... 29
Yvette Getch

4 Education, Training, and Support Programs for Caregivers
of Individuals with Disabilities.................................. 45
Sharon Goldsmith

5 Parent Caregivers of Children with Disabilities .................... 67
Karen Kuhlthau

6 Neither Prepared Nor Rehearsed: The Role of Public Health
in Disability and Caregiving ...................................... 83
John E. Crews

7 Race/Ethnicity, Culture, and Socioeconomic Status and Caregiving
of Persons with Disabilities ...................................... 99
Paul Leung

8 Faith and Spirituality: Supporting Caregivers of Individuals
with Disabilities ................................................. 117
William Gaventa

9 Family Caregivers and Health Care Providers:
Developing Partnerships for a Continuum of Care and Support ..... 135
Timothy R. Elliott and Michael Parker

10 Legal Issues Related to Caregiving for an Individual with Disabilities 153
Frank G. Bowe

**11 Long-Term Care Planning for Individuals with
Developmental Disabilities** .................................... 169
Deborah Viola and Peter S. Arno

**12 Emerging Technologies for Caregivers of a Person with a Disability**  185
Margo B. Holm and Ketki D. Raina

**13 Multiple Dimensions of Caregiving and Disability:
Supporting Those Who Care** .................................. 209
Ronda C. Talley and John E. Crews

**Index** ..................................................... 215

# About the Editors

**John E. Crews, DPA** is a Health Scientist with the Vision Health Initiative in the Division of Diabetes Translation, National Center for Health Promotion and Disease Prevention, Centers for Disease Control and Prevention.

Dr. Crews has over thirty years of experience in vision rehabilitation and disability research. He managed a clinical program for older people with visual impairments in Michigan between 1977 and 1992. He then became the Acting Director of the Rehabilitation Research and Development Center on Aging at the Department of Veterans Affairs in Atlanta. After that, he served as the Executive Director of the Georgia Governor's Council on Developmental Disabilities. In 1998, he joined the Centers for Disease Control and Prevention in Atlanta. Dr. Crews' specialties are vision impairment and aging and caregiving and disability; his research interests also include health disparities among people with disabilities and aging with a disability.

Dr. Crews has over eighty publications, including recent papers in the *American Journal of Public Health* and the *Annual Review of Public Health*. His first book, *Vision Loss in an Aging Society*, was published in 2000; it was translated and published in Japan in 2003. He has entries in the *Encyclopedia of Disability* and the *International Encyclopedia of Public Health*. He currently serves on the Editorial Board of the *Journal of Visual Impairment and Blindness,* and he serves on the National Commission on Vision and Health. He was awarded the 2007 Distinguished Alumni Award from Western Michigan University.

He may be reached by mail at 4770 Buford Highway, NE, K-10, Atlanta, GA 30341; by telephone at (770) 488-1116; or via e-mail at jcrews@cdc.gov.

**Ronda C. Talley, PhD, MPH** is Professor of Psychology at Western Kentucky University. Her prior work experience includes providing leadership on caregiving issues and organizational development as Executive Director of the Rosalynn Carter Institute for Caregiving and the National Quality Caregiving Coalition; working with national government groups to promote caregiving issues as Associate Director of Legislation, Policy, and Planning/Health Scientist for the Centers for Disease Control and Prevention, U.S. Department of Health and Human Services; and promoting the science and practice of psychology in the schools as Associate Executive Director of Education and Director of School Policy and Practice at the American Psychological

Association. She chaired the National Organization of Pupil Services Organizations and the National Education Goals Panel Committee on Safe and Drug-free Schools. Dr. Talley has more than 80 presentations and publications, including papers in the *American Journal of Public Health* and *American Psychologist.*

Dr. Talley as Adjunct Associate Professor, taught ethics and legal issues in school psychology at the University of Maryland, College Park, and directed the School Psychology Program at Spalding University; she was Professor of Psychology and Education at Georgia Southwestern State University for 5 years. Dr. Talley directed the School Psychological Services Program in the Jefferson County (KY) Public Schools for a decade. She received the Outstanding Alumni Award from Indiana University and the Jack Bardon Distinguished Service Award from the Division of School Psychology of the American Psychological Association. Dr. Talley serves on the national board of the American Association of Caregiving Youth and is Editor-in-Chief of the Springer book series *Caregiving: Research, Practice, and Policy.* She may be reached at 1906 College Heights Boulevard, GRH 3023, Bowling Green, KY 42101; by telephone at (270) 745-2780; or via e-mail at Ronda.Talley@wku.edu.

# Contributors

**Peter S. Arno, Ph.D.** an economist is Professor and Director of the Doctoral Program in Health Policy and Management at New York Medical College. Dr. Arno's recent work includes studies of regulation and pricing practices of the pharmaceutical industry; the economics of informal caregiving and long-term care; public health and legal implications of regulating tobacco as a drug; innovation, access, quality, and outcome measures related to HIV disease; and the impact of income support policies on health. Based on this work, Dr. Arno is coauthor of *Against the Odds: The Story of AIDS Drug Development, Politics & Profits*, nominated for a Pulitzer Prize. He has testified before numerous U.S. House and Senate committees. Dr. Arno can be reached at Department of Health Policy & Management, School of Health Sciences and Practice, New York Medical College; by telephone at (914) 594-4855, or via e-mail at peter_arno@nymc.edu.

**Frank G. Bowe, Ph.D. LLD** (deceased) was the Dr. Mervin Livingston Schloss Distinguished Professor at Hofstra University, where he taught special education, rehabilitation, and technology courses. During his career, Dr. Bowe was an advocate for individuals with disabilities and worked from 1975 with the U.S. Senate, the U.S. House of Representatives, and the White House. Over the past quarter century, he held positions with Congress and with the Executive Branch, including regional commissioner for RSA and director of research for the U.S. Access Board.

**Timothy R. Elliott, Ph.D. ABPP** is Professor in the Department of Educational Psychology at Texas A&M University. His research has examined adjustment processes among persons living with chronic and disabling health conditions, with particular emphasis on the role of social problem-solving abilities in adjustment. This work has resulted in more than 200 professional publications and continued federal funding for 15 years. His current work has focused on the development and study of problem-solving interventions for family caregivers of persons with severe disabilities. Dr. Elliott served as coeditor of the first edition of the *Handbook of Rehabilitation Psychology* (2000). In 2006, he was featured in the instructional DVD, *Caregiving*, as part of the Psychotherapy Video/DVD Series on Relationships published by American Psychological Association and subsequently served on the APA Presidential Task Force on Caregiving. He is Editor-in-Chief of the *Journal of Clinical Psychology*.

Dr. Elliott can be reached at 4225 TAMU, Texas A&M University, College Station, TX 77845; by telephone at (979) 862-3095; or via e-mail at telliott@tamu.edu.

**William Gaventa, MDiv** is Director of Community and Congregational Supports at the Elizabeth M. Boggs Center on Developmental Disabilities and Associate Professor, UMDNJ-Robert Wood Johnson Medical School. In his role at The Boggs Center, Gaventa works on community supports, training for community services staff, inclusive spiritual and religious supports, cultural competency, aging/end of life and grief, and supervision of a program in Clinical Pastoral Education. Gaventa served as Editor of the *Journal of Religion, Disability, and Health* for 14 years, and is now Associate Editor on *Intellectual and Development Disabilities*. He has served as Executive Secretary for the Religion and Spirituality Division of the AAIDD since 1985 and is co-coordinator for the AUCD Special Interest Group on Spiritual Supports. Gaventa coordinates a Faith Community Leadership project focused on clergy and seminarians in Pennsylvania, funded by the Pennsylvania Developmental Disabilities Council. He can be reached at The Boggs Center, P.O. Box 2688, New Brunswick, NJ 08903-2688; by telephone at (732) 235-9304; or via e-mail at bill.gaventa@umdnj.edu.

**Yvette Getch, Ph.D.** is Associate Professor in the Department of Counseling and Human Development Services at the University of Georgia. A Certified Rehabilitation Counselor, she conducts research in the areas of advocacy for persons with disabilities, sexuality and deafness, advocacy issues and accommodations for children with chronic illness in schools, and teacher education in asthma management. Dr. Getch can be reached at the University of Georgia, Department of Counseling and Human Development Services, 402 Aderhold Hall, Athens, GA 30602; by telephone at (706) 542-1685; or via e-mail at ygetch@uga.edu.

**Sharon Goldsmith, Ph.D.** is an internationally recognized expert on standards development, certification, and accreditation. She has held several academic appointments and authored more than 100 articles and papers. She was a 2003 recipient of the Distinguished Service Award from the American National Standards Institute (ANSI) in recognition of her leadership in international standards, accreditation, and certification. Dr. Goldsmith holds two masters degrees. She earned her Ph.D. in psycholinguistics from the Graduate School and University Center of the City University of New York. She may be reached at Goldsmith Associates International, 4064 Mansion Drive NW, Suite 100, Washington, DC 20007; by telephone at (202) 785-8940; or via e-mail at goldsmith99@msn.com.

**Margo Holm, Ph.D. OTR/L FAOTA ABDA** is Professor and Director of Post-Professional Education in the Occupational Therapy Department, School of Health and Rehabilitation Sciences, University of Pittsburgh with secondary appointments in the Clinical and Translational Science Institute and the McGowan Institute for Regenerative Medicine. Her research efforts primarily focus on functional outcomes of medical, psychiatric, and rehabilitation interventions utilizing the International Classification of Functioning, Disability and Health as a model to reflect the impact

Contributors xvii

of the continuum from disease/disorders/conditions to a state of health, in everyday functioning. Additional interests for Dr. Holm include evidence-based practice. Dr. Holm can be reached at 5012 Forbes Tower, University of Pittsburgh, Pittsburgh, PA 15260; by telephone at (412) 383-6615; or via e-mail at mbholm@pitt.edu.

**Karen Kuhlthau, Ph.D.** is Associate Professor of Pediatrics in the Department of Pediatrics at Massachusetts General Hospital. Trained as a sociologist and demographer, her research has examined the predictors and patterns of health services utilization for children and adolescents. This work includes studies of specialized therapies, high-cost children, and use of subspecialists and has led to several publications on aspects of managed care for children with chronic conditions, patterns of care for Medicaid-insured children with chronic conditions, and clinical characteristics of high-cost children insured by Medicaid. Most recently, Dr. Kuhlthau's work has focused on understanding how children, especially children with chronic conditions, affect families including examining the employment and well-being of parents and how public and employment policies assist families. She can be reached at Center for Child and Adolescent Health Research and Policy, Massachusetts General Hospital, 100 Cambridge Street, 15th Floor, Boston, MA 02114; by telephone at (617) 726-1885; or via e-mail at kkuhlthau@partners.org.

**Paul Leung, Ph.D.** is Professor in the Department of Rehabilitation, Social Work, and Addictions at the University of North Texas. He has held academic and administrative appointments at Deakin University (Melbourne, Australia), the University of Illinois at Urbana/Champaign, the University of North Carolina at Chapel Hill, and the University of Arizona. His interests include disability/rehabilitation from a multicultural perspective. He may be reached at P.O. Box 311456, UNT, Denton, TX 76203; by telephone at (940) 369-7939; or via e-mail at pleung@unt.edu.

**Susan H. McDaniel, Ph.D. ABPP** a family psychologist, is the Dr. Laurie Sands Distinguished Professor of Psychiatry and Family Medicine, Director of the Institute for the Family in Psychiatry, and Associate Chair of Family Medicine at the University of Rochester School of Medicine & Dentistry. She is known for her publications in the areas of behavioral health and primary care, genetic conditions and family dynamics, and doctor–patient communication. Dr. McDaniel is a member of the American Psychological Association Leadership Institute for Women in Psychology. She has published 85 peer-reviewed journal articles and coauthored or coedited 12 books. In 2012, Dr. McDaniel received a 2011 Elizabeth Hurlock Beckman Award, which recognizes educators in psychology, medicine, and law who have inspired a student or students to create an organization which has demonstrably benefited the community at large. Dr. McDaniel can be reached at University of Rochester, School of Medicine and Dentistry, 601 Elmwood Ave, Box PSYCH, Rochester, NY 14642; via telephone at (585) 275-URMC; or by e-mail at susanh2_mcdaniel@urmc.rochester.edu.

**Michael Parker, DSW, BCD,** is Associate Professor with the School of Social Work and serves as Board Member with Center for Mental Health and Aging, the University of Alabama, Tuscaloosa, AL. He holds an adjunct faculty appointment with the University of Alabama at Birmingham (UAB), Division of Gerontology and Geriatric

Medicine. Dr. Parker is a coinvestigator on an NIA-funded UAB Mobility study and was selected as a John A. Hartford Geriatric Scholar. Dr. Parker can be contacted at the University of Alabama School of Social Work, Box 870314, Tuscaloosa, AL 35487-0314; by telephone at (205) 348-7027; or via e-mail at mwparker@sw.ua.edu.

**Anthony R. Pisani, Ph.D.** is Assistant Professor of Psychiatry and Pediatrics and Clinical Translational Science Institute KL2 Scholar at the University of Rochester Medical Center. Dr. Pisani developed and tested *Commitment to Living: Understanding and Responding to Suicide Risk* (CTL), a suicide risk management curriculum that prepares mental health professionals and service agencies to competently and compassionately meet the needs of individuals at risk for suicide. He has published articles about clinician education and suicide prevention, including a definitive review describing the current state of workshop education in the assessment and management of suicide risk. Dr. Pisani can be reached at University of Rochester, School of Medicine and Dentistry, 601 Elmwood Ave, Box PSYCH, Rochester, New York 14642; by telephone at (585) 275-3644; or via e-mail at anthony_pisani@urmc.rochester.edu.

**Ketki D. Raina, Ph.D. OTR/L** is Assistant Professor in the School of Health and Rehabilitation Sciences at University of Pittsburgh. Her research interests include cardiopulmonary diseases, late-life depression, and evidence-based practice. Dr. Raina can be reached at University of Pittsburgh, 5018 Forbes Tower, Pittsburgh, PA 15260; by telephone at (412) 383-6614; or via e-mail at kraina@pitt.edu.

**Deborah Viola, Ph.D.** is Associate Professor of Public Health Practice at New York Medical College. Dr. Viola's research interests include regional health care planning, the impact of preconception on adverse birth outcomes, the economics of women as they age, long-term care for the developmentally disabled, emergency preparedness for vulnerable populations, and the impact of income support policies on population health. Dr. Voila can be reached at Department of Health Policy and Management, School of Health Sciences and Practice, Valhalla, NY 10595; by telephone at (914) 594-4855; or via e-mail at deborah_viola@nymc.edu.

# Chapter 1
# Introduction: Multiple Dimensions of Caregiving and Disability

**John E. Crews and Ronda C. Talley**

Many years ago, my wife, Nancy, and my daughter, Kate, and I moved to Atlanta, Georgia, from Michigan. Kate had belonged to the Girl Scouts in Michigan, and she joined a small troop in Atlanta once we got settled into our new home. She was about 11 then. Unlike in Michigan, Girl Scouts in Georgia not only sold cookies door-to-door but also set up stands at grocery stores.

One crisp October Saturday, Kate and her troop were stationed outside the local Kroger with stacks of unsold Do-si-dos®, Thin Mints, and Caramel deLites. Nancy and I took a seat in the grocery's deli and observed the proceedings from inside.

There was an old man, about 75, who was working as a bagger, and he helped carry groceries to customers' cars. As he walked by, he acknowledged Kate, and with each trip he engaged her more. First, he spoke to her, then he bought a box of cookies, and then he began directing shoppers to buy from the girls. This went on all morning, and the mountains of cookies declined remarkably.

At about noon, we stepped outside, and this old man came up to us and asked, "Are you that little girl's parents?"

"Yes," we replied.

He made a few general remarks complimenting her, and then he said, "I have a little girl who uses a wheelchair, too."

Nancy asked, "How old is your little girl?"

He replied, "She's 46 years old."

We then had one of those remarkably candid and honest conversations—the kind that only people with great shared experiences can have. He told us that he and his wife were having difficulty lifting their daughter, and he explained that baths were especially hard. He said he was just getting old, and he did not know how much longer he could lift her into bed. Then he said, "I only hope that I live one day longer than my daughter."

We were silent.

I never got the old man's name. I have no idea what happened to him or his family. But I think about him often. Each of us, however, could reconstruct that family's story. The old man was not out bagging groceries on a Saturday morning because he wanted something to do; he

J. E. Crews (✉)
Division of Diabetes Translation, Centers for Disease Control and Prevention,
4770 Buford Highway, NE, K-10, Atlanta, GA 30341, USA
e-mail: jcrews@cdc.gov

R. C. Talley (✉)
Western Kentucky University, College Heights Boulevard 1906,
Bowling Green, KY 42101, USA
e-mail: Ronda.Talley@wku.edu

probably needed the money. His daughter would have been born about 1946, when the only choice was to stay at home with absolutely no services or to live in the Milledgeville State Home. His daughter would have been 30 when the Individuals with Disabilities Education Act (IDEA) passed. There were no public school opportunities, and when the time came for her to move into the community, there were no community supports. So, in fact, there were no choices.

The power of this story is that we all can relate to it. While progress has been made over the past 50 years to develop support programs and services for people with disabilities and their families, an immense gulf remains.

For this old man, his wife, and their daughter, caregiving pretty much defined each of their lives. Caregiving, in this case, had lasted decades with no particular good resolution in sight. The intensity of caregiving was great. Transferring, toileting, bathing, and dressing someone with severe disabilities represent demanding physical work and taxing emotional stress.

This story—while perhaps unusual in terms of intensity and duration—serves as a paradigm for the purpose and structure of this book. We really do not need more detail to fill in the relevance of this family's experiences to inform practices and public policies associated with caregiving in the early twenty-first century.

## Definitions

For purposes of consistency throughout this book, several concepts will be defined here. First, *disability*, for our purposes, is defined as mobility, sensory, intellectual, or mental impairments that lead to activity limitations. While individuals can be born with or become disabled for many reasons, we will focus on issues related to their care rather than the cause or type of disability. Our rationale stems from the knowledge that caregivers have common needs regardless of the disability name or genesis.

There are several definitions of *caregiving*. To define caregiving, we turn to several of the well-known caregiving researchers and advocacy groups. The National Alliance for Caregiving (NAC) and AARP (2004, 2009) define caregiving as "caring for an adult family member or friend." A second definition of caregiving, promoted by the National Family Caregivers Association (NFCA), is "offering the necessary physical and mental health support to care for a family member." Among the descriptions of informal or family caregiving, one that has been widely accepted over time was offered in 1985 by Horowitz, who indicated that informal care involves four dimensions: *direct care* (helping to dress, managing medications), *emotional care* (i.e., providing social support and encouragement), *mediation care* (i.e., negotiating with others on behalf of the care receiver), and *financial care* (i.e., through managing fiscal resources, including gifts or service purchases; Horowitz 1985). The challenges of actually providing informal or family caregiving have been attributed to the level of intensity and physical intimacy required to provide care (Montgomery et al. 1985); the amount of burden, distress, and role strain that care engenders for the caregiver (Aneshensel et al. 1993; Berg-Weger et al. 2001; Seltzer and Li 2000); and the skill required to master care tasks (Schumacher et al. 2000).

Relatedly, the U.S. Department of Health and Human Services, Office on Women's Health (2008) defines a *caregiver* as "anyone who provides assistance to another in need." MetLife and NAC (2006) expand on this by offering additional qualifiers; they state that a family caregiver is "a person who cares for relatives and loved ones who are frail, elderly, or who have a physical or mental disability." Similarly, the National Family Caregivers Association (NFCA 2012) adds that family caregivers provide a vast array of emotional, financial, nursing, social, homemaking, and other services on a daily or intermittent basis. The NFCA advocates for the term *family caregiver* to be defined broadly to include friends and neighbors who assist with care by providing respite, running errands, or a whole host of other tasks that support the caregiver and care recipient. In this volume, we will use the terms *informal caregiver* and *family caregiver* interchangeably and employ the comprehensive definition of *family caregiver* that refers to caring relatives, friends, and neighbors.

One other point is worthy of note. We view caregiving as a process that occurs across the life span. It begins with infant care; progresses to child and adolescent care; changes, but continues as we enter adulthood and midlife; and may conclude with end-of-life care. When we look at caregiving across the continuum of life, it becomes easy to see why it is an issue that involves all people, people without disabilities, people with disabilities, the young and the old, regardless of race, gender, or socioeconomic status. Caregiving is an activity in which we will all engage at some time(s) in our lives. Each of us occupies a space along the continuum of care that reflects our own family and community circumstances at that point in time.

Within caregiving, we need to pay particular attention to four broad areas: (1) the characteristics, demands, and trends pertaining to caregivers and care recipients; (2) the practice of professionals who serve caregivers; (3) the public policies that support caregivers; and (4) the relationship between the quality of life of the caregiver and the care recipient. The structure of this volume roughly addresses these four issues.

While the experience of caregiving gets played out as an intensely personal, often very isolated, experience, we know much about the national experience of caregiving, thanks in part to some national surveys that have addressed and informed this concern.

We know that about 20% of adults at any given moment report that they are providing family caregiving. There is, however, great variability in this experience across multiple dimensions. It is useful to point out distinguishing concepts early in this volume.

*Relationship of Care Recipient* Research, policy, and programs have evolved to focus on the caregiving dynamics among older people or on families with a child who has early onset of a disability. This bifurcation of the constituency is not particularly useful. Caregiving can be upward as adults care for older parents; it can be lateral as older people care for one another, and it can be downward as parents care for children with disabilities. It must be said that providing care for one person does not exempt people from other caregiving responsibilities. An adult might care for both an aging parent and their own child with a disability.

*Duration* Parents of adult children with disabilities can face a lifetime of care responsibilities. As the story of the old man and his family illustrates, caregiving can last for decades. However, occasionally caregiving responsibilities can be intermittent. A person experiencing a temporary disability recovers and caregiving responsibilities cease.

*Intensity* The severity of disability, the type of disability, and the health of the care recipient all can affect the intensity of caregiving. People with severe disabilities might require considerable help with bathing, dressing, toileting, and managing daily needs and routines. These responsibilities can require many hours of work both day and night. Conversely, people with cognitive disabilities might require only direction, prompting, or standby help. The work differs in terms of intensity, and it might be measured in the number of hours of care each day. If the care recipient experiences poor health as well as limited physical capacity, the demand might be magnified.

*Caregiver-care Recipient Dyad* Often, caregiving is treated as though there is one caregiver and one care recipient. There is also an assumption that the care recipient has a disability and the caregiver does not. In some cases, these assumptions are true. But in other cases, the need for care ripples across the family with family members assuming various roles and responsibilities to make their particular system work. While women—mothers, wives, and daughters—provide the bulk of care, husbands and wives often trade off tasks to care for a child with a disability, and while one person might appear to take on the primary burden of caregiving for an older parent, it is often shared among siblings. For older spouses, they often employ complementary capacities to sustain the family unit. Each may have a disabling condition but their combined efforts allow them to continue valued social roles.

It seems fairly obvious that social policies and programs should be arrayed in a way to support caregivers. Policies among employers and state and local resources vary dramatically across the country. Robust programs that recognize the complex demands of caregiving might have the capacity to support caregivers in caregiving roles. By and large, however, many parents of children with disabilities are on their own, and policy makers, public health officials, and researchers have only the vaguest notion of how to effectively translate and disseminate what we know about the circumstances and needs of caregivers into interventions and support programs.

With that overwhelming limitation noted, we should pay attention to the other half of the caregiver-care recipient dyad. If caregivers are rested both physically and mentally, they are likely to be more effective as caregivers, and thus the health and quality of life of care recipients is likely to be improved.

Parents with intense caregiving responsibilities—parents who have stumbled through the week balancing work, lack of sleep, and household responsibilities, as well as bathing, dressing, toileting, occupational therapy, physical therapy, speech therapy, doctors appointments and surgeries, and insurance company demands—might not be the most fun people when the weekend comes. If parents are rested, they might be more likely to be involved in social activities with their children. Unfortunately, often well-meaning professionals load on additional care responsibilities rather than taking them away.

While much social research has focused on caregivers, one might ask how this book differs from others concerned about caregiving among children, working aged people, and older people. Here, we want to focus on the relationship of caregivers as it relates to disability across the lifespan. In this book, the cause of the disability is not altogether of concern because the effects on caregivers have common characteristics unrelated to the diagnosis of the person who receives care.

Lastly, one additional term must be defined. Throughout the book, we use the term *professional caregivers* to refer to paid care providers such as physicians, nurses, social workers, psychologists, case managers, hospice workers, home health aides, and many others. The designation as professional caregiver excludes those family caregivers who receive funds to provide care from new and emerging sources, such as the Medicaid Cash and Counseling Demonstration Program.

## Genesis of the Caregiving Book Series

Efforts to develop this book began in 2000, when Johnson & Johnson, an international health care business leader, and Dr. Ronda Talley, executive director of the Rosalynn Carter Institute for Caregiving, began discussions that led to the development of the Johnson & Johnson/Rosalynn Carter Institute Caregivers Program. Through this program, the Rosalynn Carter Institute convened a series of 10 expert panels over a period of several years to address a wide variety of caregiving issues. These included disability, Alzheimer's disease, cancer, mental health, life span caregiving, rural caregiving, intergenerational caregiving, education and support for caregivers, interdisciplinary professional caregiving, and building community caregiving capacity. With Springer as our partner, the RCI books were integrated into a new Springer caregiving book series, *Caregiving: Research, Policy, and Practice* with Dr. Talley as editor-in-chief. In 2011, we launched the series. This volume, *Multiple Dimensions of Caregiving and Disability*, is the fourth series volume.

## Caregiving Disability Issues

Within the area of disability, a number of critical issues were presented for inclusion in this volume. Lacking the space to include them all, 10 topics were selected and national experts were recruited to contribute to the caregiving and disability knowledge base. Summaries of the chapters presented in the book follow:

*McDaniel and Pisani* Susan McDaniel and Anthony Pisani's chapter rightly serves as the opening discussion for caregiving and disability by addressing the dynamics of families. This chapter employs conceptual frameworks well-known to practitioners in family therapy with insight into the particular circumstances of families dealing with disability. In this case the authors weave together conceptual issues and compelling narratives told by family members. These stories are compelling because they are honest and they provide insight into changing roles, coping strategies, isolation, anger, and guilt experienced by various members of the family. These lessons, which inform health care professional caregivers and policy makers, can be used to better support families and to target research that addresses points of intervention. McDaniel and Pisani make policy recommendations that are repeated in some way by several authors in this book: better access to respite and attendants at home, increased security at work so that families can balance caregiving responsibilities and work demands, more integrated healthcare systems to reduce the burden on families to be their own case managers, and affordable mental health care to facilitate the entire family's capacity to cope.

*Getch*  In her chapter, Yvette Getch focuses on the feelings of family caregivers. She paints a portrait of caregivers as often being isolated, depressed, fatigued, worried, anxious, sad, or fearful when facing the monumental tasks they are responsible for accomplishing. Frequently, caregivers also describe themselves in the same terms. Getch introduces the concept of "caregiver burden," the extent to which caregivers perceive their physical, psychological, emotional, social, and financial problems as a result of providing care for a family member. Caregivers' feelings are a "subjective" part of caregiving. She discusses the powerful impact of distress and guilt on social functioning, as well as the loss of friends and support that can occur. Getch also deals with feelings associated with maternal and paternal caregiving, as well as spousal caregiving. A section of the chapter is devoted to the issue of caring for children as a special situation that often requires extensive family interaction with professional caregivers and the attendant difficulties that can ensue.

*Goldsmith*  In her chapter on caregiver education, training, and support for caregivers of individuals with disabilities, Sharon Goldsmith provides an overview of the forces affecting these issues and the challenges in offering meaningful, transferable knowledge and skills. As Americans live longer, their educational needs will shift and grow over the coming years. Further, Goldsmith notes, the education and support offered to "sandwich generation" caregivers who have access to technology that was not available to their parents will be designed to take advantage of the newest web-based and other computer-supported opportunities. Goldsmith makes the case that appropriate curriculum and formats are needed to train both professional and family caregivers, and increase their access to care. Further, she explains, because there is no single best way to design and deliver education and support for caregivers, myriad strategies will be needed to address individual caregiver needs and goals. She summarizes the education and training literature that is devoted to addressing the needs of individuals with disabilities, and discusses caregiver certification issues.

*Kuhlthau*  This chapter provides an intense review of the literature informing caregiving among parents of children with disabilities. Karen Kuhlthau notes the driving forces, mainly increasing rates of disability among children, and the consequences in terms of employment and financial need, stress, and emotional and social demands, as well as the mental health of parents. Kuhlthau weaves together several conceptual frameworks to better understand the distinctive characteristics of family caregiving among children with disabilities and the particular experiences that define "normal" caregiving of a child from that of a child with a disability. This discussion leads to a better understanding of the multidimensional effects of caregiving for parents of children with disabilities. This rich foundation leads to suggestions regarding specific problems faced by such parents, including lack of sleep, depression, and lack of access to preventive care. These stressors are in addition to fragmented medical care, brief physician–patient encounters, and lack of sound information. Kuhlthau then identifies sound or promising practices and policies that have the capacity to support parents.

*Crews* In this chapter, *Neither Prepared Nor Rehearsed: The Role of Public Health in Disability and Caregiving*, John Crews argues that we must frame the caregiving experience as a public health concern. Much of public health is focused on epidemiology and surveillance, and there is no question that we need to understand the prevalence of caregiving in the United States as well as the characteristics of caregivers. Beyond that, Crews states, we need to think about how the concerns of public health might be congruent with the caregiving experience. Caregivers are not as likely to seek preventive care as noncaregivers. Because of the lifting, transferring, and positioning of intense caregiving, caregivers might be more likely to experience back injury or develop chronic health conditions, such as arthritis. Caregivers might not get enough sleep or get well as quickly when sick. These concerns are more likely to present themselves when someone has provided care for a lengthy period. They do, however, lend themselves to interventions that might help to sustain caregivers in their caregiving roles. The health of caregivers is becoming an increasingly important issue to protect the integrity of the family as an important national asset to provide care in the community.

*Leung* One could argue that the variability of health, knowledge, and resources of caregivers is great, indeed. Likewise, the capacity, circumstances, and needs of care recipients represent great variability. Paul Leung describes ethnic and racial dimensions of caregiving as they affect caregivers, care recipients, and their respective experiences with service providers and various professionals. He reminds his readers of the power of within-group variability. Simply knowing that someone has a disability tells us something, it does not tell us everything. Knowing that someone is African American or Hispanic provides only a starting point for understanding the richness, resilience, stress, and disadvantage of the caregiving experience among minority populations. This topic is of particular importance because prevalence of disability is generally higher among Hispanics and African Americans, and thus the caregiver responsibility is probably greater, and because of the socioeconomic circumstances of minority populations, caregiving demands fall disproportionately upon the family.

*Gaventa* William Gaventa's chapter on faith and spirituality explores the "profound spiritual questions" surrounding the birth of a child with a disability in the context of the experience of the family with faith communities. Faith communities can be either welcoming or excluding, and the effect can be profound. He begins his chapter with two simple questions that elicit powerful responses: "Would you be willing to share your church (synagogue, temple) story?" or "Would you be willing to describe how your faith or spirituality has been impacted by your experience?" Gaventa notes the spiritual questions raised by parents about themselves, their child, and their community. Gaventa chronicles several positive trends, illustrating the potential role of faith communities to support families and people with disabilities, as well as efforts to create fully inclusive congregations and community support systems that provide ongoing stable, respectful environments for people with disabilities. While the trends of inclusion and support are encouraging, they are far from universal, and Gaventa gives direction to research, education, and practice that has the potential to strengthen the faith community's responses to families and thus strengthen the capacity of families to be caregivers.

*Elliot and Parker* In their discussion of family caregivers and health care providers as care partners, Timothy Elliott and Michael Parker note that, contrary to popular opinion, the majority of American families do not abandon family members with chronic disease and disability to professional caregivers. They describe how health care providers can collaborate productively with family caregivers as partners to provide care and assistance to persons living with debilitating health conditions. They describe the growing caregiving movement among families who have a member with a disabling condition. Arguing for the development of collaborative partnerships between family and professional caregivers, they identify issues that have deterred the development of a partnership model and stress the need for the identification of critical caregiver tasks and competencies to facilitate its development.

*Bowe* Legal issues related to caregiving for an individual with disabilities are discussed by the late Frank Bowe. When introducing his chapter, Bowe notes that caregiving for people with disabilities is a field in dire need of more research, consistent standards of care, more education and training, and more sensible policies. He argues that in the United States, there is an acknowledgment of, but not support for, caregiving for individuals with disabilities, and that the country has only a patchwork of laws and policies that have caregiving provisions. And these, he notes, are often poorly funded and, in many cases, optional. To support his case, Bowe reviews the major legislation with caregiving relevance that has been enacted, such as the Americans with Disabilities Act, the Older Americans Act, Medicaid, the Individuals with Disabilities Education Act, the Public Health Service Act, the Family and Medical Leave Act, and Social Security Disability Insurance. He concludes his case by stating that a nation that values caregiving, whether provided by family members or by paid employees, would provide health insurance, retirement benefits, and financial compensation they deserve, as well as the respite care these persons need, given the often-draining nature of their work.

*Holm* This chapter focuses on emerging technologies for caregivers of persons with disabilities. Margo Holm notes that, historically, infants who needed a medical device to compensate for a vital organ or body function and who were technology-dependent, have been sent home from the hospital with their parent caregivers because of cost reductions and better developmental outcomes for the children. However, this relied on the parents' ability to work the technology devices that were sent home with the child. The same holds for end-of-life care; someone must be trained to operate the technology to support necessary care. Using the *International Classification of Function, Disability and Health* (ICF), Holm describes a variety of caregiver needs for technological devices. She devotes a substantial part of her chapter to profiles of emerging technological devices, both those in development and those in the field, and their potential uses.

## Concluding Comments

One additional item should be added to the list of concerns addressed by policy and programs: Time. We are all given the same 24 hours to conduct our day, the same 7 days to define the week. For families providing intense care, those 24 hours, those 7 days are quite unlike what many would describe as normal. Parents, spouses, and adult children use those hours to conduct their own lives, *and* to bathe, feed, dress, transfer, and toilet another. There are often doctor's appointments, medical procedures, and therapies, all of which require *time*—hours that are never given back. While public policies and robust programs cannot create time, they can provide the gift of time to caregivers by creating systems, policies, and social and economic supports that protect the time of caregivers so that, in addition to caregiving, they can participate in social roles that others take for granted.

Taken together, we anticipate that the topics introduced in this book will provide a unique framework for viewing multiple dimensions of caregiving for those with disabilities.

## References

Aneshensel, C. S., Pearlin, L. I., & Schuler, R. H. (1993). Stress, role captivity, and the cessation of caregiving. *Journal of Health and Social Behavior, 34*(1), 54–70.

Berg-Weger, M., Rubio, D. M., & Tebb, S. (2001). Strengths-based practice with family caregivers of the chronically Ill: Qualitative insights. *Families in Society, 82*(3), 263–272.

Horowitz, A. (1985). Family caregiving to the frail elderly. In C. Eisdorfer (Ed.), *Annual review of gerontology and geriatrics* (Vol. 5, pp. 194–246). New York: Springer.

MetLife & National Alliance for Caregiving. (2006). *2006 MetLife Foundation family caregiver awards program.* http://www.asaging.org/asav2/caregiver/index.cfm?CFID=12644792&CFTOKEN=19400852#definition. Accessed 20 April 2012.

Montgomery, R. J. V., Gonyea, J., & Hooyman, N. (1985). Caregiving and the experience of subjective and objective burden. *Family Relations, 34,* 19–26.

National Alliance for Caregiving (NAC) and AARP. (2004). *Caregiving in the U.S.* Washington, DC: Author. http://www.caregiving.org/data/04finalreport.pdf. Accessed 20 April 2012.

National Alliance for Caregiving (NAC) and AARP. (2009). *Caregiving in the U.S.* Washington, DC: Author. http://www.caregiving.org/pdf/research/Caregiving_in_the_US_2009_full_report.pdf. Accessed 20 April 2012.

National Family Caregiver Association. (2012). *What is family caregiving?* http://www.thefamilycaregiver.org/who are family caregivers/what is family caregiving.cfm. Accessed 20 April 2012.

Schumacher, K., Stewart, B., Archbold, P., Dood, M., & Dibble, S. (2000). Family caregiving skill: Development of the concept. *Research in Nursing & Health, 23,* 191–203.

Seltzer, M. M., & Li, L. W. (2000). The dynamics of caregiving: Transitions during a three-year prospective study. *Gerontologist, 40*(2), 165–178.

U.S. Department of Health and Human Services. Office on Women's Health. (2008). *What is Caregiving?* http://www.womenshealth.gov/publications/our-publications/fact-sheet/caregiver-stress.cfm#a. Accessed 20 April 2012.

# Chapter 2
# Family Dynamics and Caregiving for People with Disabilities

Susan H. McDaniel and Anthony R. Pisani

Caregiving is at the heart of family life. Parents care for children, spouses care for each other, and, when illness or disability occurs, family members care for each other. At least 80% of primary caregivers for individuals with severe disabilities are family members (U.S. Census Bureau 1997; National Alliance for Caregiving (NAC) and AARP 2004). Families affected by a disability experience a host of relational opportunities and challenges. In this chapter, we will discuss factors that shape family dynamics in caregiving for individuals with disabilities related to chronic illness, trauma, or congenital conditions and how clinicians, educators, researchers, and policymakers can promote health family dynamics.

The study of caregiving and disability naturally lends itself to a systemic approach (McDaniel et al. 1992; Rolland 1994; Lyons et al. 1995). All people in relationships depend on one another; disability makes interdependence explicit. Medical decisions, hygiene routines, and residential choices directly affect the caregiver as well as the disabled person. Domains that would otherwise be private become open to relational scrutiny and negotiation. For example, Manuel, an adult with quadriplegia, prefers manual, intermittent bladder catheterization to an indwelling catheter that continuously drains to a leg bag or other device. Under most circumstances, the mode and frequency of voiding is a personal, unilateral choice. But for Manuel, his personal assistants, his family, and his healthcare team must decide with him because the decision to catheterize several times a day requires significant commitment on the part of caregivers. Families such as Manuel's must strike a balance between autonomy of the individual and the sometimes competing needs of caregivers. This is a tension that exists in every family but disability highlights and amplifies these relational intricacies.

Disability is also an inherently systemic concept because it resides in the fit between the individual's needs and the physical, social, and legal environment.

---

S. H. McDaniel (✉)
School of Medicine and Dentistry, University of Rochester, 601 Elmwood Ave,
Rochester, NY 14642, USA
e-mail: susanh2_mcdaniel@urmc.rochester.edu

A. R. Pisani (✉)
e-mail: anthony_pisani@urmc.rochester.edu

Problems related to a disability often have as much to do with deficiency in the environment as with physical or mental impairment. Similarly, some of the challenging interpersonal dynamics that arise among individuals with disability and their caregivers are sometimes more accurately attributed to failings in larger system supports, rather than to the disability, per se. This contextual view of disability should inform any discussion of family dynamics and caregiving.

The "family" of an individual with disabilities often extends beyond those who are biologically related. Healthcare providers, friends, personal assistants, and community agents form an identifiable system that interacts around the disability. Anderson et al. (1986) argued that the most helpful focus of attention for family therapists is the "problem-determined system," that is, the group of people that are involved in shaping each others' experience of a presenting issue. This is certainly true when it comes to discussion of family dynamics and disability. The most meaningful focus will almost always be on the person living with disability, plus those inside and outside the family who care for and about that person. Thus, we intend our discussion of family dynamics to apply to the relationships and structures of this system as well as to the nuclear or extended family as traditionally defined.

## The Biopsychosocial Model

The biopsychosocial systems model (McDaniel et al. 1992) provides a comprehensive framework from which to understand the needs, desires, and interactions of the person with disability and the family, broadly defined. Internist George Engel (1977, 1980) first described the biopsychosocial model, an alternative to the traditional biomedical model. Engel's model takes into account different levels of a problem, ranging from molecular, genetic, and organ systems, to the individual's psychology and belief systems, family functioning, community responsiveness, and federal policies that impact the daily lives of people with disabilities and those who care for them. Biopsychosocial theory sprang from the same roots as family systems theory, that of General Systems theory from the early twentieth century (Wynne 2003). Integrating biopsychosocial and family systems theory, biopsychosocial systems theory encourages assessment of any problem at the most relevant levels of the biopsychosocial hierarchy. For people with disabilities, this always means the biological, the psychosocial, and the relational. It includes community and policy levels when disparities or discrimination are apparent. Intervention is targeted for levels that are most relevant and most likely to produce useful change. Most often, any intervention involves the family—either directly by targeting relationship problems, or indirectly as part of the care system.

The dynamic interplay between physical factors, individual psychology, and relational dynamics is the purview of the professional healthcare team, especially the medical family therapist[1] (McDaniel et al. 1992) who may provide consultation to

---

[1] In this chapter, we often refer to "illness and disability" together. These terms are not technically interchangeable. Illness does not always lead to disability, and many disabilities are not a result of

physicians, nurses, and other professional providers, as well as to the person with the disability, the family, and others caring for the disabled person. Drawing from the literature on psychology and theology (Bakan 1969), the general goals for medical family therapy are to increase both *agency* and *communion* (McDaniel et al. 1992). These goals offer a useful framework for considering the individual and family factors that influence outcomes for people with disabilities.

Agency is a sense that one can make personal choices in dealing with illness and the healthcare system. In the West, we struggle with the relationship between individual responsibility and illness: we hold people responsible for their emotional problems, while believing they are *not* responsible for physical illness. Framing a problem as "physical" can lift the burden of blame from a person's shoulders but it can also encourage a passive-dependent patient role that is socially acceptable. For patients and families facing illness and disability, agency means not remaining passive. It means coming to grips with what they must accept while discovering what action they can take. Agency is a sense of activism about one's own life in the face of all that is uncertain. Dealing with this uncertainty is part of the challenge of facing illness and disability.

Communion refers to strengthening emotional and spiritual bonds that can be frayed by illness, disability, and contact with the healthcare system. It is the sense of being cared for, loved, and supported by a community of family members, friends, and professionals. Serious illness or disability is an existential crisis that can isolate people from those who care for them with significant health consequences. Research shows lack of good social support is a stronger risk factor for illness and disability than cigarette smoking (House et al. 1988). At the same time, serious illness or disability provides opportunities for resolving old conflicts and forging new levels of healthy family bonding.

Taken together, agency and communion describe individual autonomy in a relational context. Helgeson (1994), in a review of research on agency and communion, concluded that both are required for optimal health. Unmitigated agency, or unmitigated communion is associated with increased morbidity. When illness or disability challenges functioning, individuals or families may be high on one of these dimensions and low on the other. For example, a family caregiver may be high on her sense of competence (agency) in the face of disability but low on support (communion). Unbalanced agency and communion also puts people at risk for mental health symptoms. As professional caregivers, we want to assess, increase, and balance agency and communion for people with disabilities and their caregivers. To do so, it is helpful to be aware of the patterns that define human interactions.

---

illness. We have chosen an inclusive stance toward defining our focus of study for several reasons. First, many of the family dynamics we address pertain to circumstances in which one or more individuals in a family experiences a change in physical functioning, irrespective of the source. Second, from a conceptual and political level, we believe there is much to be gained for families when those with caregiving needs unite around common concerns. Finally, much of our clinical experience and previous writing has focused on families and chronic illness and we wished to draw from that knowledge base.

## Understanding Family Systems

"Family dynamics" is a broad term that encompasses the myriad processes, which together constitute the family system. Walsh (2003) has identified three basic domains of family functioning: organization patterns, family belief systems, and communication processes. These domains help to organize any assessment of family dynamics.

*Organizational Patterns* A family is more than a collection of individual members. Families are systems that have distinct structures. Roles, boundaries, hierarchy, and connectedness yield patterns of interaction, expectation, and support. Family caregiving for an individual with disabilities challenges families to evolve patterns that are flexible enough to adapt to demands created by the disability but stable enough to provide some predictability, continuity, and room for growth. Because kin and social networks support successful family caregiving, boundaries between the family and the outside world ideally are semipermeable, allowing a system of care to develop, while protecting and demarcating core family members.

*Family Belief Systems* Just as individuals have distinct identities and worldviews, so families have shared beliefs that shape how they adapt to stress and change (Rolland 1994). Families living with disabilities must make meaning out of the challenges they face. What seems overwhelming and difficult for one family may be embraced as a valuable difference in another. Health professionals should attend to the meaning and value families assign to any difference or disability. Resilient families are able to increase agency by gaining a sense of coherence, maintaining hope, focusing on growth, and forging a group identity that includes but goes beyond the disability. For some families, spiritual beliefs and practices unite the sometimes painful realities of disability with a larger purpose or story.

*Communication Processes* Communication connects and empowers stressed families. Walsh (2006) regards clarity, open emotional expression, and collaborative problem solving as the key elements of healthy communication. Direct messages delivered in an open and collaborative environment result in increased communion for the individual and the system. Sharing care among family members often requires frequent information exchange, decision-making, and cooperation. Some disabling conditions (especially those that require physical accommodation) demand that families and care providers engage in intricate planning and coordination in order to pursue an activity that would otherwise be spontaneous. A simple outing like a family picnic, for example, can require extensive planning for transportation and access. Empathy for all involved is useful oil for the communication system that is needed to anticipate and plan for the future needs of its members.

*The Dynamics of Disabilities* Like families, disabilities have unique features that influence caregiver experience. Rolland (1994) proposed a typology of illness and disability with four key dimensions: onset (acute or gradual), course (progressive, constant, relapsing/episodic, predictable/unpredictable), incapacitation (presence or absence and severity), and outcome (fatal, shortened lifespan, or nonfatal). The matrix formed by combining these dimensions helps to predict the pattern of psychosocial and caregiving demands created by a particular disability. Cystic fibrosis, for example, has a gradual onset, progressive relapsing course, varying levels of incapacitation, and shortened lifespan. The caregiving demands and family dynamics of this disabling condition would be quite different from those associated with traumatic brain injury, which has acute onset, constant course, and nonfatal outcome.

Seaburn and Erba (2003) found that the time of onset in the history of a family also influences family dynamics. A disability that predates the inception of the family, such as when a person has epilepsy before he marries, become "nested" in family life such that roles and relationships accommodate the needs of the disabled individual and caregivers. Caregiving routines become part of the rhythm of normal family life. When a disability occurs after a family is formed, such as head trauma after a biking accident, families must reorganize and redefine themselves. Often, families have difficulty making these adjustments. They can become stuck in chronic state of crisis, so that individual and family development are disrupted or even frozen around the time of the disability.

*Disabilities and the Family Life Cycle* Individuals develop within the context of family and other systems. These systems, in turn, adapt over time in response to the developmental needs of individual members and to pressures exerted on the system from outside. Thus, families of disabled individuals experience their roles and relationships in continuously evolving context. This fluidity means that the dynamics of caregiving will be different at different times in the life cycle of a family.

Key transition points in the family life cycle include: leaving home, coupling, pregnancy and childbirth, raising young children, raising adolescents, launching children, middle-age reevaluation, retirement, and end-of-life issues (Carter and McGoldrick 2005). Obviously, many families do not follow this sequence in order; for example, many circle back to the coupling stage after a divorce while also raising adolescents. The stages in the family life cycle are influenced by culture, opportunity, and preferences and should not be viewed as prescriptive. Nevertheless, the family life cycle provides a useful lens for viewing developmental issues and family dynamics at a given point in time.

This lens may be particularly salient for families with disabilities because caregiving demands may be out of phase with the family's life cycle stage. For example, the parents of an adolescent with cognitive disabilities may need to arrange social opportunities or help with grooming during a time when other families with adolescents are preparing to launch their children and move on. This asynchrony with expected life stages can seem more pronounced if the family has other children who progress "normally." Likewise, as we will see in the case example below, physically disabled parents often need help from their children in ways that the life cycle model does not predict, such as caring for their hygiene, performing daily household tasks for them, or acting as liaison to a society that is often not equipped for their needs. (For a thorough review of disability and the family life cycle, see Marshak et al. 1999).

## "Things Aren't As They Should Be:" A Family Struggles with the Effects of Serious Illness and Disability[2]

> Mr. White, a 54-year-old German-American man, had Parkinson's Disease, which is a chronic, progressive illness. He was sick for a number of years. He lost his ability to speak, so went to communicating by laptop. His wife of 24 years requested a medical family therapy consultation with Dr. McDaniel because she was concerned about the effects of her husband's long-term illness and disability on her three daughters: Denise, 22; Jessica, 19, and Barbara, 16. At the time of the consultation, Mr. White was bed-ridden, had a feeding tube down his throat, and his tremor was so significant that he could no longer communicate by computer. Prior to his illness, Mr. White had been a prominent community leader with a highly visible counseling and consulting practice.

Mrs. White and her daughters were articulate about many of the family dynamics they experienced. The dialogue[3] from this session illustrates some of the family dynamics common to so many families facing chronic illness and disability.

### Shifting Family Roles

Barbara: ...It isn't fair that he should be going through all this.... It isn't fair for him to just stay home and not lead a normal 54-year-old life.... It's not fair that he can't go on vacation.... Denise said it isn't fair for me not to be able to lead a normal 16-year-old life. Mom, you don't have a husband... well, I mean you do have a husband, but you can't do normal things with him.

Disability can challenge long-standing family roles and patterns of family organization. In this case, the daughters express concern that their mother has lost her "companion" and all that means. Likewise, the mother set up the session because of her concern about the girls losing a functional father.

Mother: ...I noticed the other night that... when he wanted to communicate and would have difficulty, he would end up crying, you know, and that is very hard. He was never the one to cry.... That was my job. It still is.

Denise: I know the first time that I ever really saw him cry was the second time he was in the hospital.... We hadn't made it in all day to visit him... and we got there pretty late at night.... He was very upset because he was expecting us and then we didn't come.... He just broke down. That was the most disconcerting thing I have ever been through because he was... always, you know... he was the person in control when the rest of us fell apart.

Mr. White's role shifted with his increasing disability, from being the "rock" of the family to the vulnerable patient. The family finds the fact that he now cries

---

[2] Medical family therapy is an approach to working with families, rather than a distinct profession. A medical family therapist may be a social worker, psychologist, psychiatrist, or family therapist—anyone trained to do psychotherapy with families in medical settings.

[3] This description is of an actual case. Details of the family have been camouflaged to protect their confidentiality.

"disconcerting." Mom said, "That was my job. Still is," as she wiped her eyes. Progressive disabilities require family members and the disabled person to reorganize and take up new roles with regard to affective communication, instrumental chores, and functions in the family.

Of course, family dynamics shift depending on which member is disabled or ill. When a primary family caregiver becomes disabled, family roles must shift to redistribute the tasks she is unable to perform (McDaniel and Cole-Kelly 2003). Both instrumental and emotional work must be distributed across other family members, who must develop the ability to project strength in the face of adversity. It requires flexibility for a family to accommodate new realities in a respectful, unintrusive way that preserves the previous caregiver's remaining sense of agency.

When a parent is disabled, the challenge for the family is meeting the children's developmental needs while also caring for the disabled adult. Mrs. White expressed concern about striking this balance when she requested a medical family therapy consultation for herself and her daughters. Barbara also referred to this dynamic when she said it was not fair that she cannot lead a "normal" life.

When a child is disabled, from congenital defects, chronic illness, or an accident, parents are absorbed by the typical tasks of raising children *and* caregiving for someone with disabilities. Healthy siblings may also feel the strain, often feeling they must be perfect to accommodate. Maturity and caregiving come early to these children. With proper support for their developmental challenges, caregiving can be an enriching experience. If, however, their needs are overlooked or undetected, these children may develop symptoms of their own at some point.

## *The Confluence of Coping Styles*

Jessica: I talk to Barbara about... my Dad.... I don't really talk to Denise about it, and that sort of bothers me.
Dr. McDaniel: Somehow the illness has come between you, and you're kind of missing Denise.
Jessica: I think it's like Denise has a different way to deal with it.
Denise: I think sometimes I bury it so far down.... Something happens or... I react immediately, but then it gets buried and I don't even realize that it's still bothering me... on a conscious level.
Jessica: Sometimes it bothers me that it doesn't look like it's bothering her.
Denise: ...That's where the tension arises for us because sometimes people... look and think I don't care, because in an effort not to fall apart I just push it further down.

Patients and family members have to find a way to cope with chronic disability and with each other's coping styles and conflicting health beliefs. Family members often accept serious illness or disability at different points in time. It's almost as if someone in the family needs to deny the illness or disability and advocate for life to go on, and someone else needs to help the family grapple with the hard realities associated with the disability. Of course, people can get polarized and move into major conflict over this. Successful families respect each others' coping styles, and allow space for each person to grieve with his or her own rate and style.

In the White family, Denise is near the denial end of the continuum, pushing down her feelings, while Jessica is at the other end of accepting the illness. Jessica, who was very expressive and let her anger and frustration out, misinterpreted Denise's behavior as "not caring." In response, Denise described herself as just trying to get through a difficult situation. Airing these differences and normalizing them can be useful. It is also important to understand that when the coping styles of one individual changes, it may have implications for others in the family.

## *The Isolation of Illness and Disability*

Barbara: It would be nice to be able to talk to someone, like one of my good friends. I mean, it is my father [and] none of them know... a lot of the stuff... I am sure I am going to go through this whole week and none of them are going to know about what is going on.... Everybody says that I'm so happy.... It's all a front.

Dr. McDaniel: If it was one of your good friend's fathers who were in the hospital, would you want to know?

Barbara: Yeah.

Illness and disability can be a singular, lonely experience for the patient. It can also be isolating for the family, diminishing their sense of communion and community. Barbara, whose typical interpersonal style was extroverted, did not tell her friends about her father's recent decline and hospitalization. She felt that her life experience was foreign to them. At the same time, challenging this belief was easy. When she left the session, she did communicate with her closest friends and received the support she needed from them. When stressed, it is natural for a family unit to close ranks and hunker down but they then can become depleted. The community and professionals involved with patients and families with disabilities must help them access the support and resources they need for the long haul.

## *Managing Anger and Guilt*

Jessica: My main problem is... a major guilt complex.... Like [my father] will ask me to do something and I'll get frustrated... and go off stomping into my room. [I wonder] why did I yell [at him]? It's not really fair. He just asked a simple thing, and I could have said, "Well, I don't have time" and walk away. But instead I yell and stomp around and slam something down on the table because it seems... like you have to go and do so much out of your way. But he can't do it.... It's always something.

Dr. McDaniel: So, you have normal feelings that anybody would have in this demanding situation, but you don't really feel like you have a right to

|          | them because your dad has a terrible illness and is very disabled. So, what do you do with your anger? Where does that go? |
|----------|---|
| Jessica: | I take it out on him. |

Each family develops a style of managing uncomfortable feelings. Some family cultures are loud and expressive; others are quiet and conflict avoidant. Many styles can work. But illness and disability can inhibit the normal expression of feelings because people like Jessica feel they must treat the ill or disabled person with such care. Generally, this response becomes unhealthy because it inhibits the natural development of the relationship, including corrections that come from honest feedback. Negative feelings can accumulate over time resulting in a blowup or in depression or psychosomatic problems in the patient or family member. Normalizing anger, frustration, and sadness is important for everyone involved when someone's functioning deteriorates. It can be useful for the family to realize that these feelings are more about the illness or disability rather than about the person with diminished functioning him/herself. It is possible to share negative feelings about the illness or disability without mistaking the feelings for anger at each other.

## Disruption of the Individual and Family Life Cycles

Jessica: Our lives are totally different than they should be. . . .

It is a major challenge for families to tend to its members' individual developmental needs *and* meet the caregiving demands of a serious illness or disability. It is impossible during an acute or crisis phase. Some families then become frozen around the family organization at the time of the crisis, rather than being able to shift and reorganize to care for the chronic demands of an illness or disability. During the chronic phase, the family needs to be able to care for the illness and still have energy, resources, and space for the patient and other family members to meet developmental challenges that face each stage of the life cycle (Penn 1983).

### *Managing Loss*

Another challenge for families with people with disabilities is managing the loss at the onset of disability or when functioning deteriorates. It can be an ambiguous loss (Boss 1999) in the sense that Western culture has no clear rituals to handle lost dreams. When chronic illness or disability is progressive, anticipatory loss becomes another member of the family. In the White family, the children and mother have watched Mr. White's functioning deteriorate over a period of years. They know that he will die prematurely. This awareness can offer the possibility of intimate, meaningful moments between family members. However, it also puts pressure on individuals and the family so that they are at risk for other individual and relational problems. Ideally, health professionals and a caring community provide support for people with serious illness and disabilities during this time. Hospice is a wonderful example of a social response to a problem not handled well by the cure-focused traditional medical community.

## *The Response of the Extended Family*

How much family members share care can predict the degree of caregiver burden. Negotiation of shared caregiving is complicated. Some caregivers have difficulty sharing the role, even when they are exhausted. Some family members distance themselves in response to fears about an illness or disability, leaving one family member with all of the responsibilities.

Relationships can become skewed because of conflict related to caregiving tasks. These tasks need ongoing renegotiation as the demands of a disability, wishes of the disabled individual, or capacity of caregivers change. Unacknowledged feelings of sadness or anger are sometimes acted out through withdrawal—or its counterpart—smothering and infantilizing the person with disabilities. Family meetings with primary care or medical family therapy professionals can be useful at points when disability tasks are neglected or family relationships become strained. Videotaping the family meeting can be very useful for family members who are unable to come to the meeting, so that they too have the relevant information to decide how they want to respond.

## Special Issues for Families

### *Genetics and Family Caregiving*

Genes play a role in many disabilities. In some cases, such as Huntington's disease, a single inherited gene causes the disease that leads to disability. In other cases, such as cancer or heart disease, genes interact with environmental variables to increase the risk of illness and disability in some affected family members. In either circumstance, the genetic link adds a layer of complexity to the family caregiving experience (Miller et al. 2006).

First, the family may have prior experience with the illness or disability. This familiarity can equip family members to understand and anticipate the needs of the disabled individual. Caregivers can draw on collective family wisdom; extended family members can counsel each other based on their successes and struggles. Conversely, prior experience can evoke painful memories of suffering or strife related to an illness or disability. Without conscious intervention, problematic dynamics developed in previous generation of caregiving may be transmitted to the next. For example, a mother who watched her parents coddle or infantilize a sibling with sickle cell disease may replicate that dynamic in caring for her son who develops the disease.

Second, genetic disorders can evoke caregiver fear about future experiences with a heritable condition. When caregiver and disabled person share (or might share) genetic risk, the relational dynamics can be complicated and intense. One can imagine the thoughts that run through the mind of a young man as he washes and feeds his father, the most recent in a line of close relatives disabled by early-onset Alzheimer's disease. Knowledge or suspicion of genetic risk can have ripple effects in the caregiver and family system. For example, the wife and children of this young man may respond in a variety of ways—compassion, withdrawal, anger—to concerns about their own future with him.

The increasing availability of genetic testing has similar family implications. Genetic knowledge is inherently relational in that information about one person potentially affects everyone in a family. The ethical, relational, and psychological implications of genetic testing are beyond the scope of this chapter; however, readers should be aware that emerging genetic knowledge is changing practice and family experience of healthcare in the twenty-first century (for a further discussion, see McDaniel and Campbell 1999).

## *Mental Disability: The Invisible*

In the 2006 American Community Survey sample, mental disabilities affected approximately 11.5 million Americans between the ages of 5 and 64 years. This group represented about 43% of the total 26.6 million disabled individuals in that age group (U.S. Census Bureau 2006). This group included those who reported having a "physical, mental, or emotional condition" lasting 6 months or more that made it difficult to "learn, remember, or concentrate." This heterogeneous group would presumably include individuals with cognitive/intellectual impairment, serious mental health disorders, dementia, some developmental disorders, and other neurocognitive conditions.

Mental disabilities differ from many others in that they are "invisible," hidden in the brain and intrapsychic experience of the affected individual. The causes of many mental disabilities are unknown and the ways in which they impair can be subtle and unpredictable. Thus, families coping with mental disabilities face the dual stress of social stigma and ambiguous loss. For example, Jonathan and Alexis, the parents of a boy with Asperger's disorder, routinely hear comments from family members and coworkers that question their competence. "Just give him to me for a day," Jonathan's boss recently told him after the boy became nervous and refused to interact with guests at a company picnic. In addition to being hurtful, such comments occasionally cause the boy's father to question the validity of the diagnosis, leading to conflict with his wife who has become a fervent advocate for the boy and others with his disability. Like many parents of disabled children, Jonathan and Alexis had to mourn the loss of the child they had expected and begin to dream of new possibilities for their family. The invisibility of their son's disorder complicates this process; even they wonder how a boy who looks so healthy could have so many problems.

## Recommendations for Practice, Education, Research, and Policy

### *Supporting Healthy Family Dynamics in Professional Practice*

Most Western healthcare systems are organized to meet the needs of individual patients. Family-oriented healthcare has been espoused by members of the Collaborative Family Healthcare Association (for more information, see http://www.cfha.net/not.org) and by various health professionals working in Family Medicine

(Bloch 1983; McDaniel et al. 2003). When one health professional treats the person with disabilities as well as the caregivers, that professional is able to monitor the needs of the patient and caregiver and suggest individual and family-based interventions for prevention, respite, and improved management as needed.

Collaborative Family Healthcare advocates for health professionals collaborate actively with patients, families, and other health professionals. A collaborative, strengths-focused approach to people with disabilities and their caregivers supports individual and family competencies, encourages prevention, and addresses caregiver burden and other problems as early as possible. Having a family-oriented mental health professional working onsite with a healthcare team allows the inevitable stresses and strains of caregiving to be addressed throughout the course of the life cycle of the family (Olkin 2001). A medical family therapist can assist other professionals in assessing and treating problems as they arise (McDaniel et al. 1992).

While this approach to care is not yet widespread, some programs have established interdisciplinary, preventive, strengths-focused care systems. They include many hospice, respite, geriatric, and rehabilitation programs. Several model programs have integrated mental health into primary care clinics.

In summary, health professionals must work together to increase and balance agency and communion for the caregiver and the person with the disability over time. Providers should seek to: (1) deliver family-oriented healthcare, (2) assess and intervene with a family members as a matter of course, (3) focus preventively on family dynamics early in the course of a disability, and (4) assess family dynamics as the needs of the person with disabilities and caregivers change over time.

## *Supporting Healthy Family Dynamics Through the Education of Health Professionals*

Because of the individual bias of current healthcare practice, education and training generally focuses on the needs of the person with disabilities, rather than on assessment, support, and intervention for the family caregivers. However, some medical and nursing programs are infused with family systems approaches to patient care. Psychology and social work programs also exist, but they, too, are not the norm. Caring for the caregiver comes naturally when the family is the unit of care, whether the focus is on the physical or the mental health of family members (McDaniel et al. 1992, 2003).

In addition to providing insight into individual and family dynamics, family systems concepts can also be helpful in training the health professional about his/her own role. For example, *triangulation* is an interpersonal process that occurs when two people handle some stressful situation by talking or complaining about a third person. Some venting, especially in the caregiver role, is understandable as a way to support and affirm each other's efforts. However, triangulation can be toxic when it involves serious issues and avoids direct discussion between the most relevant parties. It is not uncommon for a caregiver to complain to a health professional about some issue regarding the person with the disability. It is very important that the health professional avoids any destructive triangulation, which means avoiding being drawn into siding with one party against another. Instead, that professional should detriangulate and bring the relevant parties together to discuss the problem. Similar interpersonal problems can occur with personal assistants, specialists, or extended family members. Health professionals must be close enough to patients and their families to care, while not becoming inducted into any unhealthy family dynamics. Training in family systems helps to sensitize health professionals to these common difficulties and increase a sense of agency and communion for members of the healthcare team.

## *Supporting Healthy Family Dynamics Through Research*

Research on family factors with chronic illness or disability has been growing over the past decade. A section of the Institute of Medicine report on Health and Behavior, written by the National Working Group on Family-Based Interventions in Chronic Disease, is devoted to reviewing research on families, health, and behavior (Weihs et al. 2002). This review reported that protective factors for health and mental health outcomes include: family closeness, caregiver coping skills, mutually supportive family relationships, clear family organization, and direct communication about the illness/disability and its management. Risk factors include: intrafamilial conflict and criticism, trauma related to treatment of the disease, external stress, lack of extrafamilial support, interruption of family member's developmental tasks, and perfectionism and rigidity. Nonmalleable risk factors include: low socioeconomic status, high disease severity, recent diagnosis and invasive treatment, and prior patient and family member disability and psychopathology. All these protective and risk factors are valuable variables for future research and intervention for people with disabilities and their families. While studies are badly needed for the range of disabilities in every age group, many more studies have been conducted of families of children with chronic illness and disability. Studies of disabled adults are particularly scarce.

Intervention studies to date have focused more on adherence to management plans than on family processes themselves. Preintervention and intervention research on family factors and disability is still in its infancy. Preintervention research has yet to study family characteristics and disability outcomes. Rarely is the *quality* of these relationships examined, a factor that seems crucial in disease and disability management. Research on family psychoeducational programs for a variety of problems offer a hopeful approach to improving family functioning when struggling with physical or mental disability (MacFarlane 2002). A randomized, controlled trial of family psychoeducation for caregivers of Alzheimer's patients offers a model for this approach with other disabilities (Mittleman et al. 1996). The intervention included individual and family psychoeducation groups about Alzheimer's, ongoing support groups, and crisis counseling by mental health professionals. The results were robust and cost-effective: a significant decrease in caregiver depression, a significant increase in physical health outcomes for the caregiver, and a 329-day delay in nursing home placement for the disabled Alzheimer's patient. More systematic research is needed to learn what individuals and families need and want when they are caring for people with disabilities.

## *Supporting Healthy Family Dynamics Through Policy*

An overarching theme in our discussion has been that caregivers and individuals with disabilities are embedded in a multilayered biopsychosocial system. Policymakers have a unique opportunity to support families by improving how different parts of this system work together. In this section, we identify several legislative and economic priorities that can guide public policy toward developing systems to promote agency and communion for individuals with disabilities and family members who care for them.

Providing care for a disabled family member is often a labor of love. Nevertheless, caregiving requires time, money, and social capital (Coleman 1988). Families and other "informal" caregivers contribute an estimated US$ 200–300 billion per year in uncompensated labor (Arno et al. 1999; Arno 2006). In addition to their labor, families often finance uncovered healthcare costs, such as disposable supplies, assistive devices, and therapies that are deemed "not medically necessary." Tax law often requires individuals to reach a certain percent-of-income threshold before medical expenses can be claimed as tax deductions. The time and opportunity costs are equally great. Medical appointments, unexpected care needs, and fatigue can interfere with work performance and reduce outside social opportunities. Recent evidence suggests that poorer women, who disproportionately have children with chronic illness and disability, find themselves caught between their children's caregiving needs and the increasing pressure from social service programs to secure and maintain employment (Patterson 2002).

As we have seen, families of disabled individuals must navigate complex emotional and relational dynamics. Financial strain can sap energy needed for relational work, making family strife more likely. Family-centered disability policy can promote healthy family dynamics by enhancing the economic and community resources available to caregivers.

First, families need better access to and funding for quality home health assistants and respite care. According to the U.S. Census Bureau (2005), seven million Americans have difficulty dressing, bathing, or getting around inside the home. Many more need monitoring and assistance for safety and other reasons. Many families experience frustration with the high turnover rate and lack of experience among some home health workers. Better pay and training could improve the overall quality of the workforce, thereby easing family stress. Regular respite from the demands of caregiving also promotes healthy family relationships. When fully funded, the Lifespan

Respite Care Act (Public Law 109–442 2006) is a good example of legislation that will address a portion of this need. This bill explicitly recognizes that "the family caregiver role is personally rewarding but can result in substantial emotional, physical, and financial hardship" (Sec 2801a). The bill aims to provide grants to states and other entities to develop lifespan respite programs, to evaluate such programs, to improve planned and emergency respite services, and to train and recruit respite care workers and volunteers. Initial funding came in 2009 when President Obama allocated US$ 2.5 million in the FY09 Omnibus Appropriations bill for respite care (ARCH Respite Coalition 2009).

Second, family caregivers would benefit from flexibility and security in the workplace. Disabled individuals may require care from family members during typical working hours. For example, a mentally disabled adult, Lucy, needs to be fed and driven to her part-time job each morning. Flexible work schedules ("flextime") can enable family members like Lucy's sister, a legal assistant, to provide that care by shifting her hours at the office. Flexible leave policies also support healthy family functioning by allowing a caregiver to care for a disabled family member for an extended period of time without penalty in the workplace. The Family Leave Act of 1993 (FMLA) represented a remarkable step in the right direction. However, many families cannot afford to take advantage of the leave policies provided by FMLA because of the pay and benefits (including health insurance) they would forfeit during an extended leave. Lawmakers should consider remedying this limitation by providing funding for health insurance for full-time family caregivers. A bill with this aim, the Caregivers Access to Health Insurance Act (S. 3179[107]), was introduced in 2002, but did not make it out of committee (Library of Congress 2006a, b, c).

Third, families of disabled individuals need a healthcare system that facilitates interdisciplinary care. It is common for individuals with disabilities to receive treatment from several healthcare professionals. A single individual may work with a primary care provider, several medical specialists, a physical therapist, an occupational therapist, a social worker, and a psychotherapist. Coordination among these professionals is essential for effective care (McDaniel et al. 2003; Seaburn et al. 1996). Without it, families are left to integrate complex opinions and information on their own, often leading to conflict when family members hear different opinions from providers. Yet interdisciplinary collaboration is rarely reimbursed. Third-party payors almost never compensate providers for the time and resources required to conduct care team meetings, joint visits, and multilateral written communication. Furthermore, some payors prohibit visits with more than one professional per day. Obviously, these policies are aimed at preventing fraud and abuse. Policymakers and payors should strive to develop plans that achieve that protection without undercutting interdisciplinary cooperation in the care of individuals with disabilities and their families.

Fourth, caregivers need affordable access to mental health services. Lawmakers have moved in recent years to increase parity between coverage for physical and mental disorders. The Mental Health Parity Act of 1996 took an important step forward by eliminating annual and lifetime dollar limits for mental healthcare for companies with more than 50 employees. Unfortunately, the law contains loopholes that have allowed employers to skirt the spirit of the law, for example, by placing new restrictions that do not exist for other medical conditions, such as additional limits on outpatient office visits and number of days for inpatient care. In fact, the U.S. General Accounting office estimated that 87% of employers that comply with the law have reduced other aspects of mental health coverage. Families of disabled individuals would benefit from a law requiring full parity for all aspects of coverage, including dollar limits, day/visit limits, coinsurance, deductibles, and out-of-pocket maximums. In June 2008, the House and Senate reached bipartisan agreement on a new mental health parity bill that would move the country toward true parity. At the time of writing, this law is awaiting final vote in congress.

Finally, families need comprehensive legislation specifically targeting the needs of caregivers. The National Family Caregiver Support Program (NFCSP), established in 2001 by the Older Americans Act Amendments of 2000 (Public Law 106–501), is an excellent example of such legislation. NFCSP provides money (US$ 125 million in 2001, US$ 141 million in 2002, to US$ 155.7 million in 2005, and US$ 156.1 million for 2006; Administration on Aging (AOA 2006) to states to work with local agencies and service providers to provide information and assistance to caregivers and counseling, support groups, respite, and other community-based services to families caring for frail older members. Lawmakers should consider expanding eligibility to include caregivers of all disabled individuals, regardless of age.

## Conclusion

People with disabilities exist within networks of family members, friends, and professionals. Disabilities present challenges that can strengthen as well as strain individuals and families. Family systems concepts and approaches can help to improve the quality of life of the person with disabilities, caregivers, and the professionals involved in supporting these families. Healthcare professionals will benefit from using a biopsychosocial approach. We need more government and foundation support for research on how to improve support for people with disabilities within the context of their families. And, any policy regarding people with disabilities should include consideration of how it might help or hurt families.

## References

Administration on Aging (AOA). (2006). *Legislation and budget.* http://www.aoa.gov/about/legbudg/current_budg/legbudg_current_budg.asp.

Anderson, H., Goolishian, H., & Winderman, L. (1986). Problem determined systems: Towards transformation in family systems. *Journal of Strategic and Systemic Therapies, 5,* 1–14.

ARCH Respite Coalition. (2009). *Lifespan respite to receive $2.5 million for this fiscal year.* http://chtop.org/ARCH/ARCH-National-Respite-Coalition.html.

Arno, P. S. (2006). *Economic value of informal caregiving.* Paper presented at the Care Coordination and the Caregiving Forum, Dept. of Veterans Affairs, NIH, Bethesda, MD, January 25–27, 2006.

Arno, P. S., Levine, C., & Memmott, M. M. (1999). The economic value of informal caregiving. *Health Affairs, 18,* 182–188.
Bakan, D. (1969). *The duality of human existence.* Chicago: Rand McNally.
Bloch, D. (1983). Family systems medicine: The field and the journal. *Family Systems Medicine, 1,* 1–3.
Boss, P. (1999). *Ambiguous loss.* Cambridge: Harvard University Press.
Carter, B., & McGoldrick, M. (Eds.). (2005). *The expanded family life cycle: Individual, family, and social perspectives* (3rd ed.). Boston: Allyn & Bacon.
Coleman, J. C. (1988). Social capital in the creation of human capital. *American Journal of Sociology, 94,* 95–120.
Engel, G. L. (1977). The need for a new medical model: A challenge for biomedicine. *Science, 196,* 129–136.
Engel, G. L. (1980). The clinical application of the biopsychosocial model. *American Journal of Psychiatry, 137,* 535–544.
Helgeson, V. (1994). Relation of agency and communion to well-being: Evidence and potential explanations. *Psychological Bulletin, 116,* 412–428.
House, J. S., Landis, K. R., & Umberson, D. (1988). Social relationships and health. *Science, 241,* 540–545.
Library of Congress. (2006a). Lifespan Respite Care Act of 2002 (S 2489 IS). http://frwebgate.access.gpo.gov/cgi-bin/getdoc.cgi?dbname=107_cong_bills&docid=f:s2489is.txt.pdf.
Library of Congress. (2006b). Title XXIX—Lifespan Respite Care, Ronald Reagan Alzheimer's Breakthrough Act of 2004 (S. 2533). http://thomas.loc.gov/cgi-bin/query/F?c108:20:./temp/~mdbsu0yPm4:e2490.
Library of Congress. (2006c). *Bill summary and status for the 109th Congress.* http://thomas.loc.gov/bss/abt_stat.html.
Lyons R. F., Sullivan, M. J. L., Ritvo, P. G., & Coyne, J. C. (1995). *Relationships in chronic illness and disability.* Thousand Oaks: Sage.
MacFarlane, W. (2002). *Multifamily groups in the treatment of severe psychiatric disorders.* New York: Guilford.
Marshak, L. E., Seligman, M., & Prezant, F. (1999). *Disability and the family life cycle.* New York: Basic Books.
McDaniel, S. H., & Campbell, T. L. (Eds.). (1999). Genetic testing and families: A special issue. *Families, Systems & Health, 17,* 1–144.
McDaniel, S. H., & Cole-Kelly, K. (2003). Gender, couples, and illness: A feminist analysis of medical family therapy. In L. Silverstein & T. J. Goodrich (Eds.), *Feminist family therapy* (pp. 267–280). Washington, DC: American Psychological Association.
McDaniel, S. H., Hepworth, J., & Doherty, W. (1992). *Medical family therapy: A biopsychosocial approach to families with health problems.* New York: Basic Books.
McDaniel, S. H., Campbell, T. L., Hepworth, J., & Lorenz, A. (2003). *Family-oriented primary care* (2nd ed.). New York: Springer.
Miller, S., McDaniel, S. H., Rolland, J., & Feetham, S. (2006). *Individuals, families & the new genetics: A biopsychosocial perspective.* New York: Norton.
Mittleman, M. S., Ferris, S. H., Shulman, E., Steinberg, G., & Levin, B. (1996). A family intervention to delay nursing home placement of patients with Alzheimer's disease: A randomized controlled trial. *Journal of the American Medical Association, 276,* 1725–1731.
National Alliance for Caregiving (NAC) and AARP. (2004). *Caregiving in the U.S.* http://assets.aarp.org/rgcenter/il/us_caregiving.pdf.
Olkin, R. (2001). *What psychotherapists should know about disability.* New York: Guilford.
Patterson, J. M. (2002, October 14). Personal communication.
Penn, P. (1983). Coalitions and binding interactions in families with chronic illness. *Family Systems Medicine, 1,* 16–25.
Public Law 109–442. (2006, December 21). 120 STAT. 3291. Lifespan Respite Care Act of 2006.
Rolland, J. (1994). *Illness, families & disabilities.* New York: Basic Books.

Seaburn, D. B., & Erba, G. (2003). The family experience of "sudden health": The case of intractable epilepsy. *Family Process, 42,* 453–468.

Seaburn, D. B., Lorenz, A. D., Gunn, Jr., W. B., Gawinski, B. A., & Mauksch, L. B. (1996). *Models of collaboration: A guide for mental health professionals working with health care practitioners.* New York: Basic Books.

U.S. Census Bureau. (1997, December). *Census brief* (CENBR/97–5). http://www.census.gov/prod/3/97pubs/cenbr975.pdf.

U.S. Census Bureau. (2005). Facts for features (CB05-FF.10–2). http://www.census.gov/Press-release/www/releases/archives/facts_for_features_special_editions/004998.html.

U.S. Census Bureau. (2006). http://factfinder.census.gov/servlet/STTable?_bm=y&-geo_id=01000US&-qr_name=ACS_2006_EST_G00_S1801&-ds_name=ACS_2006_EST_G00_&-_lang=en&-_caller=geoselect&-redoLog=false&-format=.

Walsh, F. (2003). Family resilience: A framework for clinical practice. *Family Process, 42,* 1–18.

Walsh, F. (2006). *Strengthening family resilience.* New York: Guilford.

Weihs, K., Fisher, L., & Baird, M. (2002). Families, health, and behavior—A section of the commissioned report by the Committee on Health and Behavior: Research, Practice, and Policy, Division of Neuroscience and Behavioral Health and Division of Health Promotion and Disease Prevention, Institute of Medicine, National Academy of Sciences. *Families, Systems & Health, 20,* 7–46.

Wynne, L. C. (2003). Systems theory and the biopsychosocial model. In R. Frankel, T. Quill, & S. H. McDaniel (Eds.), *The biopsychosocial approach: Past, present, and future* (pp. 219–230). Rochester: University of Rochester Press.

# Chapter 3
# Feelings of Family Caregivers

Yvette Getch

In recent years, more attention has been given to caregiving for persons with disabilities and/or chronic illness. Research has been conducted on different aspects of caregiving and the impact the acts of caregiving have on the person providing care. While there are many facets of family caregiving that could be investigated, this chapter will focus upon the feelings of family caregivers, what we currently know about the feelings caregivers experience, the direction of future research, and the implications for improving the quality of life for caregivers and the recipients of caregiving services.

Feelings are subjective and are often difficult to substantiate. However, the stress and lifestyle changes that occur and the stress encountered when family members become caregivers impact these individuals emotionally. The literature indicates that caregiving has numerous effects on caregivers. Some of the effects include isolation (Brody et al. 1984); depression (Dura et al. 1990; Gallagher et al. 1989; Morris et al. 1988); anger; sadness; fatigue; loss of friends, hobbies, job, and relationships; worry; fear; guilt; anxiety (Power and Dell Orto 2003; Rabins et al. 1982); and exhaustion (Chenoweth and Spencer 1986). Parents of children with disabilities vary in their emotional well-being but are more likely to experience distress and depression (Cadman et al. 1991; Kronenberger and Thompson 1992; Power and Dell Orto 2003). While these feelings are not surprising, it is important to recognize that these emotions are real and that they impact the lives of the caregiver and the person receiving care, as well as significant others.

## Caregiver Burden

Feelings of caregivers are difficult to discuss without first defining the concept of caregiver burden. "Caregiver burden" is used to refer to the extent to which caregivers perceive their physical, psychological, emotional, social, and financial problems as

Y. Getch (✉)
Department of Counseling and Human Development Services, University of Georgia,
402 Aderhold Hall, Athens, GA 30602, USA
e-mail: ygetch@uga.edu

a result of providing care for their family member (George and Gwyther 1986; Stull et al. 1994; Zarit et al. 1986). Feelings are considered to be the "subjective" part of the caregiving burden (Zarit et al. 1986). Caregivers might feel resentment, bitterness, frustration, and depression (Chenoweth and Spencer 1986; Francell et al. 1988; Marples 1986; Worcester and Quayhagen 1983). Caregiving tasks like bathing, feeding, supervising, assisting with medication, or physical therapy are considered to be the "objective burden." Also included in the "objective burden" are tasks that the caregiver must take over due to the deteriorating skills of the person being cared for. These tasks may include chores, finances, home repairs, car repairs, errands, transportation, etc. (Worcester and Quayhagen 1983).

Both the age and income status of the caregiver are associated with the subjective burden, while tasks that may limit or take the caregiver's time are associated with the objective burden (Montgomery et al. 1985). Although attention needs to be given to the "objective" burden, we must be careful not to overlook the "subjective" burden because it is central to family caregiving (Levine et al. 2003–2004). Because this chapter is dedicated to the emotional aspects of caregiving, the term caregiver burden will be used to indicate the subjective (feeling) aspect of the caregiving burden.

Caregiver distress is likely to increase if the person receiving care exhibits impaired social functioning and/or disruptive behaviors (Deimling and Bass 1986). The feelings associated with this kind of distress may include isolation, bitterness, sadness, or guilt. Caregivers may decline invitations to social events or may choose to stay at home because they are concerned that the person they are caring for may be disruptive in public or may engage in behavior that is embarrassing to them or others. Choosing to decline social invitations because of fear of disruptive or embarrassing behavior may increase feelings of isolation. A study by King et al. (1999) found that a child's behavior problems were the most important predictor of parental well-being. Even though the majority of the behaviors exhibited were not severe, the child's behavior was related to the amount of distress and depression experienced by the parents. Other researchers have found that the challenges faced by these families increase when the child has a severe emotional or behavior disorder (Friesen 1989).

Caregivers may resent missing out on social activities or events and may blame their isolation, lack of support, or loss of friends on the person they are providing care to. Regardless of whether they assign blame, family functioning and social support appear to be a significant predictor of parents' well-being. Those parents who are more satisfied with their social supports and whose families are doing well, report lower levels of stress and depression (King et al. 1999). An interesting finding is that family and friends who may be considered to be supports, may also be a source of stress as well. Caregivers reported stressful events in regard to friends, spouses, and partners (McDonald et al. 1996). Parents may also experience stress when attempting to seek support from family members. For example, parents may not reveal the severity of a child's illness or disability to grandparents for fear that the information may burden the grandparents, negatively impacting their health and well-being (Power and Dell Orto 2003).

Lack of respite care may also contribute to feelings of isolation. Caregivers who are unable to find or afford respite care may decline social invitations. It is not that the caregivers do not want to engage in social activities, but rather they may feel unable to participate because they cannot afford to pay for caregiving services and/or they have no one they trust to care for their family member. These situations may lead to feelings of helplessness. One mother of a child with a chronic illness expressed:

> It sometimes feels like you are in a bubble... the world goes on around you and nobody seems to know the conditions or how you are feeling inside... you have no resources to get you out of the bubble... you're dealing with a sick child and all that. So you don't have any social life.... It's a combination of not really having much time or if you have the time, no money, or if you have time and money, nobody to watch the kids (Getch 2002).

Not only does the inability to secure respite care lead to feelings of isolation, it may lead to feelings of helplessness as well. Caregivers may not want to "burden" others with the care of their family member or they may have exhausted their known resources by overutilizing the same relatives or friends to provide respite care. The caregiver may feel that they are unable to change the situation because even if they did locate a source of support that source would be short-lived as well. When caregivers make attempts to find respite care and their attempts fail, they may feel helpless and may evaluate the situation as hopeless. As a result, they may discontinue seeking respite and resign themselves to being isolated. Regardless of the reasons for declining social invitations, the end result is isolation. Isolation may lead to depression or a perception that others do not understand, or simply do not care. One mother explained the difficulty she had finding respite care.

> ...there is not anybody there to help me. I don't have anybody that, [to say] well, I need a few minutes can you watch the kids? I don't have that.... People are afraid to watch [my daughter]. I had a friend of mine... she wouldn't watch [my daughter] because she gets sick so easy and the fact that she goes from healthy one minute to critically ill the next... people don't want to watch her. And I can't blame them. Because it is scary (Getch 2002).

In the case above, the mother expresses that she understands why other people are reluctant to care for her daughter. However, she also expressed disappointment that a friend was unwilling to take on this responsibility to help her out or assist her. It is possible that caregivers may feel guilty asking others to care for their family member because they recognize it places an enormous responsibility on those individuals.

Family caregivers include parents of children with disabilities, siblings of individuals with disabilities, children who have parents with disabilities, spouses of persons with disabilities, and extended family members caring for persons with disabilities. The remainder of the chapter will focus upon the feelings of family caregivers with an emphasis on parents as caregivers and spouses as caregivers.

## Parents Caring for Children

Children with disabilities are most likely to be cared for by their families rather than a social institution or other form of care (Lourie 1987). Families who care for children with disabilities and/or chronic illness have a variety of special needs including respite care, provision of services, financial stress, and social education (McDonald et al. 1996). These families also interact with a variety of professionals as they attempt to provide care to their children. Interaction with professionals associated with the care of their child often becomes a large part of the caregiver's life as he or she attempts to meet the needs of the child and the needs of the family as well (Bailey and Garralda 1989; Collins and Collins 1990). Frequent interactions with professionals may not always be a pleasant experience, and researchers have proposed that parents would like to see professionals have more supportive attitudes toward them and change their attitudes. Parents have expressed that they often feel as if professionals blame them or attempt to exclude them. Parents also express a need to receive stronger commitments from professionals to assist the family in keeping the child with a disability at home (Early and Poertner 1993; Petr and Barney 1993). Many children are seen by numerous professionals including doctors, therapists, specialists, educators, and psychologists. Arranging and attending these appointments require both effort and time (Traustadottir 1993).

Although the research on childcare usage by parents who have children with disabilities is limited, data indicate that mothers of children with disabilities enter the labor force at essentially the same rate as the general population (Landis 1992 as cited in Booth-LaForce and Kelly 2004). Booth-LaForce and Kelley (2004) found that more than 58% of children in their study were in some form of nonmaternal childcare by the time they were 15 months of age. Families who have children with disabilities face a number of childcare issues including affordable care that is of good quality, location of quality care, and finding programs with staff who are trained and facilities that are equipped to meet the needs of children with disabilities (Booth-LaForce and Kelly 2004). Booth-LaForce and Kelly (2004) found that for children with disabilities, patterns of participation in childcare differed over time when compared to children without disabilities. These children often entered childcare an average of 6 months later and were in childcare fewer hours per week when compared to their peers without disabilities. Children with disabilities were also more likely to be in an informal childcare placement with most of them being cared for by relatives (Booth-LaForce and Kelly 2004). Mothers expressed several issues that were problematic for them in regard to childcare. These issues included finding good quality care, developing confidence in the staff, cost, access to special equipment, location of care (distance one must travel), and transportation concerns. The most significant issue appeared to be finding quality care. This may explain why researchers have found that childcare for children with disabilities is most often provided by relatives rather than childcare centers (Warfield and Hauser-Cram 1996, as cited in Booth-LaForce and Kelly 2004).

Childcare issues can significantly impact the families of children with disabilities. It is likely that difficulties securing quality care that is affordable increase caregiver burden, particularly "subjective" burden. One mother explained the difficulty she experienced attempting to find quality daycare for her child.

> ...I interviewed 15 daycares. I asked how they handled children with allergies and asthma and if I provided them with the proper medication and the proper tools to administer that medication, would they do it? And a lot of them told me no.... I think probably six said no and another six that said well, oh yeah, we're familiar with it...you could tell they really weren't... when we tried to have a conversation on allergy and asthma, they didn't use the right terms...they didn't know what a nebulizer was... (Getch 2002).

Many families spend enormous amounts of time locating and securing childcare. Mothers often describe this process as particularly stressful because they must consider so many other factors than most parents. The childcare provider must not only provide a clean, safe, warm, and nurturing environment, but must also be competent and willing to handle medical issues and emergencies as well.

Family caregivers of children with disabilities have described some of the most pleasant events in caring for their child. McDonald et al. (1996) found when children are able to participate in normal, everyday activities, the parents experience a great deal of pleasure. Some of these events included the child teaching the caregiver how to play a game, the child learning to fish, or the child participating in church activities. Several parents described pleasant experiences related to the child's effort and success in school. These experiences included the teacher stating the child had a good day at school, the child improving his grades, or not missing any days of school. Caregivers also stated that professionals and professional services had made a positive impact including providing respite care and receiving other needed services that made a difference in their family life. Family relations and social support were also considered to be sources of pleasure (McDonald et al. 1996).

Family caregivers are also faced with a variety of stressful or unpleasant events. These events include receiving information about their child's problems, waiting for school evaluations, difficulty obtaining needed services, feeling as if professionals did not listen to them, feeling misunderstood, dealing with school-related issues or family-related issues, and work (McDonald et al. 1996). Also, specific expectations and demands are placed on parents or caregivers of children with chronic illnesses. These include managing the illness by providing treatment, monitoring symptoms, maintaining family integrity, and insuring financial stability (Willis et al. 1982).

Caregivers must also be constantly alert regarding symptoms and often spend much time and energy monitoring the child's condition. Caregivers must watch for early symptoms of potential problems associated with the illness and make decisions regarding medical treatment (Hauenstein 1990). This level of vigilance and decision-making contributes to the stress experienced by the parents. Although it is likely that all caregivers experience stress, data indicate that mothers of children with disabilities experience more stress than their spouses. Specifically, they are reported to have higher stress levels and greater levels of depression (Lewis-Abney 1993; Little 2002).

## *Mothers as Caregivers*

Approximately, 59–75% of caregivers are women (Family Caregiver Alliance 2003; NAC-AARP 1997). Studies indicate that mothers of children with disabilities assume more responsibility for medical treatments, medically related activities, and other caregiving activities than fathers (Canning et al. 1996; Quittner et al. 1998). In a study by Getch (2002), mothers reported they felt they needed more medical training or education. As one mom said, "I feel like I need a stethoscope...." Mothers in this study also reported feeling stressed in regard to making treatment decisions. Another mom explained it in this manner: I mean, "you just got to make the call, you're not a doctor... *[but you]* make the medical decision." Clearly, these mothers expressed the stress and distress they encounter as they care for their children. Research also indicates that parents may experience guilt regarding the accurateness of the judgments and decisions they make regarding treatment. Thirty-one percent of mothers whose infants were on apnea monitoring expressed fears of waiting too long to seek medical help or fears of seeking help too early (Nuttal 1988). If the mothers waited too long to seek professional help, they could place their child in danger. Yet, seeking help too early produced fears that they would be seen as over-reactive, incompetent, overprotective, or hysterical mothers. Mothers also express fears and guilt related to making medical and treatment decisions. For example, one mom stated:

> ...What if you're not right?...I feel guilty about not being more knowledgeable...that's scary to feel like you're not doing the right thing (Getch 2002).

Mothers in this study expressed feelings of stress, uncertainty, guilt, and fear in regard to making medical or treatment decisions. Many of the mothers reported they needed medical training or should have gone to school to be a nurse. They also expressed a desire not to be placed in the position to make decisions based on their own limited knowledge regarding treatment and what they perceived as medical interventions. The fear that these mothers expressed regarding being responsible for treatment and medical decision-making is likely to contribute to their overall stress. These fears may also contribute to marital role strain, particularly if the parents disagree on treatment options or medical decisions. An example of the role strain was disclosed by a mother in the following manner:

> ...your spouse will make you feel like you're overexaggerating...then you feel bad and you start...getting that question in your head...am I overexaggerating? Or am I not? ...Sometimes he will tell me...just chill out...but gosh, if I do that though what's gonna happen? (Getch 2002).

Many children are seen by numerous professionals including doctors, therapists, specialists, educators, and psychologists. Many mothers often act as their child's "case manager" ensuring that their children receive the care they need and that the myriad of professionals actually communicates with one another. Traustadottir (1993) conducted a qualitative study and one of the mothers stated:

> Now who is going to take the responsibility for making sure that all these 17 professionals are seen? That whatever they say is followed up on? That they coordinate and talk to each other, that they are paid (Traustadottir 1993, p. 179).

Case management can include a variety of activities and may be accompanied by a variety of emotions as well. It is not unusual to hear mothers talk about their frustration regarding receiving what they consider to be good medical care or services for their children. For example, one mother talks about the frustration of receiving a referral for her child:

> She probably needs to see a specialist.... It's like an act of Congress to get that *[referral to a specialist]* done.... You need a referral from your doctor. Of course, your child has to be near dead for you to get a referral. I don't know if it is a money issue or what, but they [the primary physician] will not give a referral to a specialist (Getch 2002).

Other moms discuss the frustration of dealing with insurance companies and the red tape involved in acquiring the necessary services. This may be best exemplified by one mom's description of the necessity for mothers to be advocates for their children. "Unfortunately, how active and forceful you are determines what you get" (Traustadottir 1993, p. 179). The implication is that if the mother did not advocate or fight for what was best for the child, the child would not receive the care and services needed. These kinds of activities require much time and energy and may increase the amount of stress mothers experience as caregivers for children with disabilities.

Demands on the mother's time can seriously limit opportunities for her to engage in other things. Mothers report fewer opportunities for community and outside leisure activities (Hauenstein 1987). Even when the mothers find time to be with friends, they often find themselves worrying that necessary treatments or routines may be missed. This fear or worry often diluted the sense of fun they expected to have with friends. As one mom explained:

> ...initially you want a break but then...I would be...stressed knowing that the responsibility...you know homework...uh, that treatment...or the medication wouldn't get done...it bothers you to think it's not [getting done] so then you kind of want to leave and go home and get it done (Getch 2002).

Many mothers may experience fatigue or exhaustion. Fatigue may be due to the level of care required by the child, frequent hospitalizations, and attempts to continue to fulfill other time-demanding roles including work or managing the household. Caregiving and the vigilance required when caregiving for a child with a chronic illness and/or disability may best be understood by the following quotes:

> I mean, I don't think I slept for the first year of her life because I knew something was wrong with her...at night it just felt like she was strangling and choking every time she breathes...so I would say I didn't start sleeping through the nights until Rose was three... (Getch 2002).

Another mom expressed how fatigue had a negative impact on her marital relationship and seemed to create marital strain:

> ...I don't look tired [at my job]...well, so I look tired without makeup.... But they won't know that I am stressed or whatever. But at home my husband suffer[s] all the consequences. He always tells me you're always smiling to all your friends, to everybody. Can't you be the same way here? [I say] No. It's just that here is the real thing. I'm not that happy or energetic. I'm tired (Getch 2002).

Family members may see mothers as giving their best to others. Family members may resent or criticize mothers for appearing energetic, pleasant, and friendly toward coworkers and friends when they appear grumpy, irritable, and seem to lack energy at home. This may especially interfere with the marital relationship. Mothers express feelings of frustration, fatigue, and anger about feeling responsible for making sure their child receives the level of care they require and that everything gets accomplished. One mom expressed how she handles feeling overwhelmed with the caregiving responsibilities and how these feelings surface in her marital relationship:

...when I just can't take it anymore, I will go, that's it. You're going to take care of her this week. I'm always doing it. She's yours and I want to see [how you would handle it]...because he will say, oh, you're laying down. He will come home [and say] "you're laying down" (Getch 2002).

Since mothers are often the primary caretakers for children with disabilities (Quittner et al. 1998; Traustadottir 1993), the multiple roles moms play are likely to become overwhelming. Little (2002) speculates that mothers may experience greater caregiver burden as they may be doing most of the childcare and home maintenance, attending school meetings, advocating for various services, and dispensing mediation when difficulties arise. There is no doubt that mothers play a significant role in the lives of their children with disabilities; however, we must not ignore the role fathers play in the lives of these same children.

## Fathers as Caregivers

Although mothers are the primary caregivers, it is important to note that relatively few studies have investigated the impact of caregiving on fathers (Quittner et al. 1998; Seagull 2000). The lack of research focusing on fathers is disconcerting because there is evidence that disability and childhood illness has an impact on each member of the family system (Droter 1992; Quitttner et al. 1992; Roberts and Wallander 1992) and that having a child with a disability or chronic illness appears to generate different reactions from fathers as compared to mothers (Hanson et al. 1989; Little 2002; McKeever 1981; Seiffge-Krenke 2001, 2002).

Fathers appear to encounter greater stress in relation to finances and attachment issues with the child (Quittner et al. 1998). Fathers feel their role is to support their wives, and they tend to generate the income in the family (McKeever 1981; Seiffge-Krenke 2002). Thus, in many families who have children with chronic illnesses and/or disabilities, the role of the father as "breadwinner" may be reinforced (Seiffge-Krenke 2002).

If the father is spending much time at work or takes on a second job, he is not as able to participate in the child's care. Often, as a result, the mother and child form a bond around treatment and care issues, but the father becomes more distant and may experience feelings of incompetence regarding treatment issues. If the father begins to feel increasingly incompetent about medication and treatment issues, he may distance himself even more from the situation (Seagull 2000). In her work, Seagull (2000) has found that fathers experience deep feelings that may be difficult for them to express. They may fear for their child's future and feel helpless or intense anguish because they are unable to protect their loved ones. Even though fathers experience these feelings, research indicates that they are less likely to find professional support (counseling) helpful (Little 2002).

Quittner et al. (1998) found that fathers spend more time at work each day and were less involved with caregiving tasks. There was also evidence of increased role strain with conflicts regarding childcare issues, childcare tasks, frustration with current role division, and fewer numbers of positive interactions between spouses. Men did not appear to be as frustrated with the division of labor as women. However, husbands did report fewer out-of-home activities and less recreation time than their wives. These findings suggest that fathers experience caregiver burden in a different way than mothers. It may be that fathers feel the way they can best support their children and spouse is to insure that they are financially stable. This may place fathers in a position to be unintentionally excluded from activities that directly impact their child's care. These activities include: (a) being with the child at medical appointments and during medical procedures; (b) discussing medical treatments, medications, and therapies with specialists, pharmacists, and therapists; (c) attending school-related meetings to discuss their child's educational needs; and (d) providing direct treatment or dispensing medication to the child. When fathers are excluded from these activities, they are likely to receive less information and be less knowledgeable about their child's condition, medication, and therapies.

## Spouses as Caregivers

Marriages must contend with numerous ebbs and flows throughout the family life cycle, but a supportive spouse typically provides a buffer in negotiating life transitions and crises (Figley and McCubbin 1983; McCubbin and Figley 1983). When a spouse becomes disabled and their health, mental capacities, and/or physical capacities deteriorate to the point that they require substantial caregiving, the buffer that once existed may no longer be present.

Spouses of persons with chronic conditions may feel a variety of losses including the loss of intimacy and companionship (Jivanjee 1995; Lefley 1996), the loss of future plans that had been made but are no longer possible because of deteriorating health or mental capacities (Jivanjee 1995), the loss of predictability of behavior (Judge 1994), and the loss of a sexual partner (Martinson et al. 1993). These may be especially difficult if both spouses are older and experiencing declining health. Caregiving may be a source of significant stress and may have a marked effect on both the caregivers' emotional and physical health (Bass et al. 1994; Jivanjee 1995; Pearson et al. 1988).

The loss of intimacy and companionship may be particularly hard. Activities that a couple previously enjoyed may no longer be possible, thus creating sadness and isolation for the caregiver (Jivanjee 1995; Martinson et al. 1993). Spouses may feel tied down and unable to keep their social connections because they feel guilty about leaving their spouse in the care of someone else or they may not be financially able to pay someone to provide care while they take a break (Jivanjee 1995).

Cognitive impairments appear to impact the emotional closeness and positive bonds between caregivers and their spouses (Townsend and Franks 1997). Conflict between spouses is likely to be related to the caregiver's appraisals of caregiving effectiveness. Negative appraisals of caregiving may evoke feelings of inadequacy. These feelings may be intensified and cause conflict if the spouse's efforts to assist are misperceived or unwanted (Townsend and Franks 1997). Research by Jivanjee (1995) revealed that some spouse's feelings may become intense creating fears about their own potentially violent reactive behavior. She found that caregivers may recognize their changing emotional reactions and may take action to avoid doing harm to their spouse. One respondent in her study replied:

> I felt myself getting irritable. Then I realized the best thing to do is to put him in a nursing home. I was getting tired and irritable. I didn't want to lose my cool. I couldn't take it anymore. He didn't deserve that.... I've seen workers in nursing homes slap people. Before I get to that, I'd put him in a nursing home (p. 124).

Negative responses to the extreme stress of caregiving can be intense. Spouses need support systems to help them deal with these emotions and they need services to assist them so that the cumulative stress effects will not escalate (Jivanjee 1995).

Not all responses to caregiving are negative. Some spouses found a role for themselves as caregivers, believing they were the only ones who could provide good quality care and believing marriage was a basis for accepting this responsibility (Jivanjee 1995). Perry and O'Conner (2002) identified a number of ways that spousal caregivers may contribute to the preservation of their spouse's personhood. Caregivers may identify retained abilities and provide their spouse with opportunities to employ these retained skills. Conversely, the spouses are also careful to evaluate situations and avoid those that might expose the person's declining abilities. Caregivers protected their spouses by manipulating the environment, normalizing the partner's loss, and gradually taking control of situations without making it obvious that they had taken control (Perry and O'Conner 2002). It may be that these spouses feel that the caregiving they were providing was a continuation of the loving relationship they had developed and nurtured over the years.

In summary, spousal caregivers experience a wide range of feelings and emotions. These feelings include a sense of loss, sadness, isolation, grief, fear, regret, irritation, frustration, and accomplishment. Caregiving for a spouse changes the nature of the relationship and the roles previously played by each partner. Motivation for providing caregiving may be an important factor in response to the stresses of caregiving. Spouses who provide caregiving as continuation of their loving relationship were more gratified than those who felt obligated to provide care out of a sense of responsibility (Montenko 1989).

## Cultural and Ethnic Differences

Just as there are differences among the varying kinds of family caregivers (i.e., spouses, parents, mothers, fathers, etc.), there are cultural and ethnic differences that are likely to influence the feelings experienced by individual caregivers (see Leung, this volume). Data from the National Alliance for Caregiving and the AARP (1997) indicate that European Americans earn markedly more than African Americans and report that caregiving does not place a financial burden on them. European American caregivers are more likely to be married and be a little older on average than African American caregivers. African American caregivers are more likely to be caring for an extended family member when compared to European Americans, and they are more likely to be caring for a family member with dementia or stroke. Data also indicate that African Americans spend substantially more hours per week in caregiving activities.

Cultural and ethnic differences are important. The manner in which families support and care for their members who have disabilities or chronic illnesses vary and are influenced by culture and ethnicity as well as socioeconomic status. These factors contribute to caregiver burden and the emotions experienced by the family members providing care. For example, African American families are more likely to rely on their kin or church members for support (Foley et al. 2002). South Asian family caregiving appears to be strongly influenced by cultural beliefs and the hierarchical nature of decision-making in South Asian families who adhere to their traditional cultural values. Caregivers who adhere to South Asian cultural norms about elder caregiving appear to experience lower levels of caregiver burden (Gupta and Pillai 2002). In Latino families, there is a strong identification and attachment to nuclear and extended families (Marin and Marin 1991). Latina mothers who receive little or no help from family members may experience greater caregiver burden. These mothers may be more at risk for maternal depression, and data indicate that a lack of family cohesion may contribute to depressive symptoms (Blacher et al. 1997).

Culture, ethnicity, and adherence to cultural norms appear to play a role in caregiver burden, caregiver expectations, and caregiver experiences. Family cohesion and adherence to cultural norms regarding caregiving appears to impact caregiver burden (Blacher et al. 1997; Gupta and Pillai 2002). Even similar levels of depressive symptomology may be experienced differently by individual caregivers due to cultural context (Foley et al. 2002). Therefore, the emotions exhibited and feelings experienced are likely to be influenced by culture and adherence to cultural norms.

## Discussion

Family caregivers experience a wide range of both positive and negative emotions. Negative feelings include a sense of loss, sadness, isolation, grief, fear, regret, irritation, frustration, and anger (Brody et al. 1984; Chenoweth and Spencer 1986; Dura et al. 1990; Gallagher et al. 1989; Morris et al. 1988; Power and Dell Orto 2003; Rabins et al. 1982). Positive feelings include a sense of accomplishment, fulfillment, and purpose. The nature of the caregiving experience (spouse to partner, parent to child, child to parent, etc.) and the cultural context influence caregiver burden and the feelings experienced by family caregivers (Jivanjee 1995; McDonald et al. 1996; Montenko 1989; Perry and O'Conner 2002).

A variety of needed supports have been alluded to in this chapter. Caregivers seem to fare better when they have access to family support, education about the condition, social support, and respite care. Culture, ethnicity, and socioeconomic status also appear to impact caregiver burden and influence the feelings experienced by caregivers. Future research should focus on the cultural, ethnic, and economic factors that impact caregiver burden and provide the context for feelings experienced by caregivers. Greater attention needs to be paid to the importance of social support and respite care. The data indicate that while mothers and women tend to be the primary caregivers, each member of the family is impacted by disability or chronic illness (Power and Dell Orto 2003). Maladaptive coping by one family member increases that individual's distress and may have negative effects on other family members' psychological functioning and well-being (Kotchick et al. 1996). The emotions experienced by family caregivers may have a significant impact on family functioning and the perception of caregiver burden. The more professionals understand about the feelings experienced by caregivers, the more apt they are to understand the types of services that will benefit these families and reduce caregiver burden.

Isolation, lack of social support, and lack of respite care appear to be three significant factors that contribute to the negative feelings experienced by family caregivers. When investigating these factors it is imperative that researchers pay attention to gender, cultural, ethnicity, and socioeconomic issues as they appear to be central to the caregiving experience and the perception of caregiver burden. Services that promote emotional well-being need to be provided. Some of these services may include counseling, resource mobilization, support groups, quality respite services, and financial assistance.

Future research should also focus upon the factors that contribute to reduced caregiver burden (Committee on Disability in America, Institute of Medicine 2006). It appears that attitudes toward caregiving, adherence to cultural norms, and family cohesion reduce caregiver burden (Blacher et al. 1997; Dilworth-Anderson et al. 2002; Gupta and Pillai 2002). Studying family caregivers who appear to experience low levels of caregiver burden may provide insight into the supports needed to reduce caregiver burden for those family caregivers who experience high levels of stress, negative emotions, and depressive symptomology. Future researchers should be aware that men and women may experience caregiving differently and the supports that may be helpful to women may not be particularly helpful to men.

The feelings of family caregivers vary and can be negative or positive. Even though feelings are subjective, the feelings experienced by family caregivers are very real and are influenced by the stress and lifestyle changes that occur when a family member acquires a chronic illness or disability. Caregiving has numerous emotional effects on family caregivers (Brody et al. 1984). These emotions and the manner in which they are expressed impact the lives of the caregiver, the care recipient, and significant others. Understanding the feelings experienced by family caregivers is likely to lead to improved services for families who have members with chronic illness and/or disabilities.

## References

Bailey, D., & Garralda, M. E. (1989). Referral to child psychiatry: Parent and doctor motives and expectations. *Journal of Child Psychiatry, 30,* 449–458.

Bass, D. M., McClendon, M. J., Deimling, G. T., & Mukherjee, S. (1994). The influence of a diagnosed mental impairment on family caregiver strain. *Journal of Gerontology: Social Science, 49,* 146–155.

Blacher, J., Lopez, S., Shapiro, J., & Fusco, J. (1997). Contributions to depression in Latina Mothers with and without children with retardation: Implications for caregiving. *Family Relations, 46,* 325–334.

Booth-LaForce, C., & Kelly, J. F. (2004). Childcare patterns and issues for families of preschool children with disabilities. *Infants and Young Children, 17,* 5–16.

Brody, E. M., Lawton, M. P., & Leibowitz, L. (1984). Senile dementia: Public policy and adequate institutional care. *American Journal of Public Health, 74,* 1383–1385.

Cadman, D., Rosenbaum, P., Boyle, M., & Offord, D. (1991). Children with chronic Illness: Family and parent demographic characteristics and psychological adjustment. *Pediatrics, 87,* 884–889.

Canning, R. D., Harris, E. S., & Kelleher, K. J. (1996). Factors predicting distress among caregivers to children with chronic medical conditions. *Journal of Pediatric Psychology, 21,* 735–749.

Chenoweth, B., & Spencer, B. (1986). Dementia: The experience of family caregivers. *Gerontologist, 26,* 267–272.

Collins, B., & Collins, T. (1990). Parent-professional relationships in the treatment of seriously emotionally disturbed children and adolescents. *Social Work, 35,* 522–527.

Committee on Disability in America, Institute of Medicine. (2006). In M. J. Field, A. M. Jette, & L. Martin (Eds.). *Workshop on disability in America: A new look—Summary and background papers.* Washington, DC: National Academies.

Deimling, G. T., & Bass, D. M. (1986). Symptoms of mental impairment among elderly adults and their effects on family caregivers. *Journal of Gerontology, 41,* 778–784.

Dilworth-Anderson, P., Williams, I. E., & Gibson, B. E. (2002). Issues of race, ethnicity, and culture in caregiving research: A 20-year review (1980–2000). *Gerontologist, 42,* 237–272.

Droter, D. (1992). Integrating theory and practice in psychological intervention with families of children with chronic illness. In T. J. Akamatsu, M. A. Stephens, S. E. Hobfall, & J. H. Crowther (Eds.), *Family healthy psychology* (pp. 175–192). Washington, DC: Hemisphere.

Dura, J. R., Haywood-Niler, E., & Kiecolt-Glaser, J. K. (1990). Spousal caregivers of persons with Alzheimer's and Parkinson's disease dementia: A preliminary comparison. *Gerontologist, 30,* 332–336.

Early, T., & Poertner, J. (1993). Families with children with emotional disorders. In A. Algarin, R. Friedman, A. Duchnowski, K. Kutash, S. Silver, & M. Johnson (Eds.), *Children's mental health service and policy: Building a research base.* Tampa: University of South Florida Research and Training Center for Children's Mental Health.

Family Caregiver Alliance (2003). Fact sheet: Women and caregiving: Facts and figures. http://www.caregiver.org/caregiver/jsp/content_node.jsp?nodeid=892. Accessed 8 Aug 2008.

Figley, C. R., & McCubbin, H. I. (1983). *Stress and the family: Vol. 2. Coping with catastrophe.* New York: Brunner/Mazel.

Foley, K. L., Tung, H., & Mutran, E. J. (2002). Self-gain and self-loss among African American and White caregivers. *The Journals of Gerontology, 57B,* 14–22.

Francell, C. G., Conn, V. S., & Gray, D. P. (1988). Families' perceptions of burden of care for chronic mentally ill relatives. *Hospital and Community Psychology, 39,* 1296–1300.

Friesen, B. J. (1989). National study of parents whose children have serious emotional disorders. In A. Algarin, R. Friedman, A. Duchnowski, K. Kutash, S. Silver, & M. Johnson (Eds.), *Children's mental health service and policy: Building a research base.* Tampa: University of South Florida Research and Training Center for Children's Mental Health.

Gallagher, D., Rose, J., Rivera, P., Lovett, S., & Thompson, L. W. (1989). Prevalence of depression in family caregivers. *Gerontologist, 29,* 449–455.

George, L. K., & Gwyther, L. P. (1986). Caregiver well-being: A multidimensional examination of family caregivers of demented adults. *Gerontologist, 26,* 253–259.

Getch, Y. Q. (2002). Mothers of children with chronic medical conditions: Multicultural perspectives. Unpublished raw data.

Gupta, R., & Pillai, V. (2002). Elder caregiving in South Asian families: Implications for social service. *Journal of Comparative Family Studies, 33,* 465–576.

Hanson, C. L., Henggeler, S. W., Harris, M. A., Burghen, G. A., & Moore, M. (1989). Family systems variables and the health status of adolescents with insulin-dependent diabetes mellitus. *Health Psychology, 8,* 239–253.

Hauenstein, E. J. (1987). *Families and illness: Family function and adaptation in families of ill children*. Unpublished doctoral dissertation, University of Virginia, Institute of Clinical Psychology, Charlottesville, VA.

Hauenstein, E. J. (1990). The experience of distress in parents of chronically ill children: Potential or likely outcome? *Journal of Clinical Child Psychology, 19,* 356–364.

Jivanjee, P. (1995). *Caregiving to family members with Alzheimer's disease*. New York: Garland.

Judge, K. (1994). Serving children, siblings, and spouses: Understanding the needs of other family members. In H. P. Lefley & Y. M. Wasow (Eds.), *Helping families cope with mental illness* (pp. 161–194). Newark: Harwood Academic.

King, G., King, S., Rosenbaum, P., & Goffin, R. (1999). Family-centered caregiving and well-being of parents of children with disabilities: Linking process with outcomes. *Journal of Pediatric Psychology, 24,* 41–53.

Kotchick, B. A., Forehand, R., Armistead, L., Klein, K., & Wierson, M. (1996). Coping with illness: Interrelationships across family members and predictors of psychological adjustment. *Journal of Family Psychology, 10,* 358–370.

Kronenberger, W. G., & Thompson, R. J., Jr. (1992). Psychological adaptation of mothers with spina bifida: Association with dimensions of social relationships. *Journal of Pediatric Psychology, 17,* 1–14.

Lefley, H. P. (1996). *Family caregiving in mental illness*. Thousand Oaks: Sage.

Levine, C., Reinhard, S. C., Feinberg, L. R., Albert, A., & Hart, A. (2003–2004). Family caregivers on the job: Moving beyond ADLs and IADLs. *Generations, 27,* 17–23.

Lewis-Abney, K. (1993). Correlates of family functioning when a child has attention deficit disorder. *Issues in Comprehensive Pediatric Nursing, 16,* 175–190.

Little, L. (2002). Differences in stress and coping for mothers and fathers of children with Aspergers Syndrome and nonverbal learning disorders. *Pediatric Nursing, 28,* 565–570.

Lourie, N. (1987). Case management. In T. A. Talbott (Ed.), *The chronic mental patient* (pp. 159–164). Washington, DC: American Psychiatric Association.

Marples, M. (1986). Helping family members cope with a senile relative. *Social Casework, 67,* 490–498.

Marin, G., & Marin, B. V. O. (1991). *Research with Hispanic populations*. Newbury Park: Sage.

Martinson, I. M., Chesla, C., & Muwaswes, M. (1993). Caregiving demands of patients with Alzheimer's disease. *Journal of Community Health Nursing, 10,* 225–232.

McCubbin, H. I., & Figley, C. R. (1983). *Stress and the family: Vol. 1. Coping with normative transitions*. New York: Brunner/Mazel.

McDonald, T. P., Couchonnal, G., & Early, T. (1996). The impact of major events on the lives of family caregivers of children with disabilities. *Families in Society, 77,* 502–516.

McKeever, P. T. (1981). Fathering the chronically ill child. *American Journal of Maternal Child Nursing, 6,* 124–128.

Montenko, A. K. (1989). The frustrations, gratifications, and well-being of dementia caregivers. *Gerontologist, 29,* 166–172.

Montgomery, R. J. V., Gonyea, J., & Hooyman, N. (1985). Caregiving and the experience of subjective and objective burden. *Family Relations, 34,* 19–26.

Morris, R. G., Morris, L. W., & Britton, P. (1988). Factors affecting the emotional well-being of the caregivers of dementia sufferers. *British Journal of Psychiatry, 153,* 147–156.

National Alliance for Caregiving & the AARP. (1997). *Family caregiving in the U.S.: Findings from a national survey*. Washington, DC: Authors.

Nuttal, P. (1988). Maternal responses to home apnea monitoring of infants. *Nursing Research, 37,* 1031–1038.

Pearson, J., Verma, S., & Nellet, C. (1988). Elderly psychiatric patient status and caregiver perceptions as predictors of caregiver burden. *Gerontologist, 28,* 79–83.

Perry, M., & O'Conner, D. (2002). Preserving personhood: Remembering the spouse with dementia. *Family Relations, 51,* 55–62.

Petr, G. C, Barney, D. D. (1993). Reasonable efforts for children with disabilities: The parents' perspective. *Social Work, 38*(3), 247–254.

Power, P. W., & Dell Orto, A. (2003). *The resilient family: Living with your child's illness or disability*. Notre Dame: Sorin Books.

Quittner, A. L., DiGirolamo, A. M., Michel, M., & Eigen, H. (1992). Parental response to cystic fibrosis: A contextual analysis of the diagnosis phase. *Journal of Pediatric Psychology, 17*, 683–704.

Quittner, A. L., Espelage, D. L., Opipari, L. C., Carter, B., Eid, N., & Eigen, H. (1998). Role strain in couples with and without a child with a chronic illness: Associations with marital satisfaction, intimacy, and daily mood. *Health Psychology, 17*, 112–124.

Rabins, P. V., Mace, N. L., & Lucas, M. J. (1982). The impact of dementia on the family. *Journal of the American Medical Association, 248*, 333–335.

Roberts, M. C., & Wallander, J. L. (1992). Family issues in pediatric psychology: An overview. In M. C. Roberts & J. L. Wallander (Eds.), *Family issues in pediatric psychology*. Hillsdale: Erlbaum.

Seagull, E. A. (2000). Beyond mothers and children: Finding the family in pediatric psychology. *Journal of Pediatric Psychology, 25*, 161–169.

Seiffge-Krenke, I. (2001). *Diabetic adolescents and their families: Stress, coping, and adaptation*. New York: Cambridge University Press.

Seiffge-Krenke, I. (2002). "Come on, say something, dad!": Communication and coping in fathers of diabetic adolescents. *Journal of Pediatric Psychology, 27*, 439–450.

Stull, D. E., Kosloski, K., & Kercher, K. (1994). Caregiver burden and generic well-being: Opposite sides of the same coin? *Gerontologist, 34*, 88–94.

Townsend, A. L., & Franks, M. (1997). Quality of the relationship between elderly spouses: Influence on spouse caregivers' subjective effectiveness. *Family Relations, 46*, 33–39.

Traustadottir, R. (1993). Mothers who care: Gender, disability, and family life. In M. Nagler (Ed.), *Perspectives on disability* (2nd ed., pp. 173–184). Palo Alto: Health Markets Research.

Willis, D. J., Elliot, C. H., & Jay, S. M. (1982). Psychological effects of physical illness and its concomitants. In J. Tuma (Ed.), *Handbook for the practice of pediatric psychology* (pp. 28–66). New York: Wiley.

Worcester, M. I., & Quayhagen, M. P. (1983). Correlates of caregiving satisfaction: Prerequisites to elder home care. *Research in Nursing and Health, 6*, 61–67.

Zarit, S. H., Todd, P. A., & Zarit, J. M. (1986). Subjective burden of husbands and wives as caregivers. A longitudinal study. *Gerontologist, 26*, 260–266.

# Chapter 4
# Education, Training, and Support Programs for Caregivers of Individuals with Disabilities

Sharon Goldsmith

It is estimated that 54 million people in the U.S., or almost 20% of the general population, live with some level of disability. Of these, approximately 33 million people (12.3% of the general population) have a severe disability (McNeil 2001). The disabilities range from cognitive to emotional to physical and every combination. Some disabilities are inherited or are incurred before birth; others occur because of accidents at birth or later in life; are the results of disease and some occur just because we are living longer. Disabilities may be permanent or temporary. Some require little or no sustained caregiver support; some are so severe that they impose major limitations on activities of daily living (ADL), have a major impact on family and social relationships, and require that the individual with a disability receive continuous support from a caregiver.

"Disability" can be defined in various ways. An estimated 7.3 million people are limited in their capacity to perform one or more of the ADLs that include bathing, transferring, dressing, eating, and toileting. More than half of the individuals limited in their ADLs require the assistance of another person (Kennedy and LaPlante 1997). A related study reports that 9.5 million Americans (almost 5% of the American population over age 15) require the assistance of someone else in ADLs or in other self-care activities such as managing money, using the telephone, preparing meals, or getting around outside the house (Kay and Longmore 1997).

The impact of a disability on an individual's life is affected by many factors: age, sex, educational level, spiritual grounding, work history, and type and severity of the disability. One factor that most influences the impact of a disability is the availability of caregivers with the ability to provide the needed support. Therefore, training and education of caregivers is a critical element in an individual's quality of life, mental outlook, and prognosis.

Additionally, just as there are variations in the care needs of people with disabilities, there are also variations in the kinds of caregivers that are available to meet

S. Goldsmith (✉)
Goldsmith Associates International, 4064 Mansion Drive NW, Suite 100,
Washington, DC 20007, USA
e-mail: goldsmith99@msn.com

these needs. Caregivers include highly trained professionals with specialized expertise in education or healthcare, professional caregivers with less education, wives, husbands, children, parents, grandparents, siblings, and friends. Caregivers may be called on to provide short-term, focused intervention—such as the one provided by a physician—or provide 24/7/365 care to an individual. Caregivers may be young or old; some may have disabilities of their own (such as an elderly person trying to care for a spouse disabled by Alzheimer's, stroke, diabetes, or blindness) or a range of other possible conditions. Some, like parents or siblings of adults with chronic disabilities, have been caring for a disabled person for many years. Others, such as the growing number of "baby boomers" with aging parents, are just now facing the challenges of caring for a parent with an acquired disability.

Therefore, discussing the training and education needs of caregivers of individuals with disabilities is a formidable task. There is no single best way to design and deliver "education, training, and support for caregivers of people with disabilities." That, perhaps, is the most important point of this chapter, and it's a point worth dwelling on. As some of the examples that follow will demonstrate, it is a point often overlooked by those who design and implement education, training, and support programs for caregivers of individuals with disabilities. Training must be tailored to the needs of the caregiver. The effectiveness of the training for caregivers is dependent on several variables: matching the kind of information provided with the caregiver's needs, information that the caregiver wants, and information that the caregiver requires.

Training needs differ based on the combination of factors: the characteristics of the individual, the characteristics of the individual's disability, and the characteristics of the caregiver. These factors must always be kept in mind when designing training programs. A factor that most caregivers share is too little time to invest in training. Providing education, training, and support that is not appropriate for their needs is counterproductive and can waste the little time they have. Therefore, it is critical for program designers to invest the time and resources before any interventions to determine what the caregiver wants and needs and to assure that the education, training, or support meets those requirements. A review of the literature of caregiving and people with disabilities suggests that too little attention is invested to systematically assess caregiver education, training, and support program needs. Additionally, limited attention is paid to the critical tasks of defining the desired programmatic outcomes and assessing the actual learning and situational outcomes that result.

This chapter will discuss the principles of education, training, and support that are, in fact, important considerations, as well as some of the special needs of specific types of caregivers. It will also address the current trends in education and training and support programs for caregivers of individuals with disabilities. The chapter will conclude with a discussion of some of the currently unmet education, training, and support needs and provide recommendations regarding the research and other activities needed to improve education, training, and support for caregivers of individuals with disabilities in the future.

## Issues to Consider in Designing Education, Training, and Support Programs for Caregivers of Individuals with Disabilities

Several important elements should be considered when designing an education, training, and support program. Most training designs focus on the content of the training, (i.e., the topics that will be covered). However, in addition to the training content, there are equally important factors that will affect the outcomes of the training process and the usefulness of the training experience to the caregiver. These include:

- The characteristics of the trainer,
- The conduit for the program,
- The mix of people participating in the program,
- Where the program is conducted.
- Language and cultural issues,
- What kind of information the caregiver wants and needs, and
- How the caregiver needs to use the information.

To be most effective, education, training and support programs need to be tailored to the unique needs of the caregiver. The following issues need to be considered when designing and implementing education, training, and support programs.

### *The Nature of the Disability and the Caregiving Requirements Related to that Disability*

This is the obvious factor and the one most training programs consider when designing training. In fact, many formal training and informal training programs such as support groups are "disability centered." Local newspapers list support groups for individuals and their caregivers, most of them centered on particular disabilities. Additionally, courses offered through colleges and universities, as well as community based workshops, usually focus on a particular disability. Teacher certification titles are generally defined by disability such as "teacher of the learning disabled," or "teacher of the deaf."

*Wishes of the Individual with a Disability* The characteristics of the individual with a disability must also be considered. These include his/her wishes regarding the levels of independence desired as well as required, perceived role of his/her caretaker/personal preferences regarding styles of caregiving.

*The Level and Kind of Caregiving Being Provided* Caregiving can range from providing medical intervention (that itself can vary from routine checkups to special surgery), education, diagnostic services, therapy services (in fields as diverse as physical therapy, dietetics, speech and language therapy, and occupational therapy), vocational and personnel counseling, providing assistance with activities of daily living such as feeding, toileting, ambulation. The degree of care required is of course dependent on the needs of the individual being cared for and can range from 24/7 care to occasional interventions.

*The kind of Caregiver Participating in the Program* Similar levels of care may be provided in different settings by different caregivers. A common example is the parent or spouse may provide assistance with activities of daily living in the home, similar assistance may be provided in the home by a paid caretaker such as a personal assistant or certified nursing assistant, or may be provided in an assisted living center, a long term care facility, a rehabilitation center, or a hospital. In the latter instances, a variety of individuals with a variety of educational backgrounds and skill sets may be providing the care.

A review of many education and training programs showed similarities in the content of the programs directed to similar kind of caregivers. One typical program for parents and teachers of children with disabilities at the Center for Developmental Disabilities of the University of Connecticut offers courses covering topics that would be of particular interest to these caregivers. The topics include: *Understanding Special Education, Early Childhood Inclusion Strategies, Self-Advocacy, Becoming Community Leaders, Assistive Technology,* etc.

Example of programs directed to another audience—healthcare professionals working with individuals with disabilities—can be found on the CDC website (http://www.cdc.gov/ncbddd/women/publications.htm) that offers resources such as *Guidelines for Improving Access to Healthcare Facilities and Providers* and *Removing Barriers to Healthcare: A Guide for Healthcare Professionals.*

*The Relationship of the Caregiver to the Person with Disabilities* As mentioned above, caregiving is provided by many people, family, community caregivers, paid assistants, teachers, rehabilitation specialists, medical professionals including nurses and doctors. Some of these caregivers, especially family members and friends, have longstanding personal relationships with the individual being cared for and need education dealing with the emotional as well as technical parameters of providing care to someone with a disability.

An important but often overlooked caregiver that requires support in both emotional and technical parameters of caregiving is the sibling of the person with a disability. Siblings are often collateral caregivers, close in age to the person being cared for and have very different training needs than other family caregivers such as parents or spouses. Training for siblings appears to be overlooked. In a web site search for support groups for siblings of individuals with disabilities, only one web site, Sibnet, was identified (http://www.siblingsupport.org/). This is in marked contrast to the large number of web sites directed to parents or spouses. Interestingly, while every state education department offers programs for parents, not one of the reviewed sites appears to have any training and education activities specifically directed toward siblings.

*The Primary Language of the Caregiver* The need to conduct education, training, and support in languages other than English is growing rapidly. According to

Gesinger and Carlson (1992), 15–20% of U.S. school-age children speak a language other than English at home and do not speak English as their primary language. The number of different languages spoken in the United States is also increasing rapidly. Bracken and McCallum (1999) conducted a meta-analysis of the studies examining the languages used in U.S. public schools. They reported that children enrolled in the Chicago public schools alone speak more than 200 languages while 150 languages are spoken in the state of California public schools. Communities such as Scottsdale, AZ, Palm Beach, FL, and Prince William County, MD, report between 40 and 80 different languages spoken. Even small communities have students and caregivers speaking many languages. Bracken and McCallum (1999) refer a study that reported 30 languages being spoken in a single small high school in a rural community (Tukwila) in Washington State.

Differences in language use can include differences in vocabulary, syntax (word order in a sentence), morphology (use of word endings), grammar, pronunciation, and cultural referents. Variations in language use among speakers of the same language occur in most languages. Translations of educational and training materials and spoken instructions must be sensitive to dialectal and other variations that may occur among common language speakers. One approach is to use words that are expected to be understood by all, another is to identify and incorporate several variants of words in the translations. For some linguistic minority groups, using instructors from the same geographic region and social/cultural background as the caregiver is very important for conveying accurate and appropriate information.

Even using pictures to convey information between the instructor and the caregiver may not always be helpful. For example, in the widely used Peabody Picture Vocabulary Test that is used to assess language understanding (receptive language skills), individuals are shown a page with four pictures and asked to point to the correct picture as it is named. Several of the pictures are of items or scenes that are familiar in United States middle class culture but would not be familiar in other cultures or other environments. Simply translating a training manual or set of instructions into a caregivers' language is not sufficient to ensure understanding (Goldsmith 2003). The material presented must take into account both the linguistic and cultural background of the caregiver.

*The Cultural and Ethnic Background of the Caregiver* While cultural and ethnic backgrounds may affect such obvious issues as language, they also may affect some more subtle dynamics of the education process. For example, it may affect the type and role of the instructor. In some cultures, women are not seen as authority figures, so having female instructors would not be productive. In cultures where priests rather than physicians are the primary authority figures, the counseling, even on healthcare issues, might be more effectively provided by a priest than the physician. In this situation, educational programs will be better received if offered in the neighborhood church than in the neighborhood school or hospital. An illustration of this was reported by Slaton (2000) in discussing training provided to Native families. The report (p. 7) describes lessons learned from conducting a focus group. The organizers had planned to have the meeting in a hotel, with flipcharts and a formal agenda.

Learning from the failure of the first day activities, the organizers moved the group outdoors to a beach and threw away the time ordered agenda. Slaton concludes (p. 21) that providers of education, training, and support must respect that Native families need:

- Culturally sensitive terms,
- To identify and coordinate their own technical assistance, and
- To select their own technical assistance providers.

Some individuals may have come from backgrounds where formal education was limited. This may be particularly true for political refugees from nations whose schools were closed due to military or civil unrest. It may also be true of certain immigrants arriving from nations where certain groups are denied access to education because of their ethnicity or sex. For these individuals simply translating information into another language may not be sufficient. However, translated information may provide a gauge of their educational level and to what degree the difficulties they may be experiencing is due to language difference or educational differences.

*Educational Training and Support Needs as Expressed by the Caregiver* Regardless of the factors listed above, the most important element in determining the content and format of the training, education, and support programs offered to caregivers should always be the expressed educational needs of the caregiver. Goldsmith (2002a) conducted a survey among parents of students that had been diagnosed as having special needs by two schools districts, one in Maryland and one in Virginia. Current ages of the children ranged from preschool through adult. The survey was conducted through face-to-face open-ended interviews. Parents of 10 children participated in the survey. They were asked what education, training, and support and related support had been or was being provided to them, or offered to them, by their child's school district, their level of satisfaction with the programs provided or offered and the kind of opportunities they would have liked to been offered.

The results were disturbing:

- Most disturbing was the finding that *all* the parents indicated that this was the first time anyone had asked them what kind of education, training, and support they would have liked to have/felt they needed.
- The second disturbing finding was the disconnect that appeared between what parents wanted and what the schools provided. This finding was not influenced by when the child had attended school or where the child had attended school.
- The training offered by the schools:
  - Focused on the legal rights and responsibilities of the special education system,
  - Provided information about how parents could help their child with specific tasks, (i.e., homework assignments) or language development activities,
  - Provided insights into the nature of the child's disabilities.
- The parents reported they wanted more general kind of support including:

- More information on resources available outside the school including: appropriate camps, community activities,
- Strategies for helping siblings,
- Formal opportunities to meet and network with other parents whose children had similar challenges.

Based on the limited size and scope of the survey, one can only speculate why there was such a "disconnect" between the needs of the parents and the education and support offered by the schools. It may be that the school does not see its role as providing the kind of information the parents wanted but rather sees its role as focusing on the child and the family in the context of the experiences directly related to success in school (although one can reasonably argue that all of the issues expressed by the parents directly affect a child's success in school).

The lesson learned from this study is that there is a need to actively involve parents in the design of any training and related activities. This involvement can include conducting a formal needs assessment such as a survey sent to parents, conducting focus group of parents and routinely having parents sit on the committees that organize the educational events—as in some school districts—of giving parents the authority and the resources to design and direct the parent training activities. This study was limited to parents of children with disabilities. It would be interesting to conduct a similar study to assess the disconnects that may exist between the education, training, and support offered and the expressed education, training, and support needs of other kind of caregivers such as caregivers of spouses or caregivers of parents with disabilities.

*Commonalities in the Education, Training, and Support Needs of Caregivers* The United Cerebral Palsy Caregiving Guidelines (www.ucp.org/ucp_channeldoc.cfm/1/11/54/54-54/2839) cite six areas in which *all* caregivers providing care for a loved one needs expertise (United Cerebral Palsy Association n.d.). These include:

- Preserving the dignity of the person being cared for,
- Involving him or her in decision-making,
- Promoting independence,
- Asking for help in caregiving from others,
- Being an advocate for the person in one's care, and
- Taking care of "self."

Regardless of the unique needs of the person being cared for and the unique features of different caregivers as described above, there are certain common elements that should be included in caregiver education, training, and support programs. All of the areas listed above in the United Cerebral Palsy Caregiving Guidelines can be collapsed into three general topics that should be included in all education, training, and support offered. The three topics are education, training, and support on (1) how to care for yourself as a caregiver, (2) how to access support systems and (3) how to be a responsive caregiver. Each of these topics can be the focus of stand-alone training sessions or can be integrated as elements into more generic training sessions.

# Current Status

## *Caring for Yourself as a Caregiver*

Both professional caregivers and family member caregivers report that stress is a major impediment to effective caregiving. In fact, a report of healthcare workers *In Our Hands* released by the American Hospital Association Commission on Workforce (2002) reported that stress was a major factor in job dissatisfaction and therefore a significant contributor to the shortage of skilled caregivers in hospital settings. Similar conclusions were reported in a related study. This study, *Healthcare at Work Report* (2002), prepared for the American Society of Healthcare Human Resource Administrators, indicated that workers reported that after salary dissatisfaction, stress was the greatest reason why people left the workplace (pp. 23–24). Additionally, 52% of workers reported being dissatisfied in their supervisors' efforts to help them manage stress (p. 27). Family members who are caregivers also report that the stress associated with caregiving responsibilities is a problem. Caregiver education programs must provide information on:

- the importance taking care of one's self and one's own needs,
- the role stress plays in hampering effective caregiving and
- practical strategies to help caregivers reduce stress.

## *Knowing How to Access Support Systems*

For families and friends caregiving for others, learning what resources are available and how to access them are important skills. Presidents Bush's initiative "Fulfilling Americas Promise to Americans with Disabilities" calls for a demonstration project to fund respite care for caregivers of adults and children with disabilities. A document outlining these initiatives mentions that the lack of resources such as respite care to help caregivers is a major factor in institutionalizing individuals with disabilities. Teaching caregivers where and how to access support systems for themselves needs to be an important training initiative.

Professional caregivers must also be taught how to access resources, especially new information. As the body of knowledge is expanding, it is no longer reasonable to expect caregivers to know everything about all disabilities and how to treat them. The critical issues are to learn how to conduct the research and seek out needed information. In fact, research methodology is now a standard part of the educational curriculum for many professions. For example, the physical therapy, occupational therapy, and audiology have radically changed their curricula. In the cases mentioned before, the minimum degree required for entry into these professions was raised to provide the time to incorporate more training on research methodology in the curriculum. Similarly, several medical specialty board exams have initiated "open–book" tests, where the skills being tested are not the ability to recall information but the ability to conduct the appropriate research needed to find the correct answers.

## *Being a Responsive and Respectful Caregiver*

Caregivers need to learn how to continually assess their caregiving and to modify caregiving practices in response to feedback from the person for whom they are caring. Just as caregivers must be asked what they want and need in training, the caregivers must be taught how to ask individuals being cared for what they need, what they want, and maybe most importantly, what they don't want. Caregivers must also be sensitized to the importance of respecting the rights and wishes of the person being cared for even when it may conflict with their own views. This is particularly important when dealing with adults with disabilities. Parents of adult children with disabilities may infantilize them particularly when communication or physical limitations require that the parent provide caregiving interventions similar to those typically provided to a young child. Likewise, children of aging parents with disabilities may infantilize the parent when the child is required to provide assistance with bathing, toileting, and feeding.

A widely discussed example of the importance of being a responsive and respectful caregiver was the subject of a series of letters that appeared in *Dear Abby* columns seen in the Washington Post and other newspapers around the country. A letter published in the column described a situation in which a 40-year-old severely disabled man lived at home with his parents who were his primary caregivers. A friend of the man honored his friend's request to arrange a sexual experience for him. However, the parents objected and denied this friend further access to their son. The letter describing the parents' reactions evoked a flurry of response letters to the newspaper, especially from disability advocates, who argued that denying the man's wishes, denying his sexuality, and denying him further access to his friend was both legally and morally incorrect. This series of letters could provide the basis for some important and interesting discussions among caregivers for adults with disabilities and educators of caregivers for adults with disabilities. A controlled study of caregiver training (Singh et al. 2004) indicated that certain training can increase the happiness of individuals with profound multiple disabilities as compared with the happiness of a similar cohort whose caregivers did not participate in the training.

## Education, Training, and Support Programs

Three general sources appear to provide the bulk of the education, training, and support provided to caregivers of individuals with disabilities. The first and largest source of education, training, and support is sponsored by, or directly provided through, formal educational institutions such as colleges and universities, state departments of education, and local school districts. The second source is education, training, and support provided through the healthcare system, including hospitals, rehabilitation centers, and mental health clinics. The third source is grass root sources of education and training. This would include training offered by individuals, often caretakers themselves, who have independently organized vehicles to help educate and train other caregivers. These typically include self-help groups, chat rooms, and one-on-one counseling.

## *Education, Training, and Support Provided to Caregivers of Individuals with Disabilities Through State and Local Educational Systems*

This sector appears to be the most organized and largest supplier of education, training, and support programs addressing the disability community. The growth of educational institutions as the largest supplier of education, training, and support is a direct result of two factors:

- Federal and state legislation and regulations mandating that ongoing educational services be available to caregivers, including family and community caregivers, and
- Universal licensing which mandates specific educational requirements for professional caregivers.

The Individuals with Disabilities Education Act (IDEA) of 1975 as revised in 2004 mandates that all children with disabilities receive a free and appropriate education from their local school district. Under federal law, the "children with disabilities" are defined as infants, children, and young adults from newborn to age 22, or until graduation from high school, whichever comes first. The students with disabilities are required to be educated in their neighborhood schools to the degree possible. However, some children with disabilities require special education programs and services that can only be provided in alternative environments such as special classes within the school district, special day or residential schools, hospitals, or long-term care facilities. Regardless of where the child receives the education, the cost of arranging for and funding the education must be borne by the local school district.

Federal legislation requires states to provide training and education to administrators, teachers, support personnel, and related services personnel that work with children with disabilities. Federal law and regulation require state education agencies to develop and maintain what is referred to as a *Comprehensive System of Personnel Development* (CSPD). The purpose of the CSPD is to generate a coordinated comprehensive effort to provide education, training, and support to all caregivers. However, states have discretion in the kinds of training they support and the audiences for this training. The cost of this training is usually borne by the state education agency; however, some federal funding is provided to all states to support these efforts. Additionally, the states may have opportunities to apply for discretionary training grants from the federal government and/or may partner with local school districts, other state or local agencies or private funding sources (such as industry sponsors or philanthropic organizations) to pay for and/or provide the training.

Typically, the states direct efforts to individuals that have direct contact with children with disabilities, teachers, and related support personnel. Much of this is offered through in-service courses, workshops, and conferences. Other training for personnel is connected with colleges or universities and offers formal credit for hours of instruction that may lead to a degree. Personnel may be motivated to participate in these programs through financial incentives based on credit hours earned or stipends for participation. In many states, participation is a requirement for renewing teaching certifications and related professional licenses. Of course, it is hoped that the primary motivation for participation is the desire to enhance knowledge and skills. Some models provide a combination of formal college or university instruction and in-service education, training, and support opportunities.

For example, this author helped develop and manage a Massachusetts Higher Education/Boston public schools collaborative entitled *A Generic Teacher Training Program*. This project was designed to help neighborhood school teachers and related services personnel develop the skills to work with children with disabilities who had, up to that point, been educated in private schools or in disability-segregated schools within the city. One of the specific goals of the program was to "Retrain Boston teachers to become certified as Generic Special Teachers in accordance with Chapter 766 (Massachusetts Special Education Regulations) professional standards" (Shulman 1976, February). Teachers participated in after-school, field-based courses taught by full-time and adjunct faculty from local colleges and universities. Those courses were equivalent in content and rigor to courses being provided on campus and participants had to complete all requirements including research papers and final exams. Faculty also provided day to day in school supervision for teachers within the context of the participants regular assignments in their schools to allow them to practice and integrate skills developed through formal coursework. Teachers who successfully completed the program received a master's degree from one of the participating colleges and were eligible for certification by Massachusetts as "a teacher of children with special education needs."

This model provided many advantages; it allowed teachers to remain in their regularly assigned positions and did not deplete the number of teachers working in the district. Teachers saw it as relevant and practical as it was based in school, allowing teachers to practice skills to address real and current challenges. Cost was the major disadvantage. Another disadvantage was that the school-based, on-the-job instructional model provided teachers with less exposure to the variety of disabilities that they might see in a traditional teacher education model where students rotate between several clinical and educational sites. Although clearly very old, this model would still be an effective one to use today, almost 30 years later! This speaks both to the usefulness of the model and the limited progress that has been made in creating work-based training models regarding children with disabilities for classroom teachers.

A more common procedure is to offer a series of training workshops to teachers. For example, the author, as Director of the Massachusetts Department of Education's Bureau of Program Development and Evaluation, directed an annual series of statewide training opportunities as part of a comprehensive system of personnel development. Each year, the topics and content of the training were designed based on several data sources. These data sources included: the evaluation of the previous year's training, systematic needs assessments completed by school personnel, results of school-district-based analysis of special education outcomes, and state- and federally-defined priorities. A review of the websites of education, training, and support offered in 2006 by various state education departments revealed little change in the topics offered from state to state. These topics included:

- classroom management/modification of the classroom,
- curriculum design/effective education,
- interfacing with regular education teachers and administrators,
- accessing/utilizing community resources/legal aspects of special education, and
- current issues and trends in special education.

Various studies of the effectiveness of the training in actually changing classroom environments repeatedly indicated that teachers reported more change when teams of teachers and administrators from the same school system attended training and when they had ongoing posttraining interaction. As a result, certain training opportunities mandated participation of teams of regular and special education teachers and staff from the same school system and preferably the same school. These courses include *Curriculum Evaluation and Design, Developing Models for Professional Collaboration, Developing Social Skills in Children, Developing Effective Remediation Techniques,* and *Utilizing Consultant Services*. Additionally, some classes were designed to give school-based staff the skills to return to their systems and be able to conduct in-service training for other school staff. Massachusetts recognized that the investment in such kind of "train-the-trainer" models, while more costly initially would provide a cadre of trained personnel who could then advance the availability of training within local school districts and who could provide ongoing expertise and support for school personnel.

States continue to routinely use these various training models. The usefulness of these programs in improving the quality of services offered to students is becoming documented, especially in preschool settings where there are generally both formally trained and credentialed caregivers and caregivers who have participated only in in-service programs. One such study (Epstein 1999) reported that formal education and in-service education for teachers achieved equal levels of quality, while a related study (McCarthy et al. 1999) concluded that one of the strongest predictors of program quality is teacher preparation. Both studies support the importance of education, training, and support for caregivers.

States are also required to provide training opportunities for parents and other family caregivers. Many states (including Massachusetts) also mandate that local school districts support special education parent advisory councils. These councils often take a leadership role in assisting school districts in developing educational offerings. However as illustrated in the survey reported earlier, most of these educational offerings appear to be directed toward having parents understand the processes and systems used to screen, evaluate, identify, and provide educational and related services to children with disabilities, and the legal rights and responsibilities of parents within the educational system.

Most states also have statewide or local parent organizations that offer formal educational opportunities through workshops, websites, and newsletters. It is encouraging to see that many of these organizations offer educational opportunities for both parents and professional caregivers and also encourage parents to play a lead role in educating professionals. The Federation for Children with Special Needs provides a model for this type of education, training, and support at the national level. Headquartered in Boston, Massachusetts, the Federation (and specifically its director, Martha Zeigler) was influential in educating state legislators in Massachusetts about the needs of children with disabilities, leading to the establishment for the first state-mandated public education programs anywhere in the U.S. for all students with disabilities. The federal regulations, first Public Law 94–142, then Public Law 89–313 (which addressed the rights of preschool children) and, more recently, IDEA were, in fact, modeled on the groundbreaking legislation and accompanying regulations developed in Massachusetts. Viewing teachers and other paid caregivers as professional partners with parent caregivers, the Federation then actively provided education, training, and support programs for teachers, administrators and other school personnel as well as for parents. The Federation has received numerous grants to expand its training efforts both within Massachusetts and nationally. An example is the Early Intervention Training Center that in the spring of 2006 offered 47 workshops on a variety of topics of interest to staff and families (http://fcsn.org/education/education.php).

## *Education, Training, and Support Programs Provided to Caregivers Through the Healthcare System*

Programs provided to caregivers of individuals with disabilities through the healthcare system are not as organized or comprehensive as those provided through the education systems. Hospitals and other healthcare organizations do have—in fact are mandated to have—comprehensive systems for educating their employees who provide caregiving, less comprehensive system for patients to help them care for themselves and usually minimal education, training, and support for family caregivers. As an example, the accreditation standards of The Joint Commission (formerly the Joint Commission on Accreditation of Healthcare Organizations) require that every healthcare organization:

- identifies the competencies that staff need to perform specific job responsibilities and tasks,
- assesses whether individual staff members in fact possess the competencies needed to perform the job tasks, and
- provides ongoing staff training based on a staff member's current level of skills against the competencies needed.

The Joint Commission is the most powerful accreditor of healthcare organizations in the United States. More than 90% of accredited hospitals in the U.S. are accredited by The Joint Commission. Similar requirements exist in the standards for The Commission on Accreditation of Rehabilitation Facilities (CARF; Goldsmith 2002b).

However, there are no equivalent rigorous mandates requiring systematic and comprehensive education, training, and support programs for patients and their caregivers. As a result, the amount of education, training, and support opportunities offered to caregivers and even patients within hospitals, rehabilitation facilities, and long-term-care facilities is often sparse. Many times, education is offered in the form of support groups for individuals with disabilities, less often are there support groups for the caregivers. As a personal example, many support groups and educational materials are available for women with breast cancer through hospitals, cancer coalitions, American Cancer Society, and other resources. However, there are very few education or training opportunities or support groups for their husbands or other caregivers.

Similarly, and again from personal experience, as a caregiver to three elderly individuals with serious and debilitating mental and physical disabilities, the author was offered no training or education or support by the hospitals and long-term care facilities treating them. It is ironic perhaps that the only formal education offered was a court-mandated guardianship training course that focused solely on the legal rights and responsibilities of caregiving.

The UN International Plan of Action on Ageing (sic) cites several priorities related to the aging of individuals with intellectual disabilities. They include the educational and training needs of those providing services to older people with intellectual disabilities to ensure that quality of life is maintained at the highest level and "cultural and economic factors that support family caregiving." The World Health Organization has released a draft document that addresses aging and social policy issues for adults with intellectual disabilities (Hogg et al. 2000, January, p. 29). This report provides several recommendations related to education and training. Included among these are the following:

- The public requires education with respect to aging and disabilities.
- Staff that work with people with intellectual disabilities require training to integrate age-related information and practice into their existing practices and require training with respect to both intellectual disability and age-related issues.
- Health and social service personnel in the developing regions require training and support in identifying the specific social support and healthcare needs of older people with intellectual disabilities.

## *Education, Training, and Support Provided Through Grassroots Efforts*

Historically, most of the support available to caregivers was through grassroots efforts. Mandates for education, training, and support from federal efforts (such as

IDEA) or private accreditation efforts (such as The Joint Commission) that have resulted in formal and systematic efforts are products of the last 25 years. Caregivers depended largely on the interventions of other individuals in the community (teachers, doctors, other caregivers) to provide whatever support, training, and education was available. Toseland and Smith (2001) describe various models of education, training, and support for caregivers. They summarize research that concludes there is no evidence as to what types of education, training, and support are best, but that multicomponent programs are more effective than any single component. This might be extrapolated to suggest that education, training, and support efforts that combine some of the elements of a grass-roots model, such as training by other caregivers, and informal, less structured instruction and support systems among caregivers would be helpful even in cases where more formal educational courses and workshops are available.

In fact, it is the authors' experience that family and community caregivers provide some of the most useful training on caregiving issues not only for other family and community caregivers but also for professional caregivers of individuals with disabilities. For example, for several years this author taught a summer class on working with children with disabilities in public schools. Course evaluations consistently reported that the most valuable information was provided by the parents of children with disabilities who came in as guest lecturers.

The role of the Internet has expanded the capacity of information that can be shared through grassroot networks. This includes chat rooms and Internet support groups operated through list serves and web sites that are created by an individual or individuals with a personal interest in a particular disability or aspect of caregiving. There is concern in general about the amount of misinformation being communicated through the Internet, including information being provided to caregivers of individuals with disabilities. Such caregivers may be particularly vulnerable to rely on bad information due to physical isolation, high levels of stress, and lack of access to other sources of information. As the amount of information available through the Internet increases, the qualifications of the individuals providing this information, along with the accuracy of the information being provided, must be monitored through some mechanism. Some efforts are now being made to regulate the quality of the information being provided electronically. Another concern is the overreliance on the Internet as a source of information. Some information for caregivers is only available electronically and therefore not available to individuals who do not have access to computers and/or know how to use them.

## Research

The literature concerning effective methods of teacher preparation and medical personnel preparation is quite extensive and is beyond the physical scope of this chapter. However, there are currently very few systematic and formalized studies on best methods to address the education, training, and support needs of family and community and personal caregivers (Toseland and Smith 2001). There appear to be even less specifically addressing the needs of family, community and personal caregivers of individuals with disabilities, or the type of support and training that are most useful for family caregivers. Two exceptions are noted here because they can serve as models for other research projects. One study (McCallion et al. 2004) looked at the impact of caregiver support groups for grandparents who are providing care to children with developmental disabilities and delays versus a control group of grandparents that received no intervention. One exception is an interesting study conducted in the UK that systematically looked at the effects of caregiver training for family members providing care to individuals recovering from a stroke (Kaira et al. 2004). The study concluded that training caregivers in specific intervention techniques such as how to assist with ADL and simple nursing improved patient outcomes more than a control group of caregivers who received only social work counseling and emotional support. More studies similar to this need to be undertaken. Caregiving and the education, training, and support of family members and other individuals who provide care has been, and largely continues today to be a cottage industry, informal and local in scope.

## Policy

Most agencies that accredit colleges and universities and the educational programs offered have special standards addressing quality control for courses delivered through distance education. Additionally, national accrediting agencies such as the International Association for Continuing Education and Training (IACET) that accredit providers of continuing education programs against external standards of quality are able to accredit providers that offer courses through the Internet. There is an extensive system of private and governmental licenses, certifications, and certificates for professional caregivers of individuals with disabilities. In fact, in most states, professional caregivers must hold the appropriate credential in order to provide any service to an individual with a disability. However, there is no such parallel system of external review to assess and formally validate the quality of caregiving being provided by family and community caregivers. Only a few pilot programs currently examine this issue.

## Future Directions

### *Practice*

*New Curricula and Training Content Will be Required*  Roles and expectations for caregivers are changing as are the knowledge and skills the caregivers need to successfully respond to these new roles and expectations. Therefore, the education, training, and support provided for caregivers will need to change. We are already seeing some examples of changes in the education, training, and support in order to allow people to adapt successfully to these changing roles. This has resulted, and will continue to result, in both the content of the training provided and the type of training provided and the way outcomes of the education, training, and support are assessed.

More often, as the needs of individuals with disabilities become more complex and the care system becomes more fragmented, caregiving responsibilities increasingly involve accessing and coordinating and supervising a variety of individuals providing a variety of often disjointed services. Individuals and their caregivers must learn to be advocates for care in an increasingly difficult system to maneuver in and must learn to track and coordinate the work of others. Limited resources and limited funding and complicated and hostile insurance programs require financial acumen in order to manage. Therefore, caregiving education for families must increasingly include topics such as working with insurance companies, communicating with health care personnel, maintaining records, hiring and supervising personnel.

At the same time, formal education programs for professional caregivers in healthcare are increasingly recognizing the importance of "soft skills" in providing quality patient care. In medical schools, there is increasing focus on teaching subjects such as ethics, communication, and team building. Assessments of the education outcomes are increasing focused on assessing a clinicians' ability to communicate information to and interpret information from patients. Many of the exams used by the medical specialty boards now include less emphasis on paper and pencil multiple choice formats that assess factual recall and instead utilize professional, trained raters who watch certification candidates interact during real-time situations with live patients who have been trained to present with certain medical conditions. The skills such as patient rapport are now rated along with the more traditional technical skills (Goldsmith 2002b).

As caregivers in the healthcare community become more reliant on technology to provide patient diagnostics and interventions, the relationship of the caregiver to the patient is changing. One example is the result of practice analyses conducted for audiologists and speech–language pathologists by the American Speech Language Hearing Association. Studies showed that the "practice of the future" would shift from direct one-on-one patient interventions to supervision of support personnel (including assistants), more emphasis on being a case manager, increased use of teams, increased accountability, and increased use of technology to assist in clinical interventions and decision-making. In response to these changes in professional practice and professional role, standards for educational programs were significantly rewritten to place more emphasis in the curriculum on topics such as negotiating skills, business management, record keeping, ethics, and supervisory techniques (Rosenthal et al. 2001).

*New Ways to Provide Training will be Required* At the same time that the content of the training is changing, the format of the training is changing as well. Education, training, and support is offered in a variety of formats including formal courses, sometimes for academic or continuing education credit, support groups, mentoring and apprentice programs, workshops, conferences, and one-to-one counseling.

Training is often provided through traditional self-directed formats such as books, articles, or a set of instructions.

In recent years, however, a great deal of training has been moved to, or been created on, the Internet. The Internet has provided caregivers (and everyone else!) an unprecedented access to information and other resources. As an example, a search through the Internet via the Goggle search engine on August 1, 2008 (http://www.google.com) under the descriptors "caregiving for people with disabilities" yielded 92,200 items. Chat rooms allow historically isolated caregivers to connect with, learn from, share information with, and be supported by a network of people with common needs. The Internet has probably done more to improve access to information than all of the other formats combined. Several courses for caregivers are now available on the Internet.

The International Center for Disability Resources on the Internet (CDRI; http://www.icdri.org./about_us) is a non-profit center based in the United States. Its mission includes "the collection of a knowledge-base and quality disability resources and best practices and to provide education, outreach, and training based on these core resources."

Included in its materials is a section devoted to caregiver resources: http://www.icdri.org/resource_page.htm. As of February 28, 2007, this section links to 39 additional websites that address a variety of caregiver issues. They range in scope from websites sponsored by groups such as Accnet Care and Care There that focus on caregiving for seniors to Advocates Across America and Disability Rights Education and Defense Fund, as well as Our Kids that focus on education for parents of children with disabilities. The National Center for Children and Youth with Disabilities focuses on needs of teachers and other professionals as well as family caregivers.

The National Alliance for Caregiving has also created an Internet clearinghouse of education, training, and support materials for caregivers, as has the Institute for Caregiver Education (http://www.caregivereducation.org/) that focuses on caregiving issues for elderly.

Colleges and universities now commonly offer distance education courses for credit. It is possible to receive bachelors, masters, or doctoral degree from very prestigious and legitimate universities through distance education. This development too has had the effect of expanding education and training opportunities for caregivers, especially those whose caregiving responsibilities would not permit it then to travel to attend any training opportunities.

*New Ways of Thinking About When to Provide Training Will be Required* In addition to the content of the training and the format of the training, the timing of the training should be reconsidered. Caregivers now often receive "just in time" training paradigms, provided when caregivers are already coping with the responsibilities of caregiving. At best, they are provided early on in the caregiving process. There is a need for "proactive" caregiver education and training; training that can be available before the time individuals become actual caregivers. Of course, this proactive training paradigm forms the basis of all college and university training programs for professional caregivers. Students are introduced to subject matter and encouraged to develop and use skill sets before they actually use them in an employment setting, in anticipation of the kind of clients and patients they are likely to work with in the future.

However, no such training paradigm appears to exist for family and community caregivers. Currently most people are unprepared for their roles as caregivers; it is often a role thrust upon them suddenly and unwillingly. Training is provided in an environment of crisis.

The need for more proactive training paradigms appears to be supported by the statistics. According to the National Alliance for Caregiving, in 1996, 15% of adults were providing care to a family member who was seriously ill or who had a disability. This number is likely to increase as the population ages. According to the National Center for Health, by the time an individual reaches the age of 85 their likelihood of needing long-term care is nearly 50%. All of this suggests that more family members will become caregivers as the population ages, as more people live to be over 85, and as the number of caregivers available decrease.

Training on caregiving issues should be provided to individuals, such as children of aging parents before caregiving training needs become acute. It should also be provided as part of a school curriculum as early as grade school to educate and sensitize children to the needs of people with disabilities and teach them how they can assist classmates with disabilities in their schools and adult and elderly individuals with disabilities in their communities.

*Training Audiences Will Need to be Expanded* Training will need to be expanded to reflect new types of caregivers and new models of caregiving. This will include including training that focuses on other types of caregivers and increases the pool of potential caregivers. These would include siblings of individuals with disabilities as noted earlier in this chapter as well as friends. This might also include individuals within a community that could, with proper training, provide support to the individual *and* the caregiver through ancillary and respite caregiving services.

There should be increasing emphasis on training caregivers to be instructors for other caregivers and developing "train-the-trainer" models. Training caregivers to educate others will require providing information on best caregiving practices, conducting pre and post training needs assessments, principles of learning and instructional methodology.

## Research

There is critical need for research in this area in order to improve and expand the education, training, and support opportunities for caregivers of individuals with disabilities. It is believed that much of this research will contribute to improving education, training, and support for professional caregivers as well.

It is essential to conduct studies to assess the disconnects that exist between the education, training, and support offered and the expressed education, training, and support needs of caregivers. Such studies should focus on different cohorts of caregivers. These cohorts might include parents of children with disabilities (an expansion of the study reported earlier in this chapter), caregivers of spouses with disabilities, and caregivers of parents with disabilities. A similar study should be conducted among other cohorts of caregivers such as professionally educated/paid and non-professionally educated/paid individuals.

Research is also needed on how to define and measure best practices. These include successful models for assessing caregiver training needs including user-friendly assessment instruments that can be used when designing education, training, and support programs. Successful assessment instruments protocols should have the capacity to assess initial expectations, knowledge, and skills and whether the outcomes of the training satisfy initial expectations and if relevant, enhance knowledge and/or skills. Research into best practices should identify best practices in caregiver training: content, format, delivery models from around the country and internationally. Specifically such best practices must include best practices in education, training, and support research to determine who needs to be reached, what communication processes are most effective, and how should the information be "packaged" to be best understood and utilized (Goldsmith 1989). It should also include focused research on what constitutes effective training especially for unique groups of caregivers such as certain members of ethnic and linguistic minority groups.

## Policy/Advocacy

Increase efforts to advocate to federal, state, and private regulatory and funding authorities to increase education, training, and support efforts directed toward caregivers, especially family and community caregivers. Create and fund legislation to develop a national research and education institute and resource center that focuses on education, training, and support needs of caregivers of individuals with disabilities. Such a research institute and resource center might well be connected to an existing center within the disability, education, or caregiver support community. The activities of a national research and education institute should include research in caregiver education, training, and support issues. It could also design and teach individuals to utilize systems of continuous quality improvement, include self-assessments, systems audits, and systematic collection of information from a variety of perspectives to improve the relevancy and quality of education, training, and support provided to caregivers of individuals with disabilities. This would include selecting, developing and utilizing training and education needs assessment instruments.

It will also be important to create systems to coordinate and share information in a comprehensive and consistent way between the multitudes of training that is being provided to caregivers so that training can be built on existing information, syllabi, and best practices in delivering training. These systems should be national and international. Other countries, especially UK and Sweden, appear to be ahead of the United States in acknowledging the importance of caregivers and supporting them through education and training.

Work on developing national research and information dissemination centers has already begun but will need to be greatly expanded (U.S. Department of Health and Human Services, Administration on Aging. n.d.). However, there is a critical need to begin to develop national standards to identify what constitutes a quality caregiver and what constitutes quality training programs. It would be useful to investigate the usefulness and feasibility of formally recognizing caregivers and training programs meeting defined standards of quality. Offering a certification or similar credential to caregivers who demonstrate they have certain skills can reduce caregiving costs, including medical and insurance costs, encourage caregivers to participate in educational programs, build self-esteem and confidence for caregivers who earn the credential, and improve the quality of caregiving being provided. Accrediting training programs and materials can improve the quality and consistency of caregiver training provided and helps consumers make informed decisions about which programs to participate in and the reliability of the information he or she is likely to receive.

## References

American Hospital Association, Commission on Workforce. (2002). *In our hands: How hospital leaders can build a thriving workforce*. Chicago: American Hospital Association.

Bracken, B. A., & McCallum, R. S. (1999). International testing matters: The universal nonverbal intelligence test. *The International Test Commission Newsletter, 9*(1), 7–12. http://educ.ubc.ca/faculty/zumbo/itc/itcvol9no1.pdf. Accessed 10 July 2003.

Carter, R. (1994). *Helping yourself help others: A book for caregivers*. New York: Times Books.

Epstein, A. S. (1999). Pathways to quality in Head Start, public school, and private nonprofit early childhood programs. *Journal of Research in Early Childhood Education, 13*(2), 101–119.

Gable, S., & Hansen J. (2001). Childcare provider perspectives on the role of education and training for quality caregiving. *Early Child Development and Care, 166,* 39–52.

Geisinger, K. F., & Carlson. J. F. (1992). Assessing language-minority students. *Practical Assessment, Research & Evaluation, 3*(2). http://pareonline.net/getvn.asp. Accessed 10 July 2003.

Goldsmith, S. (1989). *Communicating results of effective practices as research*. Invited Conference on Variables that are Important to Learning. Temple University Center for Research in Human Development and Education, Washington, DC.

Goldsmith, S. (2002a). *Survey of education, training, and support for parents of children with disabilities: Needs versus realities*. Unpublished Manuscript.

Goldsmith, S. (2002b). *Issues related to skills standards in the healthcare industry*. Invited presentation to National Skills Standards Board, Washington, DC.

Goldsmith, S. (2003). Lost in translation: Issues in translating tests for limited English proficient and bilingual children. In J. E. Wall & G. R. Waltz (Eds.), *Measuring up: Assessment issues for teachers, counselors, and administrators* (pp. 127–146). Austin: PRO-ED.

Hogg, J., Lucchino, K., Wang, K., & Janicki, M. (2000). *Healthy aging-adults with intellectual disabilities: Aging and social policy*. Geneva: World Health Organization.

Individuals with Disabilities Education Act of 1997. (1975). 94–142 20 U.S.C. 1400.

Kay, H. S., & Longmore, P. K. (1997). *Disability watch: The status of people with disabilities in the United States*. Oakland: Disability Rights Advocates.

Kaira, L., Perez, I., Melbourn, A., Knapp, M., & Donaldson, N. (2004). Training carers of stroke patients: Random controlled trials. *British Medical Journal, 28*(7448), 1099.

Kennedy, J., & LaPlant, M. P. (1997). A profile of individuals needing assistance with activities of daily living, 1991–1992. *Disability Statistics Report* (11): 1–37. Washington, DC: U.S. Department of Education, National Institute on Disability and Rehabilitation Research.

McCallion, P., Janicki, M. P., Kolomer, S. R, & Allion, P. (2004). Controlled evaluation of support groups for grandparent caregivers of children with developmental disabilities and delays. *American Journal of Mental Retardation, 109,* 352–361.

McCarthy, J., Cruz, J., & Ratcliff, N. (1999). *Early childhood teacher education licensure patterns and curriculum guidelines: A state-by-state analysis.* Washington, DC: Council for Professional Recognition.

McNeil, J. M. (2001). American with disabilities: Household economics. *U.S. Census Bureau: Current population reports* (pp. 1–17). Washington, DC: U.S. Department of Commerce. http://www.census.gov/prod/2001pubs/p70-73.pdf. Accessed 10 July 2003.

Rosenthal, M., Goldsmith, S., & Reeves, R. (2001). *Defining future practice: Implications for certification and assessment.* Keynote presentation at the annual conference of the National Organization for Competency Assurance, New Orleans, LA.

Rossworm, M. A., & Larrabee, J. H. (2002). Training family caregivers of dependent elderly adults through on-site and telecommunications programs. *Journal of Gerontological Nursing, 28,* 27–38.

Schulman, B. (1976). *Memorandum to Boston Public School administrators and staff.* Boston. Unpublished memorandum to author.

Slaton, E. (2000). *Offering technical assistance to Native families: Clues from a focus group.* Alexandria: Federation for Families for Children's Mental Health.

Singh, N. N., Lancioni, G. E., Winton, A. S. W. et al. (2004). Mindful caregiving increases happiness among individuals with multiple disabilities. *Research in Developmental Disabilities, 25,* 207–218.

Toseland, R. W., & Smith, S. (2001). Supporting caregivers through education and training. *Administration on Aging Listserv: Caregiver Education, Training and Counseling.* http://www.aoa.gov/eldfam/For_Caregivers/For_Caregivers.aspx. Accessed 12 July 2003.

U.S. Department of Health and Human Services, Administration on Aging. (n.d.). National Family Caregiver Support Program resource room. http://www.aoa.gov/prof/aoaprog/caregiver/caregiver.aspx. Accessed 12 July 2003.

United Cerebral Palsy Association. (n.d.). *Caregiving guidelines.* http://www.ucp.org/ucp_channeldoc.cfm/1/11/10427/10427-10427/2839. Accessed 14 July 2003.

# Chapter 5
# Parent Caregivers of Children with Disabilities

Karen Kuhlthau

The epidemiology of childhood disability among children and adolescents age 0–21 has changed dramatically in the past three decades with many more children surviving than they did a quarter of a century ago. Improved medical and surgical technologies and access to these technologies have dramatically changed survival rates (Gortmaker and Sappenfield 1984). Improvements in care for many conditions have meant that more than 90% of children with even severe health conditions currently survive to at least age 20, although often with substantial physical or psychological morbidity (Cadman et al. 1991; Gortmaker 1985; Gortmaker and Sappenfield 1984; Gortmaker et al. 1990; Weitzman et al. 1986). This combined with increased incidence of several conditions (e.g., asthma and mental health conditions) has led to an increase in the incidence of disability among children and adolescents. National Health Interview Survey data indicate that for children under age 17 the prevalence of activity-limiting chronic conditions doubled between 1960 and 1981 and tripled by the mid-1990s (Newacheck et al. 1984; Newacheck and Halfon 2000).

With the changes in survival has come increasing interest in issues of providing more care in home and community-based settings and in directing care toward improving long-term outcomes. These changes have extended and complicated family caretaking responsibilities. Opportunities to care for children with disabilities in the home have increased (Perrin et al. 1993). Medicaid home and community care waivers provide additional services to keep individuals out of institutional facilities and in the home or community, without requiring families to "spend down" to Medicaid eligibility levels (Medicaid Source Book 1993). Increasing cost consciousness among insurers and care providers has also contributed to reduced hospital stays and a reduction in institutionalization. Several legal changes, such as the Individuals with Disabilities Education Act and the Americans with Disabilities Act, enhance the civil rights of children with disabilities (ADA 1990; Individuals with Disabilities Education Act Amendments of 1997, Public Law 105–17). These changes help children and adolescents with disabilities attend schools with their

K. Kuhlthau (✉)
Center for Child and Adolescent Health Research and Policy, Massachusetts General Hospital, 100 Cambridge Street, 15th Floor, Boston, MA 02114, USA
e-mail: kkuhlthau@partners.org

peers who do not have disabilities. They further provide for access of persons with disabilities to community services and private businesses. For example, the rights embedded in the Americans with Disabilities Act allow parents to demand communities be accessible to a child who uses a wheelchair. By promoting the ability of individuals with disabilities to live in communities these regulations support parents' desires to keep children at home. Although these changes often require parental or community activism, the legal precedent is important in facilitating change. This increased opportunity for parents and others to facilitate children and adolescents to live at home and in their communities suggests that the well-being of parental caregivers is an increasingly important public health issue.

Caregiving demands change by levels of child development and by the social and familial context in which the child lives (Bronfenbrenner 1979; Patterson and Garwick 1994). Dependency is a defining characteristic of young childhood. Since there is great variation in the amount of care any child needs, it often becomes difficult to determine when a child's needs are normative versus extraordinary. As such, it is often difficult to determine when the demands on parental caregivers are within the range of the demands on all parents and when they become unusual. Stein (2001) notes that this continuum of dependency has three consequences: (1) it creates an expectation of parental caregiving, (2) it means that measures of activities of daily living are not good indicators for children, and (3) it contributes to societal ambivalence about the public's role in care. The expectation of parental caregiving effectively suggests that parents should provide all care to their children without any additional supports. Societal ambivalence about the public's role means that parents often provide care with few public or private supports.

Raina et al. (2004) suggest a multidimensional conceptual model of caregiving. They seek to ground their theory in domains relevant in previous research including: (1) focusing on the formal and informal caregiving process, (2) incorporating new findings, (3) separating child disability and child behavior problems, (4) looking at socioecological factors (family function and social support), and (5) examining physical and psychological health. In citing Eicher and Batshaw (1993), they also introduce the notion of a "caregiver career" (albeit, a career that is often not "chosen"), the notion that caregiving is a dynamic process and that caregivers experience stages that are marked by different demands and responsibilities.

The theory focuses on five constructs: background and context; child characteristics; caregiver strain; intrapsychic factors; and coping/supportive factors and health outcomes. Their theoretical diagram is reproduced in Fig. 5.1. Background and context includes socioeconomic characteristics and the caregiving setting. Child characteristics include characteristics of the child's disability including both physical and psychological factors. Daily caregiving demands and the interaction of these demands with other roles (e.g., work) comprise the domain of caregiver strain. Aspects of the caregiver's internal state such as identification with the caregiving role comprise the caregiver intrapsychic domain. Coping factors include social support, family functioning, and ability to manage stress. The physical and psychological outcomes for the caregiver comprise the domain of caregiver health and well-being

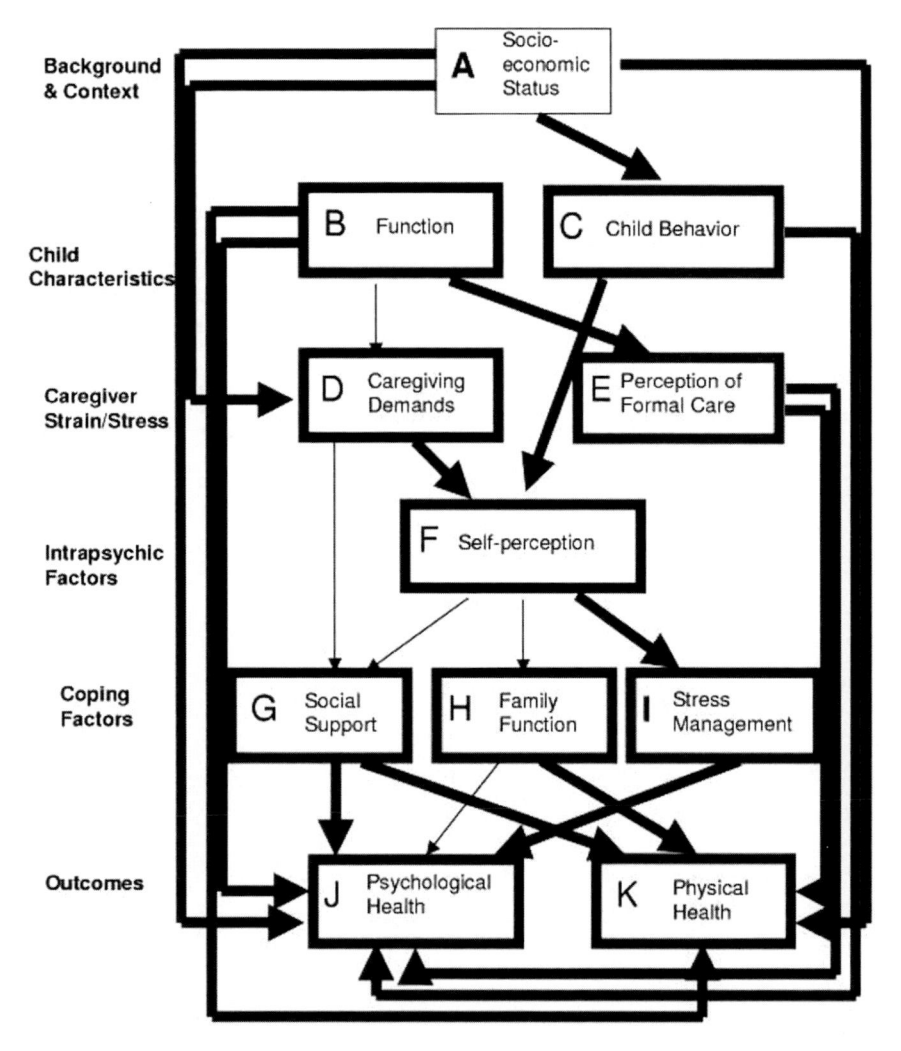

# 5 Parent Caregivers of Children with Disabilities

**Fig. 5.1** Raina's model of care: conceptual model of caregiving process and caregiver burden among pediatric population. (Reproduced from Raina et al. 2004)

(Raina et al. 2004). This framework helps define the variety of aspects that may influence parent outcomes (Fig. 5.2).

The International Classification of Functioning, Disability, and Health (ICF) framework for disability builds on the notion that changing the environment can interrupt the pathway between the impairment of a body system and limitations in functioning (ICF, http://www.who.int/icf/icftemplate.cfm?myurl=homepage.html&mytitle=Home%20Page). Borrowing from this notion, changes in the family environment can interrupt the pathway between a child's disability and a negative outcome for the caregiver. Similarly, changes in the child's environment (e.g., improving

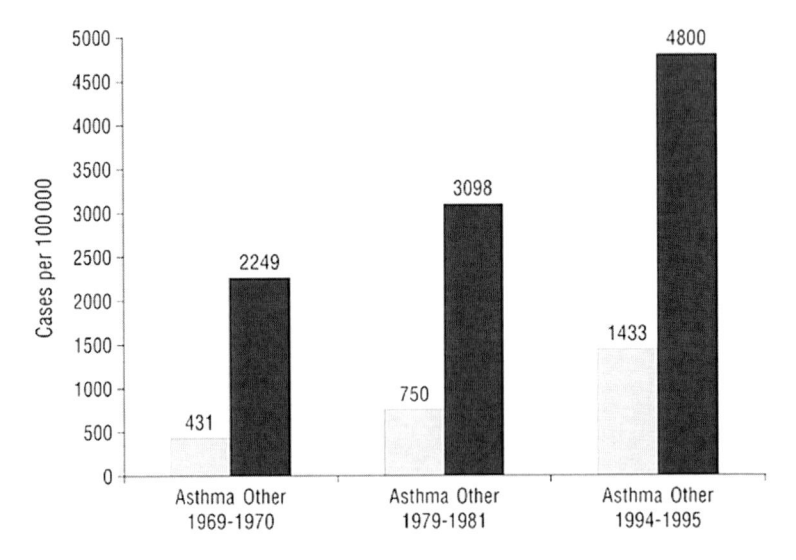

**Fig. 5.2** Trends in prevalence of disability due to asthma and other conditions among US children younger than 17 years. Prevalence data are annualized. In the National Health Interview Survey. (From Newacheck and Halfon (2000, March). *Copyright © 2000–2005 Ovid Technologies, Inc.* Version: rel9.3.0, Source ID 1.10284.1.251

school settings) may primarily serve to improve the child's well-being but may have important positive implications for the caregiver. This sort of concept is also found in Raina's model where, for example, a change in the child's environment that served to improve the child's functioning or behavior would then likely positively influence the caregiver.

Aspects of the child and family's environment may be differently amenable to change. For example, factors such as the quality of the caregiver and child's health insurance may be easier to change than the family's socioeconomic status. Thinking about the environment and what aspects are amenable to change may help focus and empower interventions. For example, changes that facilitate intergenerational care, modifying the physical environment of the home, facilitate access to nonparental caregivers, and income supports among other factors may help alleviate some of the negative outcomes for caregivers.

## How are Parents Affected?

### *Employment*

We know that having a child with a disability influences parents in a variety of ways. Having children usually decreases family employment because one parent (usually the mother) specializes in child rearing while the other parent specializes in paid employment (Sawhill 1980; Mincer 1980). The literature on labor force participation of mothers of children with disabilities generally shows decreased employment by parents of children with disabilities (Thyen et al. 1999; Salkever 1982; Breslau et al. 1982a; Hirst 1985; Wolfe and Hill 1995; Kuhlthau and Perrin 2001). Several studies with small, unrepresentative, and/or pre-1990 samples find decreased labor force participation of mothers in general and for subgroups of mothers (Breslau et al. 1982a; Hirst 1985; Thyen et al. 1999; Salkever 1982). More recent nationally representative studies also speak to these issues. They include a study that found a marginal effect on parental employment in a study of single mothers (Wolfe and Hill 1995); an effect for both mothers and fathers that increases with the intensity of the child's condition (Kuhlthau and Perrin 2001); and less full-time employment among single parents and couples (Heck and Makue 2000).

## Stress

Having a child with a disability also impacts the well-being of parents in other ways. A recent article, which received attention in the national press, documents a link between stress experienced by mothers of children with disabilities and biological indices of poor health, specifically known determinants of cell senescence and longevity (Epedl et al. 2004). The association between parental stress and caring for a disabled child is well documented for groups of children with a wide variety of disabilities (Breslau et al. 1982b; Dyson 1993; Keogel et al. 1992; McGlone et al. 2002; Miller et al. 1992; Silver et al. 1998; Sloper and Turner 1993). The kinds of stress that parents report can generally be categorized as financial, emotional, social, and care resopnsibilities.

## Financial Burden

Families with a disabled or chronically ill child experience greater financial stress that can continue even if and when the child dies (Corden et al. 2002; Leonard et al. 1992). Financial concerns are associated with increased stress (Aday et al. 1988). Recent data show that 40% of parents of children with special health care needs report having a finance-related problem during the past year (Kuhlthau et al. 2005; Strickland et al. 2004). Families also experience more out-of-pocket costs compared to other families (Hwang et al. 2001; Peter 1997; The Health Care Experiences of Families of Children with Special Health Care Needs: Summary Report of Findings from a National Survey 2000). These issues are combined with the financial burden caused by work loss and work reduction (noted above).

## Emotional and Social

Parents also experience emotional distress relating to role conflicts (how to balance the needs of the disabled child with needs of siblings and partner), parent–child interactions, child-specific concerns (e.g., concern for the child's future, particularly after the parents are gone), and marital/sibling relationships (Podolski and Nigg 2001; Smith et al. 2001). Family cohesion and fewer negative life events predict lower parent stress scores (measured at a later time) among families with children with developmental disabilities (Warfield et al. 1999). Because of a child's increased care needs, the opportunity for parents to participate in social interactions is less, causing stress and depriving the parents of often critically needed social supports.

## *Care Responsibilities*

Finally, the responsibilities of care and other parental demands such as tasks specific to the disability and other daily life demands create additional stresses for parents (Dyson 1997; Patterson et al. 1992; Smith et al. 2001).

## **Moderators and Mediators**

The literature on the relationships between caring for a child with a disability and family stress provides insight to the factors that mediate/moderate parental stress. A study examining how stress varies during the early childhood period among mothers with children with developmental disabilities indicates that family environment is important in predicting both child and parental stress (Warfield et al. 1999). The study further points to the importance of income, family cohesion, and family support in predicting stress. A longitudinal study by Hauser-Cram et al. (2001) investigated the relationship between a developmentally disabled child's cognitive and adaptive behavioral development with parental stress and found that the child's disability and the mother–child interaction were associated with parental stress. A study that examined the relationship between coping strategies and levels of stress indicates that the type of coping strategies employed by a mother affects her stress level (Miller et al. 1992). Other studies point to the importance of emotional and physical resources (Petersen 1984), a sense of coherence for parents with children with autistic spectrum disorders (Sivberg 2002), and social support networks and quality services in reducing parental stress and improving parental adaptation (McConachie 1994; Sloper and Turner 1992). Gender also plays an important role in that there are differences in the degrees to which mothers and fathers experience stress, how they respond to stress, and the types of stress to which they respond (Chesler and Parry 2001; Gray 2003; Krauss 1993).

Less is known about the specific ways in which stress affects the family. How does stress affect parent's mental and physical health and how does it influence the family's quality of life? The work done by Miller et al. (1992) indicates that higher levels of stress result in higher levels of depressive symptomatology for mothers of children with physical disabilities. Understanding the sources of stress to families is critical to designing interventions to alleviate the stress. For example, if time demands are the major issue, then services such as respite care or work-life benefits may help families better manage their time and thus reduce stress. On the other hand, if the primary source of stress is emotional issues, then parental counseling may help family members better manage their stress.

## *Mental Health*

Parents (studies are primarily of mothers) of children with chronic conditions have higher rates of mental health problems (mainly, depression) than parents in comparison groups (Aday et al. 1988; Breslau et al. 1982b; Breslau 1986; Cadman et al. 1991; Quint et al. 1990; Thompson and Gustafson 1996; Thyen et al. 1998). In another study, parents of children with chronic conditions in community-based studies have increased rates of mental health problems, particularly higher rates of depression (Cadman et al. 1991). Thyen et al.'s (1998) study comparing mothers of children with and without technology assistance indicated a strong association of poorer mental health with child health status, especially in poorer families (Thyen et al. 1998). Breslau et al. (1982a, b) and Breslau (1986) found that mothers of disabled children demonstrated higher psychological distress and more depressive symptoms than controls. Jessop and Stein (1991) found an association between the impact of the illness on the family and mother's psychiatric symptoms (Jessop and Stein 1991).

Mental health issues may be related to a specific consequence of a child's disability. Isolating these characteristics could help the process of creating effective interventions. If we knew, for example, that the mechanism through which a child's disability influenced a parent's psychological well-being was parents' lack of sleep, then designing policies and interventions that helped ease the nighttime care responsibilities for parents should improve mental health outcomes for parental caregivers. Yet we have little empirical evidence about these mechanisms. Canning found an increase in distress among caregivers of children with worse reported impairments, but once the perceived family caregiving responsibilities were held constant the rating of the impairment no longer mattered (Canning et al. 1996). Although some anecdotal information suggests that the first year after a child's diagnosis is the hardest for parents (Anderson and Elfert 1989; Thyen et al. 1998), others indicate worsening maternal mental health status over time (Quint et al. 1990).

## *Physical Health*

We know little about physical health and health behaviors among caregivers of children with disabilities. The increase in stress and mental health problems in parents, the physical demands of care, along with the time demands may limit positive health behaviors or increase negative health behaviors. This suggests that the physical health of caregivers likely suffers compared to parents of children without disabilities. On the other hand, when faced with long-term caregiving roles, parents of children with disabilities may be highly motivated to take good care of themselves so that they can assist their child in the future. As such, they may have increased incentives to improve their health status through positive health behaviors. One study shows that parents of children with a physical disability have decreased physical functioning compared with parents of children with nondisabling medical illness (Tong et al. 2002). A separate study found differences in quality of life and parental activity limitations for parents of children with activity limitations compared with other parents (Kuhlthau et al. 2010).

## Use of Health Care

We also know little about how child disability influences the health care utilization of caregivers although in general parent populations, parental and child health care utilization are associated (Hanson 1998; Minkovitz et al. 2002; Newacheck et al. 1986; Schor et al. 1987; Tessler and Mechanic 1978; Wolfe 1980). Parents' utilization of sick and prevention care among parents of children with disabilities is slightly higher than that for parents of other children (Kuhlthau et al. 2010). Differences in the physical and psychological health of caregivers will likely influence caregiver health care utilization. The evidence cited above suggests that parents of children with disabilities have more stress and worse mental health compared to parents of children without disabilities. As such, we would expect increased health care utilization by parents for their own health based on increased need for services, especially acute and chronic care. On the other hand, competing demands on parental time and money may mean that parents of children with disabilities are more likely to put off obtaining care or not obtaining some types of care at all. Alleviating competing demands on time and other resources may result in parents increasing their utilization, especially for preventive services. As noted above, when faced with long-term caregiving demands parents may seek to improve their health status so that they are able to provide care to their child for a longer period of time. Under this hypothesis, caregivers may have improved health status compared to their peers and would be expected to use more preventive health services and fewer sick care visits than other parents.

The literature on the well-being of caregivers of children with disabilities is rich in some areas and slim in others. In general, there is a need for more longitudinal studies of families of children with disabilities. This would help improve the understanding of how caregivers are affected and what factors moderate/mediate the relationship. More studies are needed in particular regarding caregiver health outcomes, especially related to the use of health care, physical health status, and health behaviors. Mapping some of these issues to developmental change of the child, caregiver, and family will help us understand how caregivers fare over the life course. The theoretical frameworks coupled with existing empirical research may provide guidance regarding where to focus interventions for families. Once we have a better understanding of outcomes for caregivers, factors that promote positive outcomes, and how these factors change over time, we will be better able to focus on interventions to help caregivers and their families. We will further be able to focus on reducing the consequences of disability for caregivers as well as the child with a disability.

## Interventions to Help Caregivers

Anecdotal evidence suggests that advice and information available at or near the time of a child's diagnosis appears to be critically important to families. Over time, families learn where to find the resources they need through family networks, providers, the Internet, and other sources. Help for families at the time of diagnosis can often be slim depending upon a number of factors (e.g., proximity and availability of resources). This is especially true for rare conditions where the provider may know little about the condition. Parents talk of being given a diagnosis for their child and told to go home and make another appointment in a few months. The structure of medical care with short office visits and difficulty integrating specialist and generalist care (in general) makes it difficult to provide helpful information through the medical system, especially at the time of diagnosis when needs are unexpected and relationships are often new.

Although parents frequently develop an expertise in caring for their child over time, families are often left with the role of coordinating care from different providers, schools, and community services. Care coordination on its own and as a component of the medical home (American Academy of Pediatrics 2002) has potential to improve the well-being of caregivers by facilitating some of the management and coordination tasks. In an early pilot study, families with children with chronic conditions were randomly assigned to an intervention—which included primary care, counseling, home visits, care coordination, parental/self-care education and support, social services, advocacy, 24-hour telephone access, and other services or to standard care in resident-run continuity clinics (Stein and Jessop 1984a, b). The intervention had important impacts on family mental health, with increased satisfaction with care, and reduced psychiatric symptoms of the mother, with some reductions persisting at 4–5-year follow-up (Stein and Jessop 1991). Households with relatively less severely ill children and with fewer community resources benefited most from the program (Jessop and Stein 1991).

In a more recent randomized control trial, a randomly selected group of families were provided social support through access to an "experienced" parent and a child-life specialist over the period of 15 months. This included seven visits of one to one and a half hours, more frequent short conversations, and other events. The intervention focused on enhancing social support. The experiment resulted in reduced maternal anxiety in the experimental group, but no change in depression (Ireys et al. 2001). Two other similar studies resulted in a decrease in anxiety that was not statistically significant, one in a sample of inner city children (Silver et al. 1995) and the other in a sample of children with arthritis (Ireys et al. 1996).

## Policy

There are many policies and programs designed to help children in general and children with disabilities. Many of these have potential direct or indirect effects on families. Since children with disabilities often have increased need for health care, access to comprehensive and affordable health insurance is critical to the health of children with disabilities and their families. Children generally either have public or private health insurance. Private insurance can be bought independently but more commonly is provided through a parent's employer. Children are often covered as dependents of the employee. Of note, some employers offer work-life or employee-assistance programs that have relevant services to parental caregivers of children with disabilities. These services are not specific to parental caregivers but are relevant to their situations. Some examples include referrals to child care centers, help obtaining services in the home, or legal services.

Public insurance may come through a variety of mechanisms and generally covers a broader scope of services compared to private insurance although accessing covered services may be a problem for some families (Perrin 1999). The major public insurance program for children is the Medicaid program. Medicaid covers low-income children and parents. Coverage is more generous for children than parents (children are generally covered at higher income levels than parents). Income cutoffs and benefits covered differ from state to state as well as between Medicaid programs within a state. Each state's Child Health Insurance Programs (CHIP) differ and generally cover income levels above that covered by traditional Medicaid. CHIP only cover children. States can design their CHIP so that children can either enroll in the State's Medicaid program, enroll in a new health insurance program, or have a hybrid approach. Several states (Alabama, California, Connecticut, and Montana) have special CHIP or augmented services for children with special health care needs (a group that includes children with disabilities) typically offering additional or enhanced services (Fox et al. 2003).

Children with disabilities can obtain Medicaid in two additional ways that are unique to the disabled population. First, there are provisions for families who incur health care expenditure such that once these expenditures are subtracted from the family income the child would be eligible for Medicaid. These families are eligible through "spend down" provisions. (In some states families are also allowed to pay a premium for the insurance if their health care spending puts them close to the Medicaid cutoff.) Second, the Supplemental Security Income (SSI) program provides Medicaid coverage (in most states) and a cash payment to families who have a child that meets disability criteria and are income eligible.

The federal and state Title V Maternal and Child Health programs provide services to families with about a third of the MCH budgets going to programs for children with special health care needs. Title V services for children with special health care needs differ from state to state, in some states children with disabilities can obtain direct services or access to health insurance through the state's Title V programs.

Of note, only the traditional Medicaid program provides health coverage for parental caregivers and this coverage is not universal. As such, although the other programs help parents by providing the child with access to care and potentially reducing the family's financial burden, parents may find themselves in the difficult situation of having insurance for their child but no insurance for themselves. Some states seek to address this issue. For example, the Michigan Medicaid program provides eligibility to parental caregivers with income limitations.

The cash benefit provided through the SSI program can provide a direct benefit to caregivers. SSI payments can help alleviate some of the financial pressures on families. The cash benefit can be used to provide relief to caregivers either directly (e.g., by paying for respite care) or indirectly by paying for children's needs, which would otherwise be paid for by the family.

Medicaid, CHIP, and SSI programs differ (to varying degrees) from state to state. Thus, families who move must understand new eligibility rules when they move to a new state. Within a state, other agencies (e.g., the mental health agency, public health, developmental disability) also have programs that differ from state to state and from program to program with services such as home health care and respite care subject to caps in coverage and changes between programs. As such, the complexity of understanding eligibility and coverage rules can be a burden for parents.

Aside from providing direct services and insurance, the federal and state Title V Maternal and Child Health programs provide supports for families. The federal Title V agency, the Maternal and Child Health Bureau provides access to parent peer support through the Family Voices Network. Title V services sometimes provide access to care (directly or though insurance) that may include: (1) personal care attendants and home care workers and (2) coverage for care coordination. Although these services are generally provided to the child and through the child's benefits, by reducing some of the caretaking demands on parents, they may provide substantial benefits to parental caregivers.

Two services sometimes provided by insurance and Title V programs that are particularly important to caregivers are care coordination and respite care. Care coordinators help families maximize the use of services for the parents and child. Without professional care coordinators, parents often fill this role, increasing the stress and time demands on parents. Care coordination gained a funding base as a service for children with special health care needs with the enactment of the Section 2176 Home and Community-Based Services Waivers of the Medicaid program (Omnibus Reconciliation Act 1981). These waivers allow states to offer expanded services to targeted recipients (aged, disabled, intellectually disabled, mentally ill) to avoid more costly institutionalization. They also allowed additional services (beyond the states' usual Medicaid services) that include case management and additional support services to help alleviate some of the problems that families experience as a result of having a health-impaired child at home (Fox 1984; Hall 1990).

Respite care as well as access to family services can help families. Analyses of the National Health Interview Survey indicate that among children with disabilities, family services (29%) and respite care (61%) are the services with the most unmet need (Maag 2000). Personal care attendant services like respite care can provide much needed assistance to the child and much needed relief to parents.

Most of the above-mentioned programs are targeted primarily at the child. These programs can substantially reduce the care responsibilities for families and thus have positive benefits for both the child and the family. However, even in this short list of federally mandated programs, there is substantial difference from state to state and families may need to tap resources from more than one of these programs. Without meaningful care coordination, the responsibility falls on families to submit applications for enrollment to the programs and for coordinating services from multiple programs.

## Future Directions

Much of what we know about parent caregivers is based on cross-sectional data and on data about mothers. Expanding the research to better understand changes over time and the roles of both mothers and fathers is needed. In addition, we need to know more about the physical health, use of health services, and health behaviors of caregivers. Furthering the research to explicitly look at positive benefits of caregiving is further warranted in order to provide a more balanced perspective to the experience of raising a child with a disability. The research on parental stress and mental health is starting to uncover protective factors for families. Further work to understand protective factors will help researchers design more targeted interventions. In addition, research needs to look at protective factors for the other parental outcomes.

Current research generally does not look at the child disability or parental caregiving in a life course perspective. As children age, their needs change with the transition to adult life being a particularly important time for all children and for children with disabilities. Young adults with disabilities lose access to age-based child and adolescent services (e.g., access to educational services) and need to transition to the adult version of other services (e.g., transition to obtaining health care from an internist). In general, young adulthood is a time when individuals start living on their own. This may be more difficult for young adults with disabilities who may be more likely to continue to live with their parents. As parents age, their ability to provide care changes. More research to understand critical life junctures and how they impact caregiving and caregivers is needed. Related to this, we need to think about the family environment and what characteristics of the family environment might reduce the negative outcomes for caregivers.

There are few intervention studies relevant to caregivers and those that exist suggest that helping families has a positive impact on parental caregivers. We need to continue to think about implementing and evaluating interventions that seek to directly help parents (as well as their children). There is very little information available regarding training of parents to act as caregivers of their child with a disability. For some parents getting information regarding their child's physiological and psychological status is difficult. Information about the consequence of a disability for the child and family is similarly difficult to obtain. Yet, we know little about what types and sources of information best help families. Anecdotal evidence suggests that some families need help to understand their child's condition and the supports available to help their family. Anecdotal evidence also suggests that peer support has a very promising role in helping families. Indeed, over time many families become experts in their child's health and related conditions and the systems that serve to support the child and family. Parents frequently report that they become resources to professionals providing information about the potential of programs or the health and medical resources available.

## References

Aday, L. A., Aitken, M. J., & Wegener, D. H. (1988). *Pediatric home care: Results of a national evaluation of programs for ventilator assisted children*. Chicago: Pluribus.
American Academy of Pediatrics. (2002). The medical home. *Pediatrics, 110,* 184–186.
Americans with Disabilities Act (ADA). (1990). PL 101-336.
Anderson, J. M., & Elfert, H. (1989). Managing chronic health conditions in the family: Women as caretakers. *Journal of Advanced Nursing, 14,* 735–743.
Breslau, N. (1986). Chronic stress and major depression. *Archive of General Psychiatry, 43,* 309–314.
Breslau, N., Salkever, D., & Staruch, K. S. (1982a). Women's labor force activity and responsibilities for disabled dependents: A study of families with disabled children. *Journal of Health and Social Behavior, 23,* 169–183.
Breslau N., Staruch, K. S., & Mortimer, E. A. (1982b). Psychological distress in mothers of disabled children. *American Journal of Disabled Children, 136,* 682–686.
Bronfenbrenner, U. (1979). *The ecology of human development: Experiments by nature and design.* Cambridge: Harvard University Press.
Cadman, D., Rosenbaum, P., Boyle, M., & Offord, D. R. (1991). Children with chronic illness: Family and parent demographic characteristics and psychosocial adjustment. *Pediatrics, 87,* 884–889.
Canning, R. D., Harris, E. S., & Kelleher, K. J. (1996). Factors predicting distress among caregivers to children with chronic medical conditions. *Journal of Pediatric Psychology, 21,* 735–749.
Chesler, M. A., & Parry, C. (2001). Gender roles and/or styles of crisis: An integrative analysis of the experiences of fathers of children with cancer. *Qualitative Health Research, 11,* 363–384.
Corden, A., Sloper, P., & Sainsbury, R. (2002). Financial effects for families after the death of a disabled or chronically ill child: A neglected dimension of bereavement. *Child Care Health Development, 28,* 199–204.
Dyson, L. L. (1993). Response to the presence of a child with disabilities: parental stress and family functioning over time. *American Journal of Mental Retardation, 98,* 207–218.
Dyson, L. L. (1997). Fathers and mothers of school-age children with developmental disabilities: Parental stress, family functioning, and social support. *American Journal of Mental Retardation, 102,* 267–279.
Eicher, P. S., & Batshaw, M. L. (1993). Cerebral Palsy. *Pediatric Clinics of North America, 40,* 537–551.
Epedl, E S., Blackburn, E. H., Lin, J., Dhabhar, F. S., Adler, N. E., Morrow, J. D., et al. (2004). Accelerated telomere shortening in response to life stress. *Proceedings of the National Academy of Sciences USA, 101,* 17312–17315.
Fox, H. (1984). *A preliminary analysis of options to improve health insurance coverage for chronically ill and disabled children*. Washington: U.S. Department of Health and Human Services, Division of Maternal and Child Health, Habilitative Services Branch.

Fox, H. B., Limb, S. J., & McManus, M. A. (2003). *Innovations for children with special needs in managed care* (SCHIP Resource Paper). Hamilton: Center for Health Care Strategies, Inc.

Gortmaker, S. L. (1985). Demography of chronic diseases. In N. Hobbs, J. M. Perrin, & H. T. Ireys (Eds.), *Chronically ill children and their families*. San Francisco: Jossey-Bass.

Gortmaker, S., & Sappenfield, W. (1984). Chronic childhood disorders: Prevalence and impact. *Pediatric Clinics of North America, 31,* 3–18.

Gortmaker, S. L., Walker, D. K., Weitzman, M., & Sobol, A. M. (1990). Chronic conditions, socioeconomic risks, and behavioral problems in children and adolescents. *Pediatrics, 85,* 267–276.

Gray, D. E. (2003). Gender and coping: The parents of children with high functioning autism. *Social Science Medicine, 56,* 631–642.

Hall, L. (1990). *Medicaid home care options for disabled children*. Washington: National Governors Association.

Hanson, K. L. (1998). Is insurance for children enough? The link between parents' and children's health care use revisited. *Inquiry, 35,* 294–302.

Hauser-Cram, P., Warfield, M. E., Shonkoff, J. P., Krauss, M. W., Sayer, A., & Upshur, C. C. (2001). Children with disabilities: A longitudinal study of child development and parental well-being. *Monograph of Social Research in Child Development, 66,* 115–126.

*The health care experiences of families of children with special health care needs: Summary report of findings from a national survey.* (2000, February). Albuquerque: Family Voices, Inc. http://www.familyvoices.org/YourVoiceCounts/sum-rep-find.html.

Heck, K. E., & Makue, D. M. (2000). Parental employment and health insurance coverage among school-aged children with special health care needs. *American Journal of Public Health, 90,* 1856–1860.

Hirst, M. (1985). Health, employment, and financial costs for family. *Child Care Health and Development, 11,* 291–307.

Hwang, W., Weller, W., Ireys, H., & Anderson, G. (2001). Out-of-pocket medical spending for care of chronic conditions. *Health Affairs, 20,* 267–278.

Ireys, H. T., Sill, E. M., Kolodner, K. B., & Walsh, B. B. (1996). A social support intervention for parents of children with juvenile rheumatoid arthritis: Results of a randomized trial. *Journal of Pediatric Psychology, 21,* 633–641.

Ireys, H. T., Robin, C., DeVet, K. A., & Young, K. (2001). Maternal outcomes of a randomized controlled trial of a community-based support program for families of children with chronic illnesses. *Archives of Pediatrics and Adolescent Medicine, 155,* 771–777.

Jessop, D. J., & Stein, R. E. K. (1991). Who benefits from a pediatric home care program? *Pediatrics, 88,* 497–505.

Keogel, R. L., Schreibman, L., Loos, L. M., Dirlich-Wilhelm, H., Dunlap, G., Robbins, F. R., et al. (1992). Consistent stress profiles in mothers of children with autism. *Journal of Autism and Developmental Disorders, 22,* 205–216.

Krauss, M. W. (1993). Child-related and parenting stress: Similarities and differences between mothers and fathers of children with disabilities. *American Journal of Mental Retardation, 97,* 393–404.

Kuhlthau, K., & Perrin, J. M. (2001). Child health status and parental employment. *Archives of Pediatrics and Adolescent Medicine, 155,* 1346–1350.

Kuhlthau, K., Hill, K. S., Yucel, R., & Perrin, J. M. (2005). Financial burden for families of children with special health care needs. *Maternal and Child Health Journal, 9,* 207–218.

Kuhlthau, K. A., Kahn, R., Hill, K. S., Srilakshmi G., & Ettner S. L. (2010). The well-being of parental caregivers of children with disabilities. *Maternal and Child Health Journal, 14*(2), 155–163.

Leonard, B., Brust, J. D., & Sapienza, J. J. (1992). Financial and time costs to parents of severely disabled children. *Public Health Reports, 107,* 302–312.

Maag, E. (2000, September). *Supportive health service needs for children with special health care needs*. Washington: The Urban Institute. http://aspe.hhs.gov/daltcp/reports/2000/suphsnd.htm. Accessed 8 May 2012.

McConachie, H. (1994). Implications of a model of stress and coping for services to families of young disabled children. *Child Care Health Development, 20,* 37–46.
McGlone, K., Santos, L., Kazama, L., & Mueller, C. (2002). Psychological stress in adoptive parents of special needs children. *Child Welfare, 81,* 151–171.
Medicaid Source Book. (1993). *Background data and analysis (a 1993 update).* Washington: U.S. Government Printing Office.
Miller, A. C., Gordon, R. M., Daniele, R. J., & Diller, L. (1992). Stress, appraisal, and coping in mothers of disabled and non-disabled children. *Journal of Pediatric Psychology, 23,* 5–15.
Mincer, J. (1980). Labor force participation of married women: A study of labor supply. In A. H. Amsden (Ed.), *The economics of women.* New York: St. Martin's Press.
Minkovitz, C. S., O'Campo, P. J., Chen, Y., & Grason, H. A. (2002). Associations between maternal and child health status and patterns of medical care use. *Ambulatory Pediatrics, 2002,* 85–92.
Newacheck, P. W., & Halfon, N. (2000). Prevalence, impact, and trends in childhood disability due to asthma. *Archives of Pediatrics & Adolescent Medicine, 154,* 287–293.
Newacheck, P. W., Budetti, P. P., & McManus, P. (1984). Trends in childhood disability. *American Journal of Public Health, 74,* 232–236.
Newacheck, P. W., Budetti, P. P., & Halfon, N. (1986). Trends in activity-limiting chronic conditions among children. *American Journal of Public Health, 76,* 178–184.
Omnibus Reconciliation Act. (1981). PL 97-35, Section 2176.
Patterson, J. M., & Garwick, A. W. (1994). The impact of chronic illness on families: A family systems perspective. *Annals of Behavioral Medicine, 16,* 131–142.
Patterson, J. M., Leonard, B. J., & Titus, J. C. (1992). Home care for medically fragile children: Impact on family health and well-being. *Journal of Developmental and Behavioral Pediatrics, 13,* 248–255.
Perrin, J. M. (1999). State and federal programs for children who have chronic conditions. In M. Green, R. J. Haggerty, & M. Weitzman (Eds.), *Ambulatory pediatrics* (5th ed., pp. 247–251). Philadelphia: WB Saunders Co.
Perrin, J. M., Shayne, M. W., & Bloom, S. R. (1993). *Home and community care for chronically ill children.* New York: Oxford University Press.
Peter, C. (1997). Paying to participate: Financial social and personal costs to parents of involvement in their children's care in hospital. *Journal of Advanced Nursing, 25,* 746–752.
Petersen, P. (1984). Effects of moderator variables in reducing stress outcome in mothers of children with handicaps. *Journal of Psychosomatic Research, 28,* 337–344.
Podolski, C. L., & Nigg, J. T. (2001). Parent stress and coping in relation to child ADHD severity and associated child disruptive behavior problems. *Journal of Clinical Child Psychology, 30,* 503–513.
Quint, R., Chesterman, E., Crain, L. S., Wrikleby, M., & Boyce, W. T. (1990). Home care for ventilator-dependent children: Psychosocial impact on the family. *American Journal of Disabled Children, 144,* 1238–1241.
Raina, P., O'Donnell, M., Schwellnus, H., Rosenbaum, P., King, G., Brehaut, J., et al. (2004, January 14). Caregiving process and caregiver burden: Conceptual models to guide research and practice. *BMC Pediatrics, 4,* 1. http://www.biomedcentral.com/1471-2431/4/1.
Salkever, D. S. (1982). Children's health problems and maternal work status. *Journal of Human Resources, 12,* 95–109.
Sawhill, I. V. (1980). Economic perspectives on the family. In A. H. Amsden (Ed.), *The economics of women and work.* New York: St. Martin's Press.
Schor, E., Starfield, B., Stidley, C., & Hankin, J. (1987). Utilization and effects of family membership. *Medical Care, 25,* 616–626.
Silver, E. J., Ireys, H. T., Bauman, L. J., & Stein, R. E. K. (1995). Psychological outcomes of a support intervention in mothers of children with ongoing health conditions: The parent-to-parent network. *Journal of Community Psychology, 25,* 249–264.

Silver, E. J., Westbrook, L. E., & Stein, R. E. (1998). Relationship of parental psychological distress to consequences of chronic health conditions in children. *Journal of Pediatric Psychology, 23,* 5–15.
Sivberg, B. (2002). Coping strategies and parental attitudes, a comparison of parents with children with autistic spectrum disorders and parents with non-autistic children. *International Journal of Circumpolar Health, 61,* 36–50.
Sloper, P., & Turner, S. (1992). Service needs of families of children with severe physical disability. *Child Care Health Development, 18,* 259–282.
Sloper, P., & Turner, S. (1993). Risk and resistance factors in the adaptation of parents of children with severe physical disability. *Journal of Child Psychology and Psychiatry, 34,* 167–188.
Smith, T. B., Oliver, M. N., & Innocenti, M. S. (2001). Parenting stress in families of children with disabilities. *American Journal of Orthopsychiatry, 71,* 257–261.
Stein, R. E. K. (2001). Long-term care for children. *Ambulatory Pediatrics, 1,* 280–288.
Stein, R. E. K., & Jessop, D. J. (1984a). Does pediatric home care make a difference for children with chronic illness? *Pediatrics, 73,* 845–853.
Stein, R. E. K., & Jessop, D. J. (1984b). *Evaluation of a home care unit as an ambulatory ICU.* Springfield: National Technical Information Service.
Stein, R. E. K., & Jessop, D. J. (1991). Long-term mental health effects of a pediatric home care program. *Pediatrics, 88,* 490–496.
Strickland, B., McPherson, M., van Dyck, P., Huang, Z. J., & Newacheck, P. (2004). Access to the medical home: Results of the National Survey of Children with Special Health Care Needs. *Pediatrics, 113,* 1485–1492.
Tessler, R., & Mechanic, D. (1978). Factors affecting children's use of physician services in a prepaid group practice. *Medical Care, 16,* 33–46.
Thompson, R. J., & Gustafson, K. E. (1996). *Adaptation to chronic childhood illness.* Washington: American Psychological Association.
Thyen, U., Terres, N. M., Yazdgerdi, S. R., & Perrin, J. M. (1998). Impact of long-term care of children assisted by technology on maternal health. *Journal of Developmental and Behavioral Pediatrics, 19,* 273–282.
Thyen, U., Kuhlthau, K., & Perrin, J. M. (1999). The effect of child health status on maternal employment. *Pediatrics, 103,* 1235–1242.
Tong, H. C., Kandala, G., Haig, A. J., Nelson, V. S., Yamakawa, K. S. J., & Shin, K. Y. (2002). Physical functioning in female caregivers of children with physical disabilities compared with female caregivers of children with a chronic medical condition. *Archives of Pediatrics and Adolescent Medicine, 156,* 1138–1142.
Warfield, M. E., Krauss, M. W., Houser-Cram, P., Upshur, C. C., & Shonkof, J. P. (1999). Adaptation during early childhood among mothers of children with disabilities. *Journal of Developmental and Behavioral Pediatrics, 20,* 9–16.
Weitzman, M., Walker, D. K., & Gortmaker, S. L. (1986). Chronic illness, psychosocial problems, and school absences. *Clinical Pediatrics, 25,* 137–141.
Wolfe, B. L. (1980). Children's utilization of medical care. *Medical Care, 18,* 1196–1207.
Wolfe, B. L., & Hill, S. C. (1995). The effect of health on work effort of single mothers. *Journal of Human Resources, 30,* 42–62.

# Chapter 6
# Neither Prepared Nor Rehearsed: The Role of Public Health in Disability and Caregiving

John E. Crews

Decades of research in social gerontology and disability have addressed the family dynamics of caregiving—characterizing family caregiving, the hierarchy of care, and the burden that caregiving responsibilities create. More recent investigations are addressing health concerns of caregiving, including caregivers' lack of access to preventive medical care and mortality related to intense caregiving. Although some health dimensions of caregiving are being identified, current approaches neglect public health principles, which are needed to address family caregiving more completely. These public health approaches can serve to organize and enhance current research, develop new and critically needed interventions, and inform policy. For example, it is critical to document the number, characteristics, and health circumstances of caregivers and care recipients at national and state levels.

By and large, the subject of disability and caregiving as a public health topic has been neglected, but increasingly rigorous investigations have been directed toward fragments of this subject so much so that we can begin to create a conceptual framework to define research, policy, and practice dimensions of caregiving and disability informed by public health (Talley and Crews 2007).

This chapter, therefore, frames caregiving and disability as a public health concern. At its core, we simply must attend to the health of families who are caring for people with disabilities over the lifespan. In order for people to remain in caregiving roles, they must remain healthy. If caregivers are no longer able to lift, transfer, and bathe the care recipient, then the independence and quality of life of the care recipient may be compromised or lost altogether; or, if the caregiver becomes depressed or overwhelmed by the long-term responsibility of caregiving, then similar declines in support are likely to occur. One would suspect that the better the health of the caregiver, the better the quality of life and the greater the social participation of the person receiving care. Moreover, if caregivers neglect their own health, they, too, may become disabled. While this topic is not well researched, there is sufficient evidence to identify the major effects of caregiving upon the health of family members.

J. E. Crews (✉)
Division of Diabetes Translation, Centers for Disease Control and Prevention,
4770 Buford Highway, NE, K-10, Atlanta, GA 30341, USA
e-mail: jcrews@cdc.gov

Several important and complex concerns must be addressed to understand the role of public health in caregiving and disability. First, there are definitional issues regarding what defines disability and what defines caregivers. Second, there are demographic contextual issues that characterize the changing population of people with disabilities and people who are in caregiving roles. Third, the roles and dynamics of families change as caregiving responsibilities span the life of the caregiver and the care recipient. Fourth, it is useful to consider a public health framework to understand disability and how that framework might be used in understand caregiving. Fifth, public health has clearly defined functions related to the health of the US population; these functions can be framed in a way to better understand disability and caregiving. Finally, some encouraging activities occurring in public health are relevant to the discussion at hand. All these concerns, then, inform the public health research, policy, and practice as they relate to caregiving and disability.

## Dimensions of Disability

Multiple factors are driving how we think about disability. These factors can be classified as demographic changes in the population, policy shifts that have altered the expectations of people with disabilities as well as their families, and conceptual changes in how we model the experience of disability. These three issues are interwoven, and they are made more complex because of confusion regarding the definition of disability. Definitional issues and population changes will be addressed first.

## Definition of Disability

There is no "gold standard" definition of disability used consistently in US data sets to characterize or estimate the population of people with disabilities. Simply put, we do not know with precision how many people experience disability, and we do not know when someone crosses a threshold into disability. Recent analysis of the 2000 census data indicate almost 50 million Americans more than the age of 5 years experience disability, representing about 19.3% of the civilian, noninstitutionalized population (Waldrop and Stern 2003). Data cited from the National Center for Health Statistics (2002) in *Enabling America* (Brandt and Pope 1997) indicate an estimated 54 million people with disabilities, and this estimate has been widely quoted. The 2007 Institute of Medicine report, *The Future of Disability in America* (Field and Jette 2007), recognizing conflicting estimates, asserts there are between 40 and 50 million people with disability in the United States. Definitions of disability generally focus upon limitations in the performance of various functional activities, such as walking, lifting, sitting down and getting up, and bathing.

While there is a lack of conceptual rigor regarding the precise definition of disability, investigations suggest that the rate of disability in the general population ranges between 15 and 20%. For example, a recent investigation of the Behavioral

Risk Factors Surveillance Survey (BRFSS) reveals a rate of disability of 19.1% for those more than the age of 18 years (Centers for Disease Control and Prevention [CDC] 2006). The definition of disability for this survey was a positive response to one or both of two questions: "Are you limited in any way in any activities because of physical, mental, emotional problems?" or "Do you now have any health problem that requires you to use special equipment, such as cane, wheelchair, a special bed, or a special phone?" As one might expect, rates of disability are higher among older populations, and the BRFSS data support that assumption; those between the ages of 18 and 44 years report a rate of 12.3%; those between the ages of 45 and 64 years report 23.6%, and those more than the age of 65 years report a rate of 32.7% (CDC).

These discussions of population estimates are made more complex in public policy, in part, because there are more than 50 definitions of disability in federal legislation (Domzal 1995). Most of these definitions are dichotomous, insofar that they are concerned with establishing eligibility for various social programs or benefits, for example, Medicaid, vocational rehabilitation, and special education. Eligibility for one program does not necessarily establish eligibility for another. As income and access to services are attached to many of these eligibility decisions, people are often required to *prove* they are "disabled." By contrast, some public initiatives, which do not have dollars directly attached to them, attend to a broader population; the Americans with Disabilities Act—which is concerned about environmental access and access to programs—casts a broad net in its definition of disability. Likewise, the concerns of public health—broadly concerned with the health and well-being of the nation—would by its nature establish a broad, inclusive definition of disability (Lollar and Crews 2003).

Disability is, of course, as varied as the human condition will allow. In addition to differences in resources and coping strategies, there are differing degrees of severity in both intellectual and physical functioning. Severity of disability becomes a critical concern in caregiving; yet severity is not consistently measured in national surveys. People with mild to moderate intellectual disabilities may not be limited in activities of daily living (ADL), and may perform physical tasks with a great deal of ease. People with severe physical disabilities, by contrast, may require around-the-clock attention that likely puts considerable stress upon caregivers. We need to consider the severity and duration of disability as well as the intensity of caregiving as dimensions of this topic.

## Increasing Population

Just as the United States is reporting significant gains in years of life, people with disabilities are living longer. Twentieth century America, as well as Europe and Japan, demonstrated remarkable gain in life expectancy. In the United States, in 1900, women at birth had a life expectancy of 50.7 years and men had a life expectancy of 47.9 years, by 2004, life expectancy for women had increased to 80.4 years, and life expectancy for men had increased to 75.2 years (Federal Interagency Forum on Aging-Related Statistics 2008). Those more than the age of 85 years represent the fastest growing cohort in the United States (Federal Interagency Forum on Aging-Related Statistics 2000). Increased longevity has, of course, created major concerns regarding caregiving of elders. A person developing a disability at the age of 65 years may live with disability for decades, and many caregivers of very old people are themselves old.

The twentieth century witnessed a remarkable 30 years of additional years of life. Much of that gain is attributable to public health, as childhood diseases were controlled and antibiotics became increasingly available to treat diseases, and as increased water and air quality and decreased injuries all combined to reduce premature death.

These advances in health also led to increases in life expectancy for people with disabilities, what Oeffinger et al. call "an epidemic of survival" (1998). For example, first-year survival rates for children with Down's syndrome increased from 50% in 1942–1952 to 91% in 1980–1996 (Yang et al. 2002). Life expectancy for people with Down's syndrome increased from 9 years in 1929 to 56 years in 1989. Now, for example, retirement programs are being designed for people with Down's syndrome. For many families of children with Down's syndrome, the parent outlived their child. That may not necessarily be the case today.

Similarly, prior to World War II people with a lower spinal cord injury had a life expectancy of 14 months (Menter 1994). Now, someone experiencing a lower spinal cord injury at age 20 (who survives the first year) can expect an average of 46 additional years of life. Someone with a high (C1–C4) spinal cord injury can expect an additional 37 years of life. These are remarkable gains. Other examples include increased survival rates and life expectancy for premature newborns. For much of the human experience, people with severe injury or diseases died; now people live, but they often live with a disability, and increasingly they experience longer life spans. These gains create substantially differing caregiving dynamics.

The absolute number of people with disabilities in the United States continues to increase among all population groups (Field and Jette 2007). In addition to increased survival rates and increased life expectancy, better methods of identification have probably led to increasing numbers. For example, increases in the number of children identified with learning disabilities may arise because parents, physicians, and teachers are more sensitive to these conditions, and thus they are identified more readily.

## Changing Concepts of Disability

In addition to increasing numbers of people with disabilities, there have been substantial changes in the expectations of people with disabilities in terms of work, education, and autonomy and self-direction; these civil rights dimensions of disability are reflected in the Americans with Disabilities Act (Shapiro 1993), but these changing views are also mirrored in evolving conceptual frameworks of disability that reflect the multi-dimensional characteristics of this complex human experience.

The conceptual framework employed to describe the onset, experience, and consequences of disability has evolved markedly in recent decades. In the middle to late

**Fig. 6.1** ICF: interaction of concepts 2001, World Health Organization, 2002

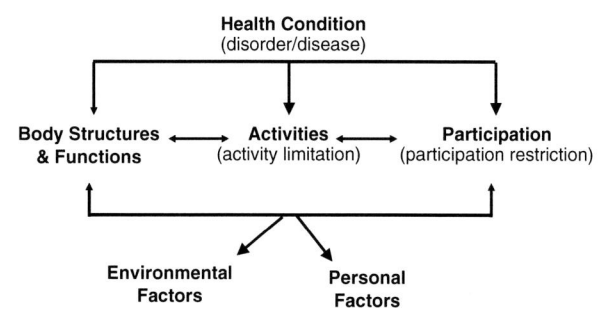

```
                    Health Condition
                    (disorder/disease)
          ┌──────────────┼──────────────┐
          ↓              ↓              ↓
   Body Structures ←→ Activities ←→ Participation
   & Functions       (activity       (participation restriction)
                     limitation)
          └──────────────┼──────────────┘
                    ↙        ↘
              Environmental   Personal
                Factors        Factors
```

Centers for Disease Control and Prevention

decades of the last century, disability was conceptually believed to reside with the person. There were things the person could and could not do, and measurement of that limitation became the defining components of disability. In addition, notions of disability were generally uni-dimensional, linear, and causal in their relations. A person had a disease or injury; that condition led to activity limitations (lifting, walking, reaching), and that in turn defined social disadvantage—the inability to work (Frey 1984). Major efforts to reconceptualize disability occurred in 1980 when Wood and Badley (1980) proposed initial drafts of the *International Classification of Impairments, Disabilities, and Handicaps* (ICIDH) for the World Health Organization (WHO 1980). Drafts of the ICIDH resulted in a refined model of disability called *the International Classification of Functioning, Disability and Health* (ICF; WHO 2001). The ICF was approved by the General Assembly of the WHO in 2001 as the companion classification to the *International Classification of Diseases* (ICD). This new framework attempted to portray multidimensional qualities of the human experience, including disability, and to recognize the role of the environment as it serves as a barrier or facilitator to people with disabilities. This new model (see Fig. 6.1) has four major conceptual components: impairments, activity, participation, and the environment:

> *Impairments* are problems in body function or structure such as a significant deviation or loss.
> *Activity limitations* are difficulties an individual may have in executing activities.
> *Participation restrictions* are problems an individual may experience in involvement of social roles.
> *Environmental factors* make up the physical social and attitudinal environment in which people live and conduct their lives. (WHO 2001, p. 10)

This framework allows one to describe or "map" human experience. The multiple arrows in the diagram illustrate that the multiple dimensions of disability are not linear or causal. A person with activity limitations may or may not have social participation restrictions, depending on the person's resources and the supports of the community. Moreover, the characteristics of the environment serve as barriers or facilitators to people with activity limitations. The obvious example would be curb cuts, but certainly accessible transportation system and employers who are accommodating increase the opportunities for people with disabilities to assume the social roles of being involved in the community and working. It is worth noting that the WHO asserts that the ICF "is about *all people*. The health and health-related states associated with all health conditions can be described using the ICF. In other words, the ICF has universal application" (WHO 2001, p. 7). The ICF taxonomy mirrors changing notions in disability rights. The focus of disability policy is upon achieving participation (work, education, relationships)—not simply the performance of various tasks.

Caregiving is modeled in the ICF as part of the environment, and the taxonomy includes specific codes for family and paid caregivers. The emphasis of the coding schema is to identify the amount of care provided not the attitudes or health of those providing services. However, as we think about this model, it is possible to describe both the health dimensions of the care recipient and the caregiver. For example, if the caregiver and the care recipient were to fall during a transfer, one could map the injury and its dimensions to the ICF.

## Impact of Disability upon the Family

Just as disability is not easily defined, case definition problems surround the concept of caregiving. Definitions of family caregiving attempt to make distinctions between normal caregiving roles, say parenting, and unexpected caregiving roles, defined by caring for a spouse with dementia or a child with disability. These distinctions are not always well circumscribed. Schofield (1998) in Australia creates a framework to define differentiating factors in family caregiving, and she notes five levels of caring, each with particular characteristics that lead to a restricted definition of family caregiving. In her model, Schofield makes a distinction between paid and nonpaid caring; among those who are not paid, some are volunteers, having "choice," or families, having no choice. Some family caregiving is reciprocal (defined by mutual dependence) and other family caregivers are "responsible for," that is, there is an "imbalance in dependence." Within the "responsible for" category, caring can be classified as parenting with "normal expectations" and "caregiving" which serves as a "transgression of normal expectations." Schofield notes, "transgression of customary expectations distinguishes parenting from caring for a person with special needs. This transgression of expectations might involve the loss of a relationship or of an expected child, the duration of care, the nature and intensity of caring tasks" (Schofield 1998, p. 13). Using these relatively narrow parameters, this investigation revealed that 5.3% of families in Australia were caregivers.

A number of national and small sample studies regarding caregiving illuminate the magnitude of the problem in the United States. A review of the literature suggests fairly consistent assessment of the burden of caregiving as well as consistent implications for the health of caregivers. A 1998 caregiving survey sponsored by the Henry J. Kaiser Family Foundation, Harvard School of Public Health, United Hospital Fund of New York, and the Visiting Nurse Service of New York (2002)—in contrast to Schofield's definition—suggests the magnitude of caregiving in the United States.

Using a very broad definition of caregiving, the Kaiser study revealed that almost one in four adults (23%) has provided caregiving within the year prior to the study. Donelan et al. (2002) noted, "The data reveal a substantial time commitment to all tasks: 20% were providing full-time or constant care, 41% had been caregivers for 5 years or more, and 37% were providing intense care with ADLs and IADLs. While caregivers report many positive experiences related to caregiving, 21% reported their health had suffered because of caregiving responsibilities." Another examination of this data set by Navaie-Waliser et al. (2002) reveals that women provide the most intense care to more severely disabled care recipients than men; moreover, 19% of women and 14% of men (16% of the total) reported their health as fair or poor, and 36% of women and 27% of men (32% of the total) report having a serious medical condition.

A more recent study conducted by the National Alliance for Caregiving and AARP (2004) reveals similar patterns and additional insights into health and caregiving. This study estimated that 21% of people more than the age of 18 years provide unpaid care—an estimated 44.4 million people. Sixteen percent of people in the general population provide care to individuals more than the age of 50 years, and 5% of people in the United States provide care to people aged 18–49 years. This study did not ask about care recipients under the age of 18 years, and therefore caregivers of children with disabilities were omitted from the study. This NAC-AARP study made distinctions regarding intensity of care and defined five levels of caregiving in a "Level of Burden Index." Level 1 caregivers provided the least amount of care and provided no assistance with ADLs. Level 5 caregivers, by contrast, helped with at least two ADLs and provided more than 40 hours of care each week. Level 1 caregivers provided a mean of 3.5 hours each week, while Level 5 caregivers provided a mean of 87.2 hours per week. Twenty-two percent of Level 5 caregivers were more than the age of 65 years, while only 12% of Level 1 caregivers were in that age group. An important finding in this investigation had to do with overall health. People providing Level 5 caregiving were three times more likely to report fair or poor health (fair = 24%; poor = 11%) than Level 1 caregivers (fair = 8; poor = 4%).

Research regarding family caregiving and disability, as one would probably expect, has become segmented in multiple ways—reflecting the interests of caregivers, investigators, or sponsors of research. While the bulk of caregiving investigations have examined experiences associated with age-related onset of disability, a growing body of research has addressed the experiences of parents caring for children over the lifespan. A large body of literature has emerged regarding the emotional adjustment of families to disabilities. Many of these investigations focus upon the early years of the families, and others have focused upon life course experiences. Considerable work has addressed lifespan caregiving for families with children and adult children with intellectual disabilities. Investigators have also examined social and economic outcomes of caregiving, and most of the findings are intuitive insofar that people required to provide significant care at home make compromises in work—promotions, moves, and amount of time dedicated to work. While the mental health of caregivers has received attention, only in recent years has attention been given to the physical health of caregivers—many of whom are required to provide care over several decades.

## Elements of a Conceptual Framework

The experience of family caring over an extended period suggests at least nine factors that define a conceptual framework:

*Dimensional Characteristics of Disability* The ICF framework embraces dimensional, fluid characteristics of disability. In addition to allowing us to characterize disability within activity and participation domains, the concept of the environment illustrates the role of caregiving. The ICF serves as the core to map disability and the role of caregiving in that framework.

*Direction of Caregiving* There is a directional quality to caregiving over the life span that seems more or less normal and is defined by the relationship of the caregiver to the care recipient. Parents care for young children; adult children care for older people, and older spouses care for each other. Some caregiving is downward, some upward, and some lateral. Research tends to divide caregivers into two broad groups: those providing care to older people—adult children and spouses—and caregivers for children with disabilities—restricted mainly to parents. Caregiving for one family member, of course, does not relieve the potential to care for others. For example, among families with a child with a disability, the care of a parent may extend from the child to the grandparent. Care, therefore, extends both upward and downward.

*Supports* Support or lack of support assumes several dimensions: informal supports may come from extended family that can provide respite and emotional understanding. Informal supports may change over time; the grandmother who provides assistance and respite in a child's early years may require assistance in her later years. Formal supports may be community day programs or employment activities. Supports may also be in the form of family wealth; families with considerable resources can purchase needed services, equipment, and home modifications.

*Domain of Disability* Disability research typically makes distinctions among three domains of disability, including intellectual impairments, sensory impairments, and mobility impairments. Intellectual impairments may manifest themselves differently among various age groups; for example, young people with Down's syndrome have a different set of experiences and a different trajectory than older people who develop dementia associated with Alzheimer's disease (AD). Moreover, sensory impairment among young people presents a constellation of experiences different from age-related sensory losses.

*Severity of Disability* Disability, of course, has multiple dimensions that predict varying demands upon caregivers. Mental illness may present unpredictable requirements from the caregiver. AD, likewise, may result in unpredictable behaviors, including outbursts of anger. Intellectual disabilities may require prompting, and severe physical disabilities may require considerable physical demands upon caregivers with daily routines of lifting, transferring, toileting, and bathing. These demands differ over time: a 30 year old parent bathing a 25 pound child is considerably different from a 70 year old parent bathing their 150 pound adult child.

*Duration* Decades of caregiving are likely to take a toll upon caregivers, and their ability to maintain physical and mental health predicts their ability to remain in caregiving roles. Schofield (1998) found that 22% of caregivers had provided care for more than 10 years; a least one had provided care for 50 years, and 46% had provided care from 3 to 9 years.

*Intensity of Care* Conceptually, there are several ways to measure intensity. One strategy might be to measure assistance with ADLs and IADLs. The greater the number would imply greater intensity. Another strategy would be to measure the number of hours of care. The work of caregiving may range from being available providing stand-by help or providing direct assistance. In each case, the caregiver is occupied in caregiving. As noted above in the NAC/AARP study, the mean number of hours for the most disabled care recipients was more than 80 hours per week.

*Dynamic Characteristics of Caregiving* As much as we are inclined to desire that situations remain stable, stability does not necessarily define caregiving relationships. As a young person grows older, parental caregiving may give way to greater paid supports in the best of circumstances. Among older people, general health may decline over time, and caregiving responsibilities may increase until perhaps the care recipient enters an institution or dies. In addition, however, as people with disabilities age, their health and capacity is likely to diminish as pain, fatigue, and weakness place increased demands upon themselves and their caregivers (Thompson 2004).

*Health of Caregivers and Care Recipients* The hypothesis of this chapter is that there are health effects related to caregiving. These health effects may take the form of chronic diseases, for example, arthritis, which may result from lifting and transferring. In addition, injuries to the caregiver and care recipients may occur during transfers or repositioning. Lack of access to preventive medical services may occur because the caregiver cannot get away for routine medical care, or they may not have time to get well when sick. These dimensions need to be measured and understood in greater detail.

## *Health of Caregivers*

Investigations into the physical and mental health of caregivers are not entirely consistent. Chen et al. (2001) examined the mental and physical health of mid-life (aged 55–64 years) and older ($\geq 65$ years) mothers caring for adult children with intellectual disabilities. Among the 108 women surveyed, findings indicated that these mothers reported physical and mental health status no worse than or better than national norms. Similarly, Seltzer et al. (2001) examined the life course and well-being of parents of children with developmental disabilities and children with mental illness. Parents were surveyed when they were in their mid-30s and 15 years later when they were in their early 50s. Using the Wisconsin Longitudinal Study, investigators examined work patterns, social participation, mental and physical health. The study revealed that mothers of children with developmental disabilities were less likely to work or worked fewer hours, and were more likely to report depression than the comparison group. However, there was no difference in reported health among parents with and without children with disabilities.

By contrast, most investigations that identified health as a variable found the health of caregivers was compromised over time. For example, Pruchno et al. (1996) examined the mental health of older women caring for chronically disabled children compared with mothers caring for children with schizophrenia. The authors used a model that characterized stressors, resources, appraisals, and outcomes. While this study did not compare these two group with older women not in lifelong caregiving roles, the authors assert the importance of health, noting, "Poor physical health and feelings of burden from the caregiving role are so powerful that not only do they increase negative psychological well-being, but they also decrease feelings of positive well-being" (Pruchno et al. 1996, p. S294).

Shaw et al. (1997) examined the health decline of spousal caregivers of older adults with AD. In this longitudinal study, 150 spousal caregivers were compared with 46 married control participants. Using survival analysis, Shaw notes, "One major conclusion for our study is that the health of spousal caregivers of AD patients may be compromised only when caregiving demands (i.e., ADLs) are great. Variability of AD family caregiving experiences has been well documented, and these differences appear to be based not only on the course of illness but on individual differences in disease manifestation. In the present study, we found that ADL assistance was predictive of poor health outcomes, but problem behaviors of the AD patients were not. The simplest distinction that could be made between these two predictor variables is that ADLs are related to greater physical demands of caregiving, and problem behaviors are related to greater interpersonal stress. Although this distinction is certainly not clear-cut, we might conclude from our results that physical demands of caregiving (bathing, toileting, feeding, lifting, etc.) have greater impact on caregiver health than the psychological stress attached to problem behaviors (repeating questions, hiding things, being agitated or argumentative, etc.). This finding provides more support for the 'physical exertion' and 'modified health behaviors' pathways than the 'depression symptoms' or 'modified autonomic control' pathways for stress-related illness" (Shaw et al. 1997, p. 107).

Similarly, Schulz et al. (1997) examining the Caregiver Health Effects Study (CHES) noted that the population-based survey provides some methodological strengths in terms of selection of subjects. Their findings indicate that not all individuals living with a spouse with a disability provide caregiving; rather, about 80% of husbands and wives provide care to their spouse with a disability, and more than half of care providers (56%) report mental or physical strain associated with caregiving responsibilities. Among these, there are substantial differences in outcome variables related to health, especially when compared with those who do not have caregiving responsibilities. This study indicates the importance of identifying the intensity of support among caregivers, and one would assume the severity of disability among care recipients. In addition, Schultz and Beach (1999) examined the same data set, the CHES, to establish the consequences upon spouses caring for their disabled partner. Among caregivers who reported mental and emotional stain associated with caregiving, they subsequently experienced significantly higher rates of mortality.

Navaie-Waliser et al. (2002) were concerned about the effects of health upon caregivers, and in a population-based study of 1,002 caregivers, they compared the caregiving responsibility and challenges of caregivers who reported their health as fair or poor or having a serious health condition (vulnerable caregivers) with caregivers without those characteristics (nonvulnerable caregivers). Some characteristics of the care recipients were gathered but not reported. The authors conclude, "Many caregivers meet the demands of caring for a relative or friend in the midst of their own deteriorating health. In this population based national survey, 36% of caregivers surveyed were vulnerable. Among these vulnerable caregivers, over half reported difficulty providing care; about half were providing care 20 or more hours per week, and over one-third reported that their physical health had suffered since becoming a caregiver. Moreover, vulnerable caregivers were more likely than nonvulnerable caregivers to be providing higher-intensity care and be aged 65 years or older. Yet vulnerable caregivers were no more likely than nonvulnerable caregivers to receive help form paid support services for their care recipients. Nearly 4 of every 5 caregivers in each category provided care without paid assistance even though vulnerable caregivers bore a heavier care burden and were in poorer health" (Navaie-Waliser et al. 2002, p. 411).

Stress is an overarching theme reported by many investigators. For example, Lieberman and Fisher (1995) reported stress and health effects throughout the family as they cared for persons with dementia. Greenburg et al. (1993) compared stress and supports among older mothers of adult children with mental retardation compared with aging mothers caring for adults with mental illness. There was no control group. Health of the mothers was not examined.

Stress is associated with depression, but is largely not associated with health outcomes. Orr et al. (1993) surveyed stress among 112 mothers using the Parenting Stress Index to measure stress of parents of preschool, middle school, and high-school students with developmental delays. This Ontario study found that all mothers reported high levels of stress with mothers of middle schoolers reporting the most stress. The investigators note, "Although the passage of time will likely mitigate the effects of some stressors and make responses to them more routine, it is also likely that the changing nature of the child and the increasing expectations associated with growing older should generally increase the magnitude of stress that parents experience" (Orr et al. 1993, p. 171). The high stress among middle-school mothers was unexpected. Finally, Heller et al. (1997) note that mothers provide most of the care and feel most of the stress.

In a 4-year longitudinal study, Cannuscio et al. (2002) compared rates of depression among women with and without spousal caregiving responsibilities. The study identified four groups, those without caregiving responsibility, those who were no longer caregivers, those with continuing spousal caregiving responsibility, and those new to caregiving. Nearly half those new to spousal caregiving reported decline in mental health.

A promising line of research is occurring in Australia where a group of investigators is examining a variety of health issues of caregiving of people who are older and/or have disabilities. Much of this research is framed as a public health concern. Schofield et al. (1998) have developed a comprehensive instrument to measure the personal characteristics of care providers, care recipients, and severity of disability. In their research, 946 caregivers and 219 noncaregivers were surveyed in a population based, longitudinal, cross diagnostic study: "(i) to create a socio-demographic profile of caregivers in the state of Victoria, Australia; (ii) to assess the effects of caregiving on their physical and emotional well being; and (iii) to explore their needs, informal and formal supports" (Schofield et al. 1998, p. 648).

Schofield's research may be instructive for guiding US investigations. The Australian study sampled 26,000 households to identify 1,000 caregivers. The screener's caregiving question was, "Do you or does anyone in your household take the main responsibility on caring for someone who is aged or has a long-tem illness, disability or other problem?" (Schofield et al. 1998, p. xxii). Using this question, caregivers were identified in only 5.3% of households, contrasting with rates ranging between 21 and 24% in US surveys. Schofield examined demographic characteristics of caregivers, use of services, employment and finances, as well as health and well-being of caregivers. Given that only 5.3% of the population identified themselves as caregivers, her findings suggest that these individual are involved in more intense caregiving roles than perhaps other boarder definitions of caregiving would imply. Her findings regarding health and well-being are particularly striking:

> A third of carers reported major problems with their own health over the past year.... Almost half were on medication and over a quarter rated their overall health as only fair or poor. Over half agreed that they were exhausted when they went to bed at night, around half felt they had more things to do than they could handle and not time just for themselves. At the same time, a high 86% were satisfied or very satisfied with their life as a whole, and around 80% were similarly content with their health, their personal and emotional life, the respect or recognition they get and their independence or freedom; a somewhat lower 87% expressed satisfaction with their financial situation. (Schofield et al. 1998, p. 20)

In addition to injury, depression, and overall poorer health, it appears that caregivers may be neglecting preventive medical care. For example, Schulz et al. (1997) analyzing—if possible the CHES, examined those caregivers who report mental and physical strain associated with caregiving. Those who reported strain were nine times more likely to report not having enough rest, five times more likely to report not having enough time to exercise, and ten times more likely to report not having enough time to rest when sick. In a companion study, Burton et al. (1997) found that spouses caring for a disabled partner were less likely to participate in preventive health behaviors, including enough sleep, time to recuperate, exercise, missed meals, missed medical appointments, missed flu shots, and lack of ability to refill medicines.

## Directions for Research, Policy Development, and Interventions

Caregiver research is well established in social gerontology, and investigators in disability studies recognize the complex consequences of raising a child with a disability. That foundation informs research, policy, and practice regarding the health effects of caregiving and disability. This review underlines the importance of the health of caregivers and suggests the importance of the health in sustaining the well-being and social participation of care recipients. Substantial gaps in knowledge remain. We do not know at the state level the number of caregivers, their health, or the potential of interventions to sustain the health of caregivers. State-level data are essential for planners in aging and disability to respond to the particular needs identified within the state. The prevalence of disability varies considerably from state to state, and those differences likely drive varying prevalence of caregiving. In 2004, investigators at the University of Florida developed a caregiving module as part of the Behavioral Risk Factors Surveillance Survey. The module was field tested in North Carolina (Neugaard et al. 2007), and in 2007, five additional states implemented offered as a module to the BRFSS and a core caregiver question were included in the 2009 BRFSS. This survey may create a method to measure the magnitude of caregiving and the health consequences of caregiving at the state level.

Moreover, the caregiver questions in national and community surveys are not consistent and therefore, there is some variation in the number of caregivers. In addition, surveys need to track who provides care to whom as caregiving often is upward, downward, lateral, or some combination.

In addition, we have only vague notions about how existing knowledge can be translated into actions to potentially improve the health of caregivers. As the knowledge base is refined, it is increasingly imperative that interventions be developed, tested, and implemented to improve overall health of caregivers and care recipients. For example, would it be useful to pay for respite care so that a caregiver could be assured to have an annual physical?

## Conclusion

Perhaps one in four or one in five Americans provide care to others. For some, this experience is short term, causes modest disruption, and quickly becomes a memory. For others, caregiving is brutal work, occupying more than 80 hours a week over decades. The intensity of caregiving takes its toll on the health of caregivers as they neglect their own health care, injure themselves in lifting or transferring, or accelerate diseases like arthritis by placing undue strain on backs and joints. These circumstances argue for us to treat caregiving as a public health concern.

## Appendix A

Schofield caregiving question: "Do you or does anyone in your household take the main responsibility in caring for someone who is aged or has a long-term illness, disability or other problem?" (Schofield 1998, p. xxii) Response rate is 5.3%.

National Alliance for Caregiving-AARP: "In the last 12 months, have you or anyone in your household provided unpaid care to a relative or friend 18 years or older to help them take care of themselves? Unpaid care may include help with personal needs or household chores. It might be managing a person's finances, arranging for outside services, to visiting regularly to see how they are doing. This person need not live with you" (NAC-AAPR 2004, p. 18). Total response rate is 21%; 16% care for people aged 50+ years and 5% care for people aged 18–49 years.

## References

Brandt, E. N., & Pope, A. M. (1997). *Enabling America: Assessing the role of rehabilitation science and engineering*. Washington: National Academy Press.

Burton, L. C., Newsom, J. T., Schultz, R., Hirsch, C. H., & German, P. S. (1997). Preventive health behaviors among spousal caregivers. *Preventive Medicine, 26,* 162–169.

Cannuscio, C., Jones, C., Kawachi, I., Colditz, G. A., & Berkman, L. (2002). Reverberation of family illness: A longitudinal assessment of informal caregiving and mental health status in Nurses' Health Study. *American Journal of Public Health, 92,* 1305–1311.

Centers for Disease Control and Prevention. (2006). *Disability and health state chartbook, 2006: Profiles of health for adults with disabilities*. Atlanta: Centers for Disease Control and Prevention.

Chen, S. C., Ryan-Henry, S., Heller, T., & Chen, E. H. (2001). Health status of mothers of adults with intellectual disability. *Journal of Intellectual Disability Research, 45,* 439–449.

Donelan, K., Hill, C. A., Hoffman, C., Scoles, K., Feldman, P. H., Levine, C., et al. (2002). Challenged to care: Informal caregivers in a changing health system. *Health Affairs, 21,* 222–231.

Domzal, C. (1995). *Federal statutory definition of disability*. Washington: U.S. Department of Education, National Institute on Disability and Rehabilitation Research.

Federal Interagency Forum on Aging-Related Statistics. (2000, August). *Older Americans 2000: Key indicators of well being*. Washington: U.S. Government Printing Office.

Federal Interagency Forum on Aging-Related Statistics. (2008, March). *Older Americans 2008: Key indicators of well being*. Washington: U.S. Government Printing Office.

Field, M. J., & Jette, A. L. (2007). *The future of disability in America*. Washington: National Academies Press.

Frey, W. D. (1984). Functional assessment in the '80s: A conceptual enigma, a conceptual challenge. In A. S. Halpern & M. J. Fuhrer (Eds.). *Functional assessment in rehabilitation* (pp. 11–44). Baltimore: Brookes.

Greenberg, J. S., Seltzer, M. M., & Greenley, J. R. (1993). Aging parents of adults with disabilities: The gratification and frustration of later life caregiving. *Gerontologist, 33,* 542–550.

Heller, T., Hsieh, K., & Rowitz, L. (1997). Maternal and paternal caregiving with mental retardation across the lifespan. *Family Relations, 46,* 407–415.

Lieberman, M. A., & Fisher, L. (1995). The impact of chronic illness on the health and well being of family members. *Gerontologist, 35*(10), 94–102.

Lollar, D. J., & Crews, J. E. (2003). Redefining the role of public health in disability. *Annual Review of Public Health, 24,* 195–208.

Menter, R. (1994). Spinal cord injury and aging: Exploring the unknown. *Journal of the American Paraplegia Society, 16,* 179–189.

National Alliance for Caregiving, ARRP. (2004). *Caregiving in the U.S.* Bethesda: National Alliance for Caregiving. http://www.caregiving.org/datat04execsumm.pdf. Accessed 19 April 2012.

National Center for Health Statistics. (2002). *National vital statistics reports, 51*(3). http://www.cdc.gov/nchs/fastats/pdf/nvsr51_03t11.pdf. Accessed 19 April 2012.

Navaie-Waliser, M., Feldman, P. H., Gould, D. A., Levine, C., Kuerbis, A. N., & Donelan, K. (2002). When the caregiver needs care: The plight of vulnerable caregivers. *American Journal of Public Health, 92,* 409–413.

Navaie-Waliser, M., Spriggs, A., & Feldman, P. H. (2002). Informal caregiving: differential experiences by gender. *Medical Care, 40,* 1249–1259.

Neugaard, B., Andresen, E. M., Talley, R. C., & Crews, J. E. (2007). The characteristics and health of caregivers and care recipients—North Carolina, 2005. *MMWR, 56,* 529–532.

Oeffinger, K. C., Eshelman, D. A., Tomlinson, G. E., & Buchanan, G. R. (1998). Programs for adult survivors of child hood cancer. *Journal of Clinical Oncology, 16,* 2864–2867.

Orr, R. R., Cameron, S. J., Dobson, L. A., & Day, D. M. (1993). Age-related changes in stress experienced by families with a child who has developmental delays. *Mental Retardation, 31*(3), 171–176.

Pruchno, R. A., Patrick, J. H., & Burant, C. J. (1996). Mental health of aging women with children who are chronically disabled: Examination of a two-factor model. *Journals of Gerontology: Series B, Psychological Sciences & Social Sciences, 51*(6), S284–S296.

Schofield, H. (1998). *Family caregivers: Disability, illness and ageing.* St Leonards: Allen & Unwin.

Schofield, H. L., Murphy, B., Herrman, H. E., Bloch, S., & Singh, B. (1998). Family caregiving: Measurement of emotional well-being and various aspects of the caregiving role. *Psychological Medicine, 27,* 647–657.

Schulz, R., Newsom, J., Mittelmark, M., Burton, L., Hirch, C., & Jackson, S. (1997). Health effects of caregiving: The Caregiver Health Study: An ancillary study of the cardiovascular health study. *Annals of Behavioral Medicine, 19,* 110–116.

Schultz, R., & Beach, S. R. (1999). Caregiving as a risk factor for mortality: The Caregiver Health Effects Study. *Journal of the American Medical Association, 828,* 2215–2219.

Seltzer, M. M., Greenberg, J. S., Floyd, F. J., Pettee, Y., & Hong, J. (2001). Life course impacts of parenting a child with a disability. *American Journal on Mental Retardation, 106,* 265–286.

Shapiro, J. P. (1993). *No pity: People with disabilities forging a new civil rights movement.* New York: Random House.

Shaw, W. S., Patterson, T. L., Semple, S. J., Ho, S., Irwin, M. R., Hauger, R. L., et al. (1997). Longitudinal analysis of multiple indicators of health decline among spousal caregivers. *Annals of Behavioral Medicine, 19*(2), 101–109.

Talley, R. C., & Crews, J. E. (2007). Framing the public health of caregiving. *American Journal of Public Health, 97,* 224–228.

Thompson, L. (2004). Functional changes affecting people aging with disabilities. In B. J. Kemp & L. Mosqueda (Eds.), *Aging with a disability: What the clinician needs to know* (pp. 102–128). Baltimore: Johns Hopkins Press.

Waldrop, J., & Stern, S. M. (2003). *Disability status: 2000.* Washington: U.S. Department of Commerce, U.S Census Bureau.

Wood, P. H. N., & Badley, E. M. (1980). *People with disabilities: Toward acquiring information which reflects more sensitively their problems and needs* (World Rehabilitation Fund Monograph No. 12). New York: World Rehabilitation Fund.

World Health Organization. (1980). *International classification of impairment, disabilities and handicaps: A manual of classification relating to the consequences of disease.* Geneva: World Health Organization.

World Health Organization. (2001). *International classification of functioning, disability and health: ICF.* Geneva: World Health Organization.

Yang, Q., Rasmussen, S., & Friedman, J. M. (2002). Mortality associated with Down's syndrome in the USA from 1983–1997: A population based study. *The Lancet, 359,* 1019–1025.

# Chapter 7
# Race/Ethnicity, Culture, and Socioeconomic Status and Caregiving of Persons with Disabilities

**Paul Leung**

While caregiving has universal characteristics, ethnicity and culture have more impact on how caregiving is valued and how families engage the experience.

> Though I live in Texas, the phone call for assistance came from an insurance case manager in the Midwest at wits end about what to do with a thirty-four year old Chinese American chef who sustained a traumatic brain injury 2 years before. The chef was living with his brother and sister-in-law in a small Midwestern community where he had worked in a Chinese restaurant. After his accident, initial hospitalization, and several months of rehabilitation, the sister-in-law assumed the role of primary caregiver even though her brother-in-law was able to take care of many of his own needs. The insurance case manager believed the chef was able to go back to work. However, the sister-in-law insisted her brother-in-law was ill and needed care, and she resisted efforts to relinquish her caregiving responsibilities.

This example illustrates the complex and often frustrating task of coping with disability, culture/ethnicity, and caregiving. People from different cultures perceive ability and disability in substantially different ways, and caregiving expectations differ as well. In this example, differences in interpretation of how disability was defined and what constituted care required resolution if the Chinese chef were to return to work. Ethnicity and culture were significant variables that affected caregiving and created fundamentally different notions of acceptable outcomes for rehabilitation and continuing family support. The chef obviously had some residual functional limitations affecting his capacity to care for himself and perhaps work, but in the familial context, he was perceived as "sick," needing continuing care and support from the family. Similar situations occur in a variety of cultural contexts everyday and are likely to increase as America's population continues to diversify.

The Family Caregiver Alliance noted in a recent report that caregiving "will preoccupy American families well into the twenty first century" (Feinberg et al. 2002, p. 1) because of the needs associated with the increasing number of persons over the age of 65 years and the disabling conditions that often accompany the aging process (Pfizer Journal 1997). The National Alliance on Caregiving and AARP (NAC-AARP 1997) in a national survey predicted caregiving to become a "prevalent and a

---

P. Leung (✉)
University of North Texas, P.O. Box 311456, Denton, TX 76203, USA
e-mail: pleung@unt.edu

normative experience" in the United States. The Family Caregiving Alliance (2008) estimates that some 52 million caregivers provide formal and informal caregiving to persons who are ill or have disabilities. Caregiving may be more likely among minority populations because disability is more prevalent among minority groups. Included in these estimates are African Americans, Hispanic Americans, and Asian Americans—groups that all represent growing US populations. Each of these groups holds values and traditions that influence how caregiving is played out by the family.

The task of exploring the intersection of ethnicity/race, caregiving and disability is complex and variable. This chapter provides a framework for understanding the impact that ethnicity, socioeconomic status, and disability have on the caregiving process, and this chapter highlights the general lack of knowledge about the role of ethnicity/race and culture on caregiving for persons with disabilities, and thus it points to directions for research, interventions, and policy.

## Disability Defined

The circumstances that require caregiving include a very wide range of conditions including mobility impairments (spinal cord injury and cerebral palsy) cognitive impairments (traumatic brain injury, stroke, and intellectual disability) and sensory impairments (vision and hearing loss). While there is no gold standard definition of disability, it is often defined by particular legislation and specific program requirements. Definitions of disability have evolved from a "medical model" concerned with treatment and cure to a "social model" that recognizes the person in the context of social roles and the environment. The addition of cultural descriptions to disability further recognizes the dimensional characteristics of this complex human experience. Definitions are important because they may determine the response to disability and whether or not informal caregiving or formal services are sought (Ory et al. 1999).

The recent adoption by the World Health Organization of a functional classification scheme was in part due to an American "cultural" objection from persons with disabilities to the use of the term "handicap" and the perspective that people do not have handicaps but that society imposes handicaps on people. *The International Classification of Functioning, Disability and Health* (ICF; World Health Organization 2000) that replaced a 1981 framework is an attempt to provide a unified and standard language related to disabling conditions. The ICF is instructive because it illustrates how disability is defined. Moreover, the ICF allows us to better understand the "contexts" in which disability occurs, namely the overarching role of the environment (built, attitudinal, and policy) as it serves as a barrier or facilitator for people with disabilities to participate fully in society. Thus, "a person's functioning and disability is conceived as the dynamic interaction between health conditions and contextual factors" (p. 8). In addition, disability is interpreted within the context of the family's cultural and ethnic beliefs and traditions.

Caution must be used in the interpretation related to a particular individual, family, or cultural/ethnic group. The nuances of language and cultural meaning of disability are further complicated by translations that do not capture subtleties in meaning. Contrasting perspectives between groups may depend on whether an individual or family adheres to traditions and cultures of their origin, or whether the individual or family has become acculturated or assimilated into mainstream American culture. The primary language used by the individual or family may contribute to their identity. The particular circumstances of geographic isolation from others of the same ethnic/racial background may play a role in cultural identity. An American family of Chinese descent living in a Midwestern community insulated from other Asian families may live in quite a different milieu from a similar Chinese American family living in southern California in an enclave such as Monterey Park.

## Caregiving and Race/Ethnicity

A review of current government policies related to caregiving and disability suggests the lack of integrated national policy, and it implies that the responsibility for caregiving falls to the family. Family caregiving occurs because there are few or no other options. The burden falls especially hard on families from ethnic/cultural minority groups because they are not aware of or inclined to use the few available resources, or because of poverty, they cannot afford paid help. The cornerstone of current federal disability policy, the New Freedom Initiative, focuses on choice, independence, and integration in the community for persons with disabilities. A recent update on the New Freedom Initiative confirms that the "vast majority of direct care (about 64%) is provided by families, friends, and neighbors" (U.S. Department of Health and Human Services 2002, p. 24).

The NAC-AARP (1997) studies note that caregiving varies considerably by ethnicity or race. While the NAC-AARP (1997) studies may have "disfavored the Hispanic and Asian/Pacific Islander populations" (John 1999, p. 3) since they were conducted only in English and by telephone, those studies illustrate the current knowledge related to race/ethnicity and caregiving for persons with disabilities. The 2004 NAC-AARP study attempted to use Spanish, but the Spanish option was ultimately abandoned before the completion of the study. The National Center for Health Statistics (2003) indicates that Hispanic persons and Black non-Hispanic persons are more likely to need help with personal care from others than White non-Hispanic persons. Navaie-Waliser et al. (2001) reported that Black caregivers were more likely to have unmet needs than White caregivers.

While culture may dictate "how to be healthy, how to behave when ill, how to care, and how to cure" (Pask 2000, p. 67), there is "pressing need for cross cultural research on caregiving" (Aranda and Knight 1997, p. 352) to include ethnic and cultural differences in terms of illness, appraisal of stressors, and use of specific coping behaviors. Young and Kahana (1995) described a conceptual model of race, caregiving context, and outcomes having the potential for informing issues of ethnicity, race, and caregiving. While the significance of culture to the caregiving process seems logical, the historical response of human service programs has been to assume that American culture is homogeneous, often synonymous with White values and beliefs. Consumers were expected to adjust to programs offerings rather than programs being sufficiently flexible to respond to specific consumer needs (Dunlop et al. 2001). As a result, little empirical knowledge is available about how to tailor caregiving for persons with differing disabilities, cultures, and race/ethnicities.

## *Culture Defined*

Culture is defined as the sum total of the values, beliefs, rules, and practices of a group including commonly used customs, communication systems, and artifacts produced or used by the group (Rosenthal 1986; Valle 1998; Sue and Sue 2002). Culture refers to "the shared, and largely learned, attributes of a group of people" (U.S. Department of Health and Human Services 2001, p. 9). Moreover, "People who are placed, either by census categories or through self-identification into the same racial or ethnic group are often assumed to share the same culture. This assumption is an over generalization because not all members in a given category will share the same culture" (U.S. Department of Health and Human Services 2001, p. 9). Culture is not static but a changing and evolving process. The Surgeon General noted:

> Immigrants from different parts of the world arrive in the U.S. with their own culture but gradually begin to adapt. The term 'acculturation' refers to the socialization process by which minority groups gradually learn and adopt selective elements of the dominant culture. Yet that dominant culture is itself transformed by its interaction with minority groups. And to make matters more complex, the immigrant group may form its own culture, distinct from both its country of origin and the dominant culture. The Chinatowns of major cities in the United States often exemplify the blending of Chinese traditions and an American context. (p. 9)

Culture filters out elements that make an impact.

## Race and Ethnicity Defined

Ethnicity has been defined as "a group's shared sense of peoplehood based on a distinctive social and cultural heritage passed from generation to generation" (Gordon 1964) and involves a connotation of belonging to a specific cultural group or active expression of culture (Rosenthal 1986; Valle 1998). Ethnicity involves a sense of identity or belonging by individuals who may have the commonalities of a particular culture.

Race and ethnicity are often used interchangeably and will be in this chapter. The major groups found in the United States Census (2000) are (1) African Americans, (2) Hispanic Americans, (3) Asian Americans, and (4) Native Americans or American Indians. While each of these groups shares some characteristics and concerns, they also differ, sometimes greatly. The abbreviated summary below provides a glimpse into these ethnic populations.

## African Americans

African Americans currently make up approximately 12% of the US population or approximately 34 million people. African Americans have been subjected to a history of slavery, exploitation, and discrimination with the majority of today's African American population having ancestors who were slaves. The African American population has become increasingly diverse with immigration from Africa and the Caribbean. African Americans have demonstrated a resiliency and cultural/social ties that have enabled their survival. More than 68% of African American elderly are poor with limited health care (U.S. Department of Health and Human Service 2002; retrieved from Barressi and Stull 1993, p. 75; U.S. Department of Health and Human Services 2001). The Surgeon General's Report (U.S. Department of Health and Human Services 2001) noted that African Americans bear a disproportionate burden of health problems with diabetes occurring more than three times that of Whites and heart disease higher by 40%. African Americans are 1.5 times less likely to have health insurance than White Americans (Brown et al. 2000).

## Hispanic Americans

Hispanic Americans are the largest ethnic/racial group in the United States having surpassed the number of African Americans (U.S. Census 2000). The primary tie between Hispanic Americans is generally assumed to be the Spanish language and associated culture. However, there is much heterogeneity among Hispanic Americans that is often overlooked. Mexican Americans are quite different than Cuban Americans in terms of their immigration and political beliefs and social status within American society. Hispanic Americans overwhelmingly assert that each Hispanic country has its own culture and traditions (Pew Hispanic Center 2000). Hispanic Americans, similar to African Americans, have higher rates of health disorders than White Americans. For example, Hispanic Americans are twice as likely to die from diabetes as White Americans and have higher prevalence of high blood pressure and obesity (U.S. Department of Health and Human Services 2001). Overall, Hispanics have been found to be the most disadvantaged with regard to access to health insurance and health care (Brown et al. 2000). In particular, Hispanic Americans are often ignored in social programming because of the large numbers who are not U.S. citizens. The CDC (2005) estimates that Hispanics were more likely to need help with care related to chronic conditions than other population groups.

## Asian Americans

Asian Americans represent the fastest growing ethnic/racial group in the U.S. accounting for some 4% of the total US population. A large majority (64.5%) of Asian Americans were born abroad, more than any other group. Asian Americans come from more than 20 countries representing more than 60 different ethnicities (Joo and Price 2002). Different immigration patterns as well as languages are particularly important issues for the Asian population. And, while reports often suggest that Asian American health status to be on par with or better than White Americans, "an overall assessment of the AA/PI ethnic category leads to simple but misleading conclusions" (U.S. Department of Health and Human Services 2001). For example, Vietnamese women are five times more likely to have cervical cancer than White women. Other Asian groups experience differential access to health insurance and care. Over one-third of Korean Americans are not covered by health insurance (Brown et al. 2000).

## *American Indians and Alaskan Natives*

American Indians and Alaskan Natives are the indigenous population in the United States having settled in North America long before Europeans arrived. They comprise 1.5% of the US population or a little more than 4 million people. The U.S. government has a specific trust responsibility for the health care needs of American Indians and Alaskan Natives. The historical interference of the federal government with American Indians has changed educational and developmental profiles and has resulted in stressful living environments and consequent negative health effects (U.S. Department of Health and Human Services 2002). Health status indicators for American Indians are often lacking, though the Surgeon General's report (U.S. Department of Health and Human Services 2001) suggests a "constellation of problems similar to that of rural communities and includes serious mental illness, alcohol and substance abuse, alcohol and substance dependence, and suicidal ideation" (p. 83).

## *Diversity Within Groups*

Each of the populations described has a cultural history and tradition that is unique. There is sometimes a tendency to describe each of these groups as homogeneous; however, variability within each group may actually be greater than that between ethnic/cultural groups. Recognizing this distinction is essential to fully understand individuals and families, and consequently their behavior. For example, the category Asian Americans is made up of groups with very different languages, history, culture, and traditions as well as immigration patterns. Some Asian Americans come from countries that have traditionally been in conflict with each other.

Hispanic Americans come from Mexico, Puerto Rico, Central America, and South America. American Indians include more than 500 U.S. recognized tribal entities, many that have their own language and traditions. African Americans, though often seen as homogenous by others, include new immigrants from Africa, the Caribbean, and South America. African Americans also differ by religious orientation. NCHS

(National Center for Health Statistics) (2003) data show that Puerto Rican Americans have poorer health and greater activity limitations than other Hispanics. Recent refugee immigrants from Cambodia are much different in their educational and health status than fourth generation Japanese Americans. Describing the various ethnic/cultural populations as homogeneous limits the potential for designing and implementing programs that are effective.

## Contrasting Perspectives

At the risk of over-generalizing, there are some broad differences inherent to all of these ethnic/racial groups in contrast to the more western European based "American values." These differences are often crucial for deciphering and describing cultural/ethnic groups and ultimately being able to provide supports needed to enhance caregiving. The reader may note the hesitation to use the term "minority" in describing the different populations because projections of America's future demography strongly suggest no group will be "majority" for much longer.

Often available data about these ethnic/cultural groups have often been presented only in comparison to the majority population with the implicit notion that "minorities" need to meet the "majority" standard (Stanford and Yee 1991). This perspective suggests that there are preconceived expectations for behaviors, and these perspectives may not allow for differences to be appreciated as differences and nothing more.

With the preceding caution noted, a major contrast that these groups seem to have in common is the more collectivistic orientation as opposed to the more individualistic orientation of White American families (Laungani and Palmer 2002). The social structure and decision-making perspective of a collectivistic orientation goes beyond the individual. In contrast to the perspective of whether an individual makes and benefits from a decision, the collectivistic perspective considers how any decision affects the family, including those beyond the immediate family members. While difficult for an individual to understand from a western approach, this type of decision-making is often taken for granted in Asian and Hispanic cultures. Thus, individuals rely upon the extended family in the decision-making process. While substantially different from the more individualistic view of American society, there needs to be a tempered appreciation of the notion of importance of the extended family so that an idealized or romanticized perspective of ethnic families does not dominate (Rosenthal 1986; Aranda and Knight 1997).

A second major difference between ethnic/racial populations and more typical western orientation is that ethnic/racial groups generally approach life with a more fatalistic viewpoint. Fatalism should be viewed as a continuum and not an absolute. The general American perspective is to control the environment rather than merely accepting it. This is perhaps typified by the medical approach of western medicine to cure rather than to allow time for healing from a disease. This perspective treats disability in a similar manner. The focus is on treating illness "as an episodic, intrapersonal deviation" that is "person-centered, temporally bounded and discontinuous" (Landrine and Klonoff 1992, p. 267). African Americans or Hispanic Americans are more likely to perceive disabling conditions as a natural part of life. Landrine and Klonoff (1992) characterize the perspective of many ethnic cultural groups to treatment of disease "as a long term, informal, highly personal and cooperative process" (p. 268). While little empirical evidence is available in the literature regarding disabling conditions, it is perhaps not unreasonable to extrapolate similarities that may exist. In fact, some Hispanic families see having a child with a disability as something of an honor that has been bestowed on them because they inherently may have the strength to handle such a child. This does not mean that there may be negative aspects related to disability within the family. There may be feelings of guilt that disability results from a family member's behavior or previous life.

A third notion that differs significantly from more mainstream America is particularly relevant to caregiving. The issue of independence is often seen as the primary objective of the rehabilitation process. American culture, following the notion of individualism, places great value on an individual being independent and self-sufficient. Within the disability context, independent living has become a permanent part of the rehabilitation lexicon. Yet the notion of independent living can be confusing to persons from cultures that do not value independence as a primary objective or goal.

## *Socioeconomic Status*

Socioeconomic status further confounds much of what is known about ethnic groups and disabilities because many individuals and families in ethnic groups have lower incomes and fewer resources than White Americans. Indeed, some researchers have suggested that socioeconomic status is a better predictor of filial support than cultural background (Rosenthal 1986). Socioeconomic factors may override culture for purposes of predicting behavior related to caregiving because poverty rates are higher among minority cultures (U.S. Census Bureau 2000), lack of resources to purchase formal support can result in increased reliance upon the family. The relationship between socioeconomic status, disability, and impact on ethnicity and caregiving remains generally unknown.

Sorting out factors related to caregiving and socioeconomic status from other cultural variables requires substantial attention, but has yet to be addressed (Valle 1998; Young and Kahana 1995). Evaluating a person in terms of economic status to the exclusion of cultural dimensions detracts from understanding complex family dynamics (Valle 1998). Individuals who cannot afford external resources may be forced to provide care not because of a cultural belief but because of economic necessity. Whether caregiving is predicated on ethnicity/culture or on socioeconomic status is currently unknown (Tennstedt and Chang 1998). Tennstedt and Chang (1998) investigated differences in need for and receipt of informal care among African Americans, Puerto Ricans, and non-Hispanic Whites in the northeastern U.S. Their study suggests that ethnicity played an important role in explaining an older person's need for and receipt of long term care assistance and that socioeconomic status did not seem to play as important a role.

## Caregiving

Caregiving has received increasing attention during the last few years in the United States as the costs of health and medical services increase. Crews and Talley define caregiving in the introductory chapter to this volume. The focus of this section is on caregiving and disability within the context of racial/ethnic groups, taking into account socioeconomic status.

Armstrong (2001) reporting on a National Institute of Nursing Research session indicated a number of factors that lead to informal care. Chronic illnesses affect about 100 million people in the U.S. and include elderly persons with two or more chronic illnesses that limit function. An estimated 4.1 million persons aged 21–64 need personal assistance; 6.8 million persons aged 65 and older have mobility and self-care limitations. In addition, an estimated 30 million persons discharged from hospitals need postacute care assistance each year (Armstrong 2001).

Persons with chronic disease with poor health and low incomes are least likely to report having adequate social support from family and friends (Bethell and Lansky 2001). Hispanics and Asian Americans with chronic illness are less likely to receive care to manage their conditions (Collins et al. 2002). These studies suggest ethnic or cultural groups often have more complex health needs and caregiving requirements compared to Whites.

Wood and Wan (1993) categorize caregiving as instrumental and expressive. Instrumental caregiving involves assistance with personal care functions and activities of daily living; whereas, expressive caregiving involves sharing in social activities, emotional support, and just "being there" (Wood and Wan 1993). Instrumental and expressive caregiving are played out within a sociocultural context tempered by socioeconomic status.

## Caregiving and Culture

Since caregiving within cultural groups has not been the subject of many empirical studies, little data are available. What is known suggests culture has a significant impact on the caregiving roles. These roles may be complex and convoluted, and subject to a host of variables. Cultural attributes of any particular group are dynamic and evolving. For example, what is passed down from generation to generation may reflect the broader majority culture and may be based on interpretations of culture that become for individual a tradition that is passed down and thus quite idiosyncratic. Immigrant families struggling with day-to-day survival may have limited exposure to the culture of their country of origin. Therefore, the practice of using respite services may be interpreted as shirking responsibility.

## *Differences Between Groups*

The prevalence of caregiving among different ethnic populations related to disability is not well investigated. Many surveys target specific groups, such as persons aged 50 and older who may need care or persons who may have Alzheimer's. Some researchers indicate the field of caregiving to be "plagued by a limited number of longitudinal studies" (Hooyman and Gonyea 1995, p. 155). Kommenick (2002), in reviewing 300 articles on informal caregiving, concluded that despite increasing studies across ethnic groups, the variables for comparative analysis were not clearly specified. Most of the available data relate to specific groups and not persons with disabilities.

The NAC-AARP survey (1997) found the prevalence of caregiving for the elderly to be higher among Asian (31.7%) and Black (29.4%) households than among Hispanic (26.8%) or White (24%) households. Analysis of the AARP survey data (1997) by Ory et al. (1999) suggested that when dementia is the disabling condition, Blacks were more likely and Asians were less likely to care for elders. The particular disabling condition drives the decision to provide care, although available data are incomplete. Overall, there is generally higher prevalence of disability within ethnic populations, and therefore, one would expect a greater need for caregiving (NCD 1993; Smart and Smart 1997). Documented health disparities also add to the higher risk for disability for ethnic groups.

Ethnic groups vary in their perception of the burden of caregiving. These perceptions may be dictated by a sense of belonging within their own communities. Black and Hispanic caregivers report less sense of seclusion than White caregivers (Cox et al. 1993). Hispanics depend more on formal services for assistance than Blacks (Cox et al. 1993). Race may have both positive and negative influences on how caregiving is perceived (Young and Kahana 1995).

Other surveys on ethnicity and persons with mental illness who live at home also suggest differences associated with ethnicity. For example, three-quarters of Hispanic American persons with mental illness live at home with their families and 60% of African American families in contrast to one-third of European American families (Lefley 1996). Lefley further indicated that Hispanic and Asian families were more likely to keep an individual with mental illness at home than other groups. African American elderly are more likely to live in an extended family household than Whites (Angel and Tienda 1982). Cantor reported higher support among Hispanics than either Whites or African Americans. Lubben and Becerra (1987) found that Hispanics were more likely to help elderly family members and that the extended family remains "one of the most structural components of Hispanic culture."

Kosloski et al. (1999), in a review of the literature on the role of cultural factors in caregiving, indicated that caregivers from ethnic cultural groups "cannot be expected to view their caregiving responsibilities in the same way because cultural and background differences are likely to moderate perceptions of need" (p. 241). Ethnicity and culture, thus, can even moderate whether caregiving is needed or required. Young and Kahana (1995) in a study on disability and caregiving pointed out the complexity of the interactions between culture and caregiving. Ethnic differences also influence expectations of assistance as well as perception of whether caregiving is perceived as strain or burden (Mui et al. 1998). Among some American Indian groups, persons who vary either physically or intellectually are afforded "slightly greater leeway in their behavior because with the Indian culture is recognition that having disabilities is beyond an individual or family's control" (Pengra and Godfrey 2001). They further note that "some physical variations may lead to the need for assistance from others. However, the need for assistance does not lead to a handicap, that is, to the person being marginalized or disempowered, because these physical variations are not within the control of the individual. They just 'are' and must therefore, be dealt with" (p. 6). These beliefs may lead to a tendency to keep someone at home without benefit of formal and other needed services (Aranda and Knight 1997). This perspective is perhaps not unlike ethnic or cultural groups where a more fatalistic acceptance of illness occurs as the norm. Davis et al. (1993) described the role that perceived cause of illness play in caregiving, citing a 74-year-old female who said, "I can put up with the pain because arthritis runs in the family and all of us get it when we reach our fifties" (p. 78). The individual chose to live without assistance knowing that her situation was considered to be "normal" and expected.

Viewing disability as the result of punishment or sanction for personal behavior is common to many ethnic populations (Landrine and Klonoff 1992). While these beliefs are not unique to ethnic cultural populations (Landrine and Klonoff), the belief that disability results from the behavior of an individual or family member may dictate family response. Guilt associated with concepts of sanctions for misbehavior may reinforce caregiving as an obligation or perhaps atonement for a transgression.

Obligation is often found in Asian American families as a motivating force and especially with the Chinese where there is the expectation that one's children will be the source of long term care for the elderly. Yu et al. (1993) suggest that cultural belief goes beyond issues of affordability or economics to include "what should be even when reality ... cannot be fulfilled" (p. 96). Changes brought about through acculturation may further mitigate expectations.

Perception of whether caregiving is a burden may also vary as a function of race and ethnicity. Marks (1995) found that in the greater New Orleans area that African-American caregivers indicated the lowest level of perceived burden and White caregivers indicated the highest level. At the same time, Marks (1995) and Mui et al. (1998) found that cognitive status of the care recipient is not significantly associated with perception of burden. Among the American Indian, Pengra and Godfrey (2001) noted that persons who have disabilities often receive assistance as part of a family's normal routine. "Kinship responsibilities are an indivisible and un-defined force" (p. 6) and as such are not considered to be "help" (Pengra and Godfrey). Assistance or care is not perceived as burdensome for the caregiver. Further, Pengra and Godfrey suggest that the assistance provided by family members does not make the recipient feel powerless or pitied as the recipient is always seen as loved and part of the family.

Understanding perception of disabling conditions as well as cultural and/or traditional roles of family and family members is critical to understand the caregiving process within ethnic groups. A 2001 AARP survey of multicultural boomers highlighted additional differences in ethnic/racial groups (AARP 2001). For example, the survey reported that Hispanic boomers have a heavier caregiving role given the combination of high expectations of their culture. Hispanic Americans also expended more effort to care for their family members than some other groups. Asian American boomers were the most apt to confess guilt for not doing more caregiving and also most likely to indicate that they experience stress as result of caring for family members. African Americans, more than any other group, include siblings as part of their definition of family. African American reliance on informal caregiving may stem from the many years in which they were isolated from mainstream health care (Davis et al. 1993), and they were required to rely on internal resources.

## Future Needs/Directions

Caregiving for persons with disabilities in ethnic populations in many respects is not that different from mainstream groups with similar concerns. At the same time, a more tailored approach to caregiving, one that is flexible and open to individual and cultural variations will undoubtedly be more effective and acceptable to minority populations. Racial/ethnic groups have much to teach others about ways to improve caregiving, regardless of ethnicity. The ability of diverse groups to garner support and survive often against tremendous odds suggests strengths that need to be better understood and utilized.

There has been a general lack of attention in practice, research, and policy related to caregiving among ethnic and cultural populations and disability. Given the complexity of what constitutes disability, who needs care, and the cultural and socioeconomic context, the gaps of knowledge are understandable. Yet, these gaps need to be understood given the importance and projected increases in caregiving in American society.

Caregiving must be given the same priority that other human service programs have in adopting a culturally competent model. Caregiving practice must be viewed from a similar perspective. Families are primarily responsible for the care of their family members who have disabilities. Despite emphasis and growing awareness of disability and caregiving, little attention has been focused on the fastest growing segments of American society—African Americans, Hispanic Americans, Asian Americans, and the American Indians.

### *Practice*

The practice of caregiving within ethnic/racial populations shares the same needs as any population providing care. However, because persons from ethnic/racial groups are more likely to have fewer resources, those who design and implement support programs need to understand the dynamics of diverse families. Moreover, the distinction between socioeconomic status and culture must be better understood. The motivations of ethnic families for providing care, in the context of their support systems, may be quite different from those found in more White families. Ethnic/racial groups may perceive the process of caregiving in ways that may not seem logical to observers outside of those groups. Service providers seeking to engage families with disabilities from diverse populations should appreciate these differing perspectives.

In addition, there is need to recognize and assess what has been called the acculturation continuum. Programs need to understand where any particular individual or family stands with regard to their acceptance and adoption of "American" values. Valle (1998) suggested that providers learn to assess how an individual or family regards their acculturation into American society. Ethnic groups continue to evolve following their initial migration. Where a family is on the acculturation continuum may have implications for their caregiving behavior. Ethnic groups exist within a host society that influences their values and interactions. There may be a strong countervailing force to preserve authentic primary cultural group orientations affecting the caregiving process. An awareness and understanding of the multidimensionality of acculturation (Aranda and Knight 1997) assists these ethnic populations utilize community supports to enhance their ability to provide care to persons with disabilities. Pinquart and Sorensen's (2005) meta-analysis of 116 studies suggested that all ethnic minority caregivers had worse physical health compared to Whites further suggesting that intervention needs varied from one group to another.

## *Education/Training*

Training and education models that better fit a variety of learning styles within varying cultures need to be developed. Perceptions of burden and guilt, patterns of stress and its manifestations, and how services are accepted and adopted are essential for understanding the dimensional experiences of diverse populations. For training and education to have impact on nontraditional participants requires new and creative strategies (Dunlop et al. 2001). Ethnic/cultural populations, especially those who struggle to survive on minimal resources, may not have the energy or time to participate in conventional programs. The demands of employment and day-to-day tasks may require different incentives to free up the time and energy to understand the need for training.

## *Research*

There has not been a systematic study of caregiving for persons with disabilities within the context of ethnic/cultural populations. Knowledge is incomplete, perhaps, because research has focused upon only one family member, addresses only negative aspects of caregiving, and lacked longitudinal characteristics (Hooyman and Gonyea

1995). Much of the literature has addressed mental health service provision and caregiving related to older individuals.

There is a need to better understand the dynamics of culture on families and caregiving process, including acculturation/generational changes, perceptions of disability, and role of the family in caregiving. Stanford and Yee (1991), though speaking primarily of the elderly, assert that researchers should not ignore the need for basic research as well as exploratory and descriptive studies. A National Institute on Nursing Research panel (Armstrong 2001) pointed out the need for research on caregiving and ethnic groups with emphasis on adequate, affordable, accessible, and culturally sensitive programs.

## *Policy*

It has been said that much of current policy within human service arena was developed on an Anglo male model (Stanford and Yee 1991) and what policies there are regarding caregiving have been predicated on a similar paradigm. In spite of the general lack of research and models related to caregiving for persons with disabilities within ethnic/cultural groups, inclusive policies and programs need to be addressed. Policy development needs to take into account differences of family structure, family tradition, and family decision-making processes.

Policies that may work for White families fully acculturated into American society may not work for families who are recent immigrants, who do not speak English as their first language, who adhere to traditions of their country of origin, and who are still in survival mode. For example, payment to family caregivers to care for their own may have very different meaning for various ethnic groups than similar payments to a White family. Very little research informs these practices. Self-help is often the model of support but very little is known about the use of self-help with populations other than those who are White (Lefley 1996). Seeking help to find resources and respite is behavior typical of western educated populations but is not a behavior necessarily found among many ethnic populations. The Family Leave Act was passed by Congress in part to allow families to care for family members with disabilities; families in the lower socioeconomic status from minority populations may not be able to afford to take time off even if allowed by employers. There is a need for legislative policy that ensures benefit to all segments of American society to provide care for their family members who have disabilities.

Because of the growing population of persons who have disabilities, caregiving needs will increase among families of diverse racial/ethnic backgrounds, and simultaneously there will be a need for "new solutions that affect the social structure and function of society" (Hooeyman and Gonyea 1995, p. 103). They noted that the underlying conflicting values of individualism, familism, and societal good (p. 103) will continue to need attention along with ways to better operationalize behaviors reflecting these values. Gelfand and Yee (1991) emphasized the importance of language and acculturation in service provision for the elderly. Similar attention is needed for ethnic/racial groups and caregiving for persons with disabilities. Acknowledgement of the role of culture and ethnicity in caregiving can open the possibility of informing increased knowledge and competence in understanding cultural and ethnic perceptions that allow professionals and systems to better serve these emerging populations. Moreover, this knowledge and competence has much to inform the general population as more is learned about the strength, resilience, and traditions of cultural minorities.

## References

AARP. (2001). *In the middle: A report on multicultural boomers coping with family and aging issues. A national survey*. http://www.aarp.org/research/housing-mobility/caregiving/aresearch-import-789-D17446.html. Accessed 20 Oct 2011.
Angel, R., & Tienda, M. (1982). Determinants of extended household structure: Cultural pattern or economic model? *American Journal of Sociology, 87*, 1360–1383.
Aranda, M. P., & Knight, B. G. (1997). The influence of ethnicity and culture on the caregiver stress and coping process: A sociocultural review and analysis. *Gerontologist, 37*(3), 342–354.
Armstrong, N. (2001). *Research in informal caregiving: State of the science workgroup meeting*, it National Institute of Nursing Research. http://ninr.hih.gov/ninr/research/dea/workgroup_chronic_conditions.html. Accessed 26 May 2008.
Barressi, C. M., & Stull, D. E. (1993). *Ethnic elderly and long-term care*. New York: Springer.
Bethell, C., & Lansky, D. (2001). *A portrait of the chronically ill in America 2001*. Princeton: Robert Wood Johnson.
Brown, E. R., Ojeda, V. D., Wyn, R., & Levan, R. (2000). *Racial and ethnic disparities in access to health insurance and health care*. Los Angeles: UCLA Center for Health Policy Research and Henry J. Kaiser Family Foundation.
Centers for Disease Control and Prevention. (2005). www.cdc/gov/omhd/po.
Collins, K. S., Hughes, D. L., Doty, M. M., Ives, B. L., Edwards, J. N., & Tenney, K. (2002). *Diverse communities, common concerns: assessing health care quality for minority Americans*. New York: Commonwealth Fund.
Cox, C., Monk, A., Barresi, C. M., & Stull, D. E. (Eds.). (1993). *Black and Hispanic caregivers of dementia victims in ethnic elderly and long term care*. New York: Springer.
Davis, L. H., McGadney, B. F., Barrasi, C. M., & Stull, D. E. (Eds.). (1993). *Self-care practices of black elders in ethnic elderly and long term care*. New York: Springer.
Dunlop, B. D., Seff, L. R., & Moreno C. (2001). *Assessment of service needs among caregivers*. Miami: Florida International University.
Family Caregiving Alliance. (2008). *Selected caregiver statistics*. http://www.caregiver.org/caregiver/jsp/content_node.jsp?nodeid=439. Accessed 21 Oct 2011.
Feinberg, L. F., Gray, L., & Kelly, K. A. (2002). *Family caregiving as a grantmaking area: Current focus and future trends*. San Francisco: Family Caregiver Alliance.
Gelfand, D., & Yee, B. Y. K. (1991). Influence of immigration, migration and acculturation on the fabric of aging in America. *Generations, 15*(40), 7–10.
Gordon, M. (1964). *Assimilation in American life*. New York: Oxford University Press.
Hooyman, N. R., & Gonyea, J. (1995). *Feminist perspectives on family care*. Thousand Oaks: Sage.
John, R. (1999, October 11). *Testimony at field hearing of the U.S. Senate*. Presented at Special Committee on Aging, Monroe, LA.
Joo, E., & Price, C. (2002). *Asian American older adults* (SS-194-02). Columbus, OH. http://ohioline.osu.edu/ss-fact/0194.html. Accessed 20 Oct 2011.
Kommenick, P. (2002). *Poster presentation: An integrative analysis of informal caregiving research literature, variables and findings*. http://stti.confex.com/stti/sos13/techprogram/paper_11756.htm. Accessed 21 Oct 2011.

Kosloski, K., Montgomery, R. J., & Karner, T. X. (1999). Differences in the perceived need for assistive services by culturally diverse caregivers of persons with dementia. *Journal of Applied Gerontology, 18*(2), 239–256.

Landrine, H., & Klonoff, E. A. (1992) Culture and health-related schemas: A review and proposal for interdisciplinary integration. *Health Psychology, 11*(4), 267–276.

Laungani, P., & Palmer S. (Eds.). (2002). *Understanding mental illness across cultures in multicultural counseling*. London: Sage.

Lefley, H. P. (1996). *Family caregiving in mental illness*. Thousand Oaks: Sage.

Lubben, J. E., & Becerra, R. M. (1987). Social support among Black, Mexican, and Chinese elderly. In D. E. Gelfand & C. Barressi (Eds.), *Ethnic dimensions of aging* (pp. 130–144). New York: Springer.

Marks, R. (1995). *Various aspects of caregiving with an aged population in the greater New Orleans area*. New Orleans: Tulane Center for Aging. http://www.tulane.edu/~aging/caremark.html.

Mui, A. C., Choi, N. G., & Monk, A. (1998). *Long-term care and ethnicity*. Westport: Auburn House.

National Alliance for Caregiving (NAC) and American Association for Retired Persons (AARP). (1997). *Family caregiving in the U.S.: Findings from a national survey*. Bethesda: Author.

National Center for Health Statistics. (2003). http://www.cdc.gov/nchs/fastats/disable.htm and http://www.cdc.gov/nchs/about/major/nhis/released200212/figure12_3.htm. Accessed 22 Oct 2011.

National Council on Disability. (1993). *Meeting the unique needs of minorities with disabilities: A report to Congress*. Washington, DC: Author.

Navaie-Waliser, M., Feldman, P., Gould, D., Levine, D., Kuerbis, A. N., & Donelan, K. (2001). The experiences and challenges of informal caregiving: Common themes and differences among Whites, Blacks and Hispanics. *Gerontologist, 4*, 733–741.

Ory, M. G., Hoffman, R. R., Yee, J., Tennstedt S., & Schultz, R. (1999). Prevalence and impact of caregiving: a detailed comparison. *Gerontologist, 39*(2), 177–185.

Pask, E. G. (2000). Culture: caring and curing in the changing health scene. In J. D. Morgan (Ed.). *Meeting the needs of our clients creatively: impact of art and culture on caregiving* (pp. 67–76). Amityville: Baywood.

Pengra, L. M., & Godfrey, J. G. (2001). Different boundaries, different barriers: disability studies and Lakota Culture. *Disability Studies Quarterly, 21*(3), 36–53.

Pew Hispanic Center. (2000). *2002 National Survey of Latinos*. Washington, DC: Author.

Pfizer. (1997). *The Pfizer Journal, 1*(3), 1–35. New York: Author.

Pinquart, M., & Sorensen, S. (2005). Ethnic differences in stressors, resources and psychological outcomes of family caregiving: A meta-analysis. *Gerontologist, 45*, 90–106.

Rosenthal, C. J. (1986). Family supports in later life: Does ethnicity makes a difference? *Gerontologist, 26*(1), 19–24.

Smart, J., & Smart, D. W. (1997). The racial/ethnic demography of disability. *Journal of Rehabilitation, 63*(4), 9–15.

Stanford, E. P., & Yee, D. (1991). Gerontology and the relevance of diversity. *Generations, 15*(4), 11–14.

Sue, D. W., & Sue, D. (2002). *Counseling the culturally diverse* (4th ed.). New York: Wiley.

Tennstedt, S., & Chang, B. (1998). The relative contribution of ethnicity versus socioeconomic status in explaining differences in disability and receipt of informal care. *Gerontologist, 53B*(2), 561–570.

U.S. Census Bureau. (2000). *Population by race and Hispanic or Latino origin, for all ages and for 18 years and over, for the United States: 2000*. http://www.census.gov/population/cen2000/phc-t1/tab01.pdf. Accessed 20 Jan 2012.

U.S. Department of Health and Human Services. (2001). *Mental health: Culture, race, and ethnicity. A supplement to mental Health: A report of the surgeon general*. Rockville: Author.

U.S. Department of Health and Human Services. (2002). *Delivering on the promise*. http://www.hhs.gov/newfreedom/final/hhsappenda.html.

Valle, R. (1998). *Caregiving across cultures*. New York: Taylor and Francis.
Wood, J. B., & Wan, T. T. H. (1993). Ethnicity and minority issues in family caregiving to rural black elders. In C. Barresi & D. Stull (Eds.), *Ethnic elderly and long term care* (pp. 39–56). New York: Springer.
World Health Organization. (2001). *International classification of functioning, disability, and health*. http://www.who.int/classifications/icf/en/.
Young, R. F., & Kahana, E. (1995). The context of caregiving and well-being outcomes among African and Caucasian Americans. *Gerontologist, 35*(2), 225–232.
Yu, E. S., Kim, H., Liu, W. T., & Wong, S. (1993). Functional abilities of Chinese and Korean elders in congregate housing. In C. M. Barresi & D. E. Stull (Eds.), *Ethnic elderly and long term care* (pp. 87–100). New York: Springer.

# Chapter 8
# Faith and Spirituality: Supporting Caregivers of Individuals with Disabilities

**William Gaventa**

The relationship between caregiving, supports for caregivers, spirituality, and faith/faith communities is both powerful and complex. The power has been evident in a simple question one can ask family caregivers of persons with disabilities: "Would you be willing to share your church (synagogue, temple, etc.) story?" or "Would you be willing to describe how your faith or spirituality has been impacted by your experience?"

The answers are rarely lukewarm or neutral. Families and other caregivers of individuals with disabilities will share, on the one hand, how important their faith or faith community has been to them or how this experience has transformed their understanding of themselves and life. Conversely, on the other, they will talk about the ways that their faith, hope, and/or caregiving role has been negatively impacted by the lack of response, or a hurtful response, from their faith communities or tradition. As a powerful tool, spirituality can be tapped for good, for ill, or as professional caregivers have sometimes chosen to do, avoided altogether.

For example, a Catholic mother once answered that question by telling about the priest's refusal to allow her disabled son to receive first communion, "When the church rejected my son, they rejected me." The pain and frustration she was expressing was not just that her faith community and cultural tradition were rejecting her son, but also her whole family. The theological dimension of this experience only deepened the pain. In this mother's story, the response of the priest was also interpreted as the response of the church and of God. That experience was later reversed, with the help of professional caregivers in a public service system that advocated and collaborated with the local diocese. When her son received first communion at the hands of the bishop of the diocese, and continued to be included in religious services and activities, the family experienced both a sense of reconciliation with their spiritual and cultural tradition and an ongoing sense of affirmation, acceptance, and support.

---

W. Gaventa (✉)
The Boggs Center, P.O. Box 2688, New Brunswick, NJ 08903-2688, USA
e-mail: bill.gaventa@umdnj.edu

Robert Wood Johnson Medical School, UMDNJ, New Brunswick, NJ, USA

Three roles are crucial in that story: (1) the family, and their willingness to tell their story and advocate for their son, (2) the professional caregiving system which supported their son and the professionals who collaborated with the faith community, and (3) the clergy and faith community, who responded in ways that reopened a whole dimension of support and participation for the young man and his family. All of those perspectives impact the role that faith and spirituality can have, both for good and for harm, in supporting caregivers of individuals with disabilities.

## Disability, Spirituality, and Families

The experience of giving birth to a child with a disability or the experience of acquiring a disability by a family member at some point in their lives through either accident, illness, or aging, can raise profound spiritual questions and issues for parents, family members, and/or the individuals themselves (Bolduc 1999, 2001; Gaventa 1997; Reynolds 2008; Walsh et al. 2008). The questions can involve ones of identity (Who am I as parent? Who is this child that was unexpected? Who will we be?), responsibility and purpose (Why did this happen? What's the reason? Why this child? Why me?), and community (Who will support us? How will this impact our family's life?).

A number of researchers have indicated the power of spirituality and religion in the lives of families with members with disabilities (Haworth et al. 1996; Miltiades and Pruchno 2002; Olson et al. 2002; Poston and Turnbull 2004; Rogers-Dulan 1998; Carter 2007; Gaventa 2008a). Some researchers have noted that families describe their faith and spirituality (practices such as prayer and belief) as a crucial source of support, but that their faith community was not that helpful (Skinner et al. 2001). Others have pointed to the importance of both spiritual beliefs (faith, prayer, and attribution of meaning) and religious participation (Poston and Turnbull 2004). Clergy have pointed to the ways that clergy and congregations have been and can be sources of support, through presence, counseling, advocacy on behalf of families and individuals with disabilities, and the mobilization of supports within a congregation as well as making sure individuals and families are included in ongoing congregational activities (Gaventa 1986, 1997; Webb Mitchell 1994). The power of spiritual and religious supports also comes from two other characteristics: (1) the capacity of congregations and faith communities to be sources both of "spiritual" and "natural" supports, i.e., a source of friendship, social supports, financial support, respite care, etc., as well as being a community of meaning and (2) the potential for congregations and faith to be a support over the life span of an individual and family (Bolduc 2001).

The potency of spiritual supports is not just evident in events like religious rites of passage such as first communion, baptism, bar and bat mitzvahs, and other celebrations of identity, growth, and community membership (Hornstein 1997). The symbolic and real power is even starker in questions of cause and purpose (Why did God do this?) and questions of support and healing (Can God heal? If so, why not now?) (Black 1996; Block 2002; Yong 2007; Reynolds 2008). When theological interpretations get misused, such as blaming a disability on the "sins of the parents," justifying exclusion on the basis of one scriptural text (e.g., the Leviticus passages that exclude a person with a disability from being a priest), or explaining the lack of healing by the inadequacy of a person or family's faith, then the power of religious supports is again evident in their misuse. It can lead to avoidance of people with disabilities and their families ("We don't have any here"), and, at times, outright discrimination, rejection, or abuse.

However, while it is important to acknowledge that congregations and religious traditions have a mixed history (as do many other community organizations!) in their response to people with disabilities and their families, that history also includes pioneering supports, such as role of Jean Vanier (Downey 1986) in founding the L'Arche communities (intentional spiritual communities with people with disabilities at their center), the role that some faith groups have taken in residential supports for people with disabilities, and the growing development of inclusive ministries and supports within congregation life as they have responded to families and individuals who have asked and advocated to be included in the typical, normal life of a given faith community and the way it supports everyone.

## The Interplay of Spirituality and Religion

The complexity also comes from the variety of ways spirituality and faith are understood and used, the great diversity of religious and cultural traditions that express and shape spirituality, faith, and caregiving, and the relationship between those issues for all parties involved, i.e., families, professional caregivers, people with disabilities themselves, clergy and congregations, and other sources of spiritual supports (Gaventa 2008b). Fortunately, the last decade has seen increasing amounts of research into the role of spirituality and spiritual supports in health and human services (Larson and Larson 1994; Matthews et al. 1993; Puchalski and Romer 2000). There is a growing consensus and body of knowledge about how spirituality and spiritual supports can be assessed and utilized in ways that address the expressed needs of individual families and caregivers, and also build bridges of understanding between "secular" and "spiritual" supports (Fitchett 1993; Gaylord 2002; Carter 2007).

All of those questions point to one dimension of a definition of spirituality: the human need to find meaning in our existence. The second dimension is that spirituality is the way we describe or name our experience of what is sacred and holy (Fitchett 1993). That two-fold definition both differentiates spirituality from religion and also points toward how one's spiritual life may be expressed through a specific religion, faith tradition, or community. Religion, while related to spirituality, is thus defined as a particular framework of beliefs, practices, and traditions that are used to define and practice a communal way of understanding the meaning and sacred dimensions of life. Spirituality can be expressed, learned, and practiced within a religious faith or community, but there are multiple other ways in which spirituality and spiritual practices can be expressed outside of a particular religion (Fitchett 1993; Gaventa 2009a).

For example, many support groups, advocacy groups, and self-advocacy organizations have often taken the place of a faith community as a source of meaning and spiritual support for individuals with disabilities and their families. Sometimes that involvement complements the supports found within a religious community or faith tradition; at others, families turn to those groups because of a lack of support in other circles, including congregations. It can also be because families feel safe and supported in a support group or advocacy organization. Families who are 24/7 caregivers often have little energy left when it comes to the simple logistics of participation in churches, synagogues, or mosques. When that lack of energy is compounded by feeling like they have to ask or fight for inclusion or support within their faith community, then religious faith and practice may lose its power. A support group that offers understanding, acceptance, hope, and united commitment to action becomes a ready alternative.

## Spiritual Supports and Other Supports

That mixed history and personal experience of individuals with disabilities, their families, and professional caregivers with religious caregivers and communities is just one of the reasons for a number of barriers that have impeded more effective collaboration between spiritual supports and other kinds of caregivers and supports. More than 2 decades ago, researcher Lou Heifitz compared the side by side experience of spiritual/religious supports and "secular/public" supports in the lives of families and individuals with disabilities to the phenomenon of "parallel play," i.e., the description given by researchers to the way children might play side by side in a room of toys but not with each other (Heifitz 1987). That parallel play, and lack of collaboration and partnership, has been shaped by a number of factors (Gaventa 2002):

(1) The question of responsibility? While many health and human services had their origin in faith communities and traditions, in the last century health and human services have increasingly been seen as the responsibility of the state and public as the government became the major funder of professionalized health, educational, and social services. The era of institutionalization also led to a perception that people with disabilities were the responsibility of the state or public systems rather than the religious community. A fundamental spiritual question of belonging, "Whose are we?" translates into a policy question of "Whose people are they?" (Gaventa 2009b).

(2) Other barriers to collaboration came from evolving understandings (or the lack thereof) between science and religion and between church and state. As scientific helping professions blossomed, questions arose about the role of personal faith in professional practice. That often came from mistrust between the perspectives of science and religion, but also from fears of abuse of religion through proselytizing by professionals, and the equation of spiritual beliefs with delusions and other symptoms in mental illness. Professional caregivers, such as nurses, social

workers, and doctors, were taught to separate their own values or spirituality from their professional practice, in order to be objective, fair, and unprejudiced. The political separation of church and state also led many professional caregivers and systems, funded by the government, to believe they could not address the role of faith and spirituality because it would be a violation of the separation of church and state. Thus, until recently, professional caregivers lacked the tools to assess or utilize the spiritual dimensions of coping or caregiving and the ways that caregivers could be supported by their spirituality or faith communities.
(3) Congregations and spiritual communities have often been excellent sources of support in an acute crisis, such as an illness, accident, or death, but sometimes not as helpful in providing sustained care over long periods of time (Gaventa and Berk 2001).

As the focus of researchers, practitioners, and advocates has shifted in the past decade to the support and strengthen the role of both "formal" and "informal" caregivers, there has been increased recognition of the importance of the spiritual dimensions of caregiving and the role generic community services (which has to include faith communities as major community resources). New models have emerged for partnership and collaboration between faith based caregiving and professional services (Carter 2007). With that shift has come the prospect of changed roles for professional caregivers in an era of person-centered planning, family-centered care, and community-based supports. Professional caregivers are challenged to develop and incorporate new roles in community building as facilitators of more effective natural supports (Gaventa 2001). Faith communities, at both national and local levels, have also developed a wide variety of resources and strategies to provide more inclusive supports to people with disabilities and their families. It is time to turn our attention to current practices, education, research, and policy.

## Current Trends in Faith Based Caregiving and Spiritual Supports with People with Disabilities and Their Families

### Trends in Practice

#### In Faith Communities

Congregations in many different religious traditions have gone through an evolution in their caregiving supports to families with disabled members over the past decades in ways that mirror some of the developments in public education and in adult residential programs. In broad strokes, the movement has been from little or no focus within a given congregation to the development of "special ministries" to more inclusive ministries and religious supports (Gaventa 1986). "Special ministries" often involved a special religious education program, the use of the church building for a program run by a religious or secular organization, or the development of faith based group homes or residential programs. Large residential institutions run by religious organizations have downsized like their public counterparts, and begun to develop and coordinate smaller residential programs in collaboration with community congregations. Rather than focusing solely on development of "specialized" and "segregated" ministries or programs within a congregation or religious network (e.g., a local Jewish Community Federation), more and more congregations are seeking ways to include children and adults with disabilities, and their families, in typical ongoing services and supports.

There are growing numbers of positive stories coming from families and individuals with disabilities about the response of their faith community and its support (Gaylord 2002; Poston and Turnbull 2004; Walsh et al. 2008; Carter 2007). Families seeking religious education experiences for their children with disabilities have encountered congregations that have set up inclusive classes with "buddy" supports and other strategies to help children be included with typical peers. Others have at least found religious educators saying, "We are not sure what to do, but we are willing to learn." Young people with disabilities are being included in important rites of transition in faith communities, such as bar and bat mitzvahs, first communion, confirmation, and baptisms (Hornstein 1997). The power of those coming of age rituals to build community inclusion is evident in the wonderful 2007 documentary, *Praying with Lior* (www.prayingwithlior.com). Respite care ministries and services, recreation and youth programs, assistance with transition into adulthood, and development of opportunities for young people and adults with disabilities to contribute to the life of the congregation are all emerging trends. The shift has been from ministries to people who are different and special to inclusive supports that build on communal models of welcoming and celebrating diversity, hospitality to the stranger, and ministry to the whole family.

Faith communities have also begun to see the similarity in supports needed for caregivers at whatever age or from whatever cause. That support has taken a variety of forms. One is a growing model of congregational health ministries, such as the parish nursing role, which explores and develops ways to support health and human service needs within congregational settings. The Mennonites have a model for congregational "circles of support," building on the potential natural networks and relationships within that setting (Preheim-Bartel and Neufeld 2011). It also begins to address the role that faith communities could play in answering the primary question faced by many caregivers, "Who will watch and care after I am gone?" Others are programs like respite nights or Saturdays, family retreats, or simply making sure that a caregiver can be relieved so they can participate in activities that refresh their spirit while someone else, either at the congregation or at home, takes responsibility for the caregiving. One way to frame the question theologically is that everyone has need of a "Sabbath," a time to refresh and renew, wherever and whenever it happens (Gaventa 1990).

Initiatives by local and regional faith communities have also been led and supported by a variety of faith based networks and resource offices within religious organizations focusing on ministries with people with disabilities and their families. Many are led by family members or people with disabilities. These include:

(1) Networks within religious groups, such as the National Catholic Partnership with Disabilities, the Presbyterian Disabilities Network within the Presbyterian Health, Education, and Welfare Association, a new national initiative within the Reform branch of Judaism, a trans Lutheran network, a Baptist network, and many more.
(2) Networks across ecumenical lines, such as the National Council of Churches Committee on Disabilities, and the Consortium of Jewish Special Educators.
(3) Regional and national organizations focused on ministries with people with disabilities, such as Joni and Friends, Inc. and Bethesda Lutheran Homes and Services, Inc.

**Collaborative Advocacy and Support Development**

The growing awareness of the impact of spirituality on health and coping, and the potential role of congregations as "generic, natural supports" has led to new examples of collaboration between advocacy/professional organizations and faith communities. The Accessible Congregations Campaign of the National Organization on Disability and the Faith in Action program funded by the Robert Wood Johnson Foundation are two examples of national collaborative and interfaith initiatives that bridge advocacy organizations, congregations, and public service providers and funders. The Religion and Disability Program of the National Organization on Disability spearheaded a collaborative Accessible Congregations Campaign that enlisted more than 2,100 congregations that have committed themselves to moving toward full accessibility and inclusion of people with disabilities and their families (www.nod.org). The Faith in Action initiative of the Robert Wood Johnson Foundation provided seed grants in the 1980s and 1990s to ecumenical and interfaith collaborative initiatives within communities to mobilize interfaith volunteer caregiving supports to people who are elderly and/or disabled *and their family caregivers* as determined by the focus of each individual project (www.rwjf.org). More than 1,000 programs began across the country through that initiative.

A final trend worth noting has been an increasing awareness of, and advocacy for, the importance of spiritual supports by public providers of services and/or advocacy and professional organizations. The Religion and Spirituality Division of the AAIDD (American Association on Intellectual and Developmental Disabilities) has bridged professional disciplines, families, and systems of support, whether "religious" or "secular." There is increasing focus on spiritual supports as a quality of life issue (Gleeson 2002; Poston and Turnbull 2004; Gaventa 2009b). Projects have grown from response by support agencies and advocacy networks to concerns expressed by families about the lack of support from their clergy, as in New Jersey where two statewide collaborative projects have occurred, one focusing on clergy education and people with brain injury and their families (Gaventa and Berk 2001) and a second on autism and faith (Walsh et al. 2008). The Atlanta Association for Persons with Disabilities developed, in collaboration with an interfaith network, an Interfaith Disabilities project that works with congregations to support families and people with disabilities (Landes 2002).

## Current Trends: Education

**Clergy and Laity**

Most of the education for clergy and congregation members around caregiving for people with disabilities and their families has emerged from the national resource offices within religious organizations and those crossing faith lines, as cited above. National conferences, newsletters, and websites are some of the growing methodologies. Other clergy education programs have come from local initiatives by organizations serving people with disabilities such as the Atlanta Interfaith Disabilities Network (Landes 2002) or a "That All May Worship" conference cooperatively sponsored by a variety of religious and disability service organizations in collaboration with the National Organization on Disability. Many family caregivers hope that their faith communities will simply provide "respect, recognition, respite, and resources" (quote from a conversation between Ginny Thornburgh and the author). National advocacy and resource organizations are recognizing this crucial role. For example, the National Family Caregivers Association has developed a suggested service of worship to honor family caregivers during National Family Caregivers Month in November (www.nfca.org).

Those educational initiatives with clergy and congregations are important but they have, for the most part, not been complemented with systematic initiatives in seminary education or in clinical or continuing education programs for clergy and other religious professionals. There have been sporadic initiatives in some seminaries around the country that have led to courses on ministries with people with disabilities, a module within a course, a conference, or a few field education or clinical training options. For the most part, however, pastoral and theological issues around caregiving with people with disabilities and their families have not received the same kind of attention as other issues related to diversity and minorities, such as gender and race. The numbers of educational initiatives within seminaries is gradually growing as seminaries respond to the growing number of congregational supports, a growing number of seminarians with disabilities, and increased interest by faculty members. A policy statement from the Association of Theological Seminaries about disability is one initiative as well as a week long Summer Institute on Theology and Disability that has been designed to enhance the capacity of seminaries to address theology and disability through many of the traditional theological disciplines (Anderson 2003b).

**Education for Professional Caregivers and Families**

If future clergy are receiving little introduction to issues around caregiving and disabilities, future professionals in other health and human service disciplines are receiving even less in relation to understanding the importance of spiritual supports and their potential role in facilitating those supports. Some interdisciplinary training programs (such as those offered through University Centers of Excellence in Developmental Disabilities, www.aucd.org) are beginning to develop initiatives in this area. In general, however, professional development and training programs in disciplines in disability services are lagging behind the work being done on spiritual assessments and supports in other areas of healthcare and human services, such as medicine and nursing. The publication of *Including People With Disabilities In Faith Communities: A Guide For Service Providers, Families, And Congregations* (Carter 2007), by Paul Brookes Publishing, a publisher primarily focused on secular supports, represents an important recognition of the need for this kind of training and collaboration.

The area that has seen the most growth is the quantity and quality of written and video resources available for clergy, congregations, service providers, and families who develop an interest in strengthening faith based caregiving with people with disabilities and their families. There may be a limited number of resources within any particular network or organization, but if clergy, congregations, service providers, and families are willing to look across ecumenical, interfaith, and religious/secular lines, the potential barrier of "no resources or models" is simply not there. An interfaith bibliography and resource guide published by The Boggs Center on Developmental Disabilities and the Religion and Spirituality Division of the AAIDD includes sections on resources for respite care ministries and resources for families (Gaventa 2009b, http://rwjms.umdnj.edu/boggscenter).

## *Current Status: Research*

Much of the growth in resources available to congregations has come out of work in both theory and practice. That includes explorations of the importance of theological and spiritual issues related to disability, reflections on personal and congregational experience, and descriptions of strategies and models for inclusive ministries, religious services and program development. Before 2005 there were books that explored theological issues (Block 2002; Eiesland 1994; Webb-Mitchell 1994), guidebooks for accessible and inclusive ministries and religious education (Benton and Owen 1995; Thornburgh 1994), books exploring Biblical and scriptural issues (Abrams 2000; Black 1996), and books focusing on spirituality and caregiving from the perspective of individuals with disabilities and their families (Bolduc 1999).

Since 2007 and 2008, there has been an "explosion" of new, significant books on theological and practical issues, many written by theologians who happen to be family members (Hubach and Tada 2007; Reinders 2008; Reynolds 2008; Yong 2007). All of them integrate learnings from the disability movements, current understandings of disability, and explorations of classical religious understandings from the perspective (and contribution) of people with disabilities and their families. Most of this is coming from within the faith communities or religious traditions.

There are signs of growing interest in exploration of issues of spiritual and religious supports from researchers in other disciplines. Erik Carter's book has already been noted. Articles on families and spiritual supports have appeared in the *American Journal of Mental Retardation* (Skinner et al. 2001), *Mental Retardation* (Haworth et al. 1996; Hornstein 1997; Rogers-Dulan 1998), and other professional journals in recent years. Family oriented magazines and newsletters have published focal issues or columns on religious and spiritual supports (*Exceptional Parent* 1993; *Disability Solutions* 1996; The Arc newsletter, *Insight*). The publication of a feature issue of the *Impact* newsletter of the Institute on Community Integration at the University of Minnesota on "Faith Communities and Persons with Developmental Disabilities" illustrates some of this interest (Gaylord 2002). The Foundation for Learning Disabilities in the United Kingdom funded a 3 year research project on the role of spirituality in the lives of people with intellectual disabilities. The first report on this project, *Spirituality: A Place to Listen* (Swinton 2001), emphasizes the importance of involving people with disabilities, their families, and service providers in understanding and addressing the issues of policy and practice that need to be addressed to strengthen spiritual supports *by both religious and secular caregivers*. The research was funded by a grant from a family member, a fact that points to their desire for both faith communities and service providers to take more responsibility in this area of support.

However, when one looks at the chronicled summaries and collections of research done on spiritual supports in other areas of healthcare like aging, addiction, and general health care from researchers like David Larson (Larson and Larson 1994), Harold Koenig at Center on Spirituality, Theology and Health at Duke Medical School (Koenig 2001, and http://www.dukespiritualityandhealth.org) and Christina Puchalski at the George Washington Institute on Spirituality and Health (www.gwish.org), there is comparatively little in the area of disabilities. Sometimes researchers who have been interested in this area have encountered unexpected barriers. The Beach Center on Disabilities, known for its research on quality of life issues and families with disabilities, found many families reluctant to talk about issues of spirituality as a separate domain because the families felt like that was an invasion of privacy (Poston and Turnbull 2004), i.e., a very powerful and important area that was hard to talk about. There are, however, other promising developments. *The Journal of Religion, Disability, and Health*, published originally by Haworth Press, now under Taylor and Francis, has attempted to be one vehicle for dissemination of research from any discipline that explores issues of spiritual supports. That journal includes studies focusing on congregational accessibility, spiritual supports for people with developmental disabilities (Shogren and Rye 2005) spiritual supports for families (Olson et al. 2002), and many other areas. A disability interest group is now part of the American Academy of Religion. The growth of disability studies programs and new focus on arts and humanities has promising possibilities for including research related to spirituality and religion.

## *Current Trends: Policy*

### Religious and Public Advocacy and Policy

There are many more positive and encouraging trends in the area of policy within both faith communities and public organizations. These include:

(1) Many national religious bodies and some ecumenical, interfaith organizations have adopted policy statements about the importance of welcoming, including, and supporting people with disabilities and their families both within congregational life. Those policy statements include:

- *Disabilities, the Body of Christ, and the Wholeness of Society*, from the National Council of Churches Committee on Disabilities, adopted by the NCC General Board in 1995 (www.nccc.org).
- An updated version of the Bishop's Pastoral Letter from 1978 called *Welcome and Justice for Persons with Disabilities: A Framework for Access and Inclusion*, adopted by the National Catholic Conference in 1998 (www.ncpd.org).
- *The Accessible Church*, a very fine and thorough policy statement adopted jointly by the Councils of Churches of Massachusetts and Rhode Island in 2000 (www.masscouncilofchurches.org/docs/accessibility.htm).

(2) A joint policy statement on *Spirituality and Religious Freedom* has been adopted by both the AAIDD and The Arc of the USA (www.aamr.org). It arose out of the concern that many service providers and professional caregivers either overlooked the importance of spiritual supports or had agency policies which professed religious freedom for its consumers but provided little in the way of choice and support to people with disabilities and their families who wanted to be more involved in their faith communities.

(3) The growing interest in "faith based supports" and "faith based caregiving" and their connection to public policy and funding is still in its early stages. My hope is the important debates and discussions in this area will lead to effective policies that both tap the power and potential of spiritual supports and faith based caregiving while also protecting religious freedom and providing appropriate boundaries between "church" and "state."

**Caregiver Advocacy and Policy**

This discussion on policy has all focused on the "macro" level, while perhaps the most important developments have been at local levels in congregations and other support organizations. It is crucial to recognize the important role that advocates have played within many faith communities around new and expanded spiritual supports for people with disabilities and their families. Those advocates have often been family members, as they claim a place and right to belong with their faith communities, and help congregations and people of faith "practice what they preach," or, as stated in secular terms, turn policy and theory into action. While they have sometimes drawn upon the policy statements cited above, more often families and other advocates are simply drawing upon their own understandings of scriptural and religious tradition and promise and their desire to support a person or family in their congregation or community. Some examples, in addition to the theologians/family members mentioned earlier, include:

- Katherine Bolduc's book, *His Name is Joel: Searching for God in a Son's Disability*, which links anecdotes from her family life with scriptural passages and prayers.
- When one hears that families are saying, "Do not offer to baptize my child unless you are really planning to support him/her in their growth and development, as the congregation vows in the ceremony," that is an application of policy to practice.
- When families question why a parochial school will not admit children with disabilities, citing that the public system has that responsibility, which is a challenge to policy and practice. One family member cited, in return, that the church took that responsibility when it baptized their child.
- Havorah, a Jewish program in Westchester County, New York has sponsored a significant number of paired bar and bat mitzvahs, linking a young person with a disability with one without, in preparation and celebration of that ceremony. In another, a bar mitzvah for a young boy with Down syndrome celebrates his gifts to the whole community (www.prayingwithlior.com).

## Hopes and Needs for the Future

### Future Needs in Practice

#### The Challenge for Faith Communities

In the broad arena of public policy, there is growing awareness of the linkage between issues impacting people with disabilities and people who are elderly. That policy has yet to be defined in many areas of policy, but the congregational arena is one area where it is happening, and could greatly expand, as faith communities explore how to welcome and support family members who are supporting people with disabilities or infirmities that come from birth, accident, disease, or aging.

Another role for congregations and spiritual supports is to recognize that faith based supports for people with disabilities can powerfully address changing needs over the life span of an individual and his or her family, as explored in other chapters of this book. It can evolve from pastoral and congregational supports to a family at time of birth, diagnosis, or onset through inclusive supports for a child within the congregational setting to assistance with a person's transition from school to work. Congregations and advocates have only just begun to realize their potential as a source for helping families as their young adults with disabilities find employment and other valued social roles. Some faith groups are also developing residential supports that link group homes with individual congregations, and others are recognizing their role as advocates and supports for individuals who have grown up within their congregation or tradition but have had to move into public residential programs. Getting a congregational representative involved in circles of support, a school based IEP (individual education plan) or an adult IHP (individual habilitation plan) or an FSP (family support plan) could be a powerful way for initiating and building collaboration between spiritual and public supports. One mother reported the impact of her pastor's presence in her daughter's IEP by saying, "It was wonderful. We got everything we wanted ... they thought he was our lawyer!"

Clergy and congregations are also significant resources for assisting people with disabilities and their families to deal with the grief and loss that is part of everyone's life but sometimes exacerbated by frequent changes of staff or program or loss of caregivers. Adults with disabilities often have few people in their lives who are friends, other than families or paid caregivers. Congregations offer one source for ongoing relationships. Faith and clergy are also resources that can be used in addressing ethical issues that face families and service providers.

Beyond meeting needs of people with disabilities and their families, a key area for practice in the future is for congregations to help find ways for individuals and families to make contributions to their congregation and community. No one likes to be on the receiving end of supports and care all of the time. Everyone has a gift (McKnight 1996). It is in and through congregations and faith communities that many are called by their understanding of their faith and religious tradition to serve God through serving and helping others. (Gaventa 2006) Many congregations who have developed inclusive and accessible ministries will tell you how that work has been a "blessing" to the whole church. There are hundreds of roles and jobs within any given congregation offering ways to contribute to the life of the congregation and community. The challenge for future practice in congregations is to focus on helping people with disabilities and their families find those gifts and interests, and figure out ways to use them, rather than focusing solely on what the congregation can do for the families and individuals with disabilities.

**The Challenge to Providers and Professional Caregivers**

For public providers and professionals in other systems of care and support, the future challenge is learning how to honor and address the spiritual needs, interests, and gifts of people with disabilities and their families. What kinds of spiritual assessments are included in ongoing support planning? Ignoring the role of spirituality or the power of congregational participation and supports fails to address a huge and important area in the lives of many families (Gaylord 2002; Carter 2007). How might clergy or congregational members be involved in interdisciplinary treatment teams, "care plans," or "circles of support?" Can formal planning processes be changed to draw people in who may be potential support providers (Gaventa 2001). That involves a new kind of attitudinal accessibility on the part of professionals to respecting and including spiritual issues.

The challenge also extends to what professionals do with that awareness and respect. For example, assume that a social worker serving in an intake or case manager role has developed a format for spiritual assessment, what will he or she do with that knowledge? Or, assume that a special education teacher, or group home manager, realizes there are ways that a child's or adult's faith community could be more supportive. What do they do? The challenge here for many professionals is one of reframing their roles and arena of practice.

In addition to serving and treating people within their service setting, the professional role of community building also helps discover and build supportive and caring communities. It is a paradoxical role change, for instead of saying, "Come to us, because of our specialized knowledge," professionals are now having to say "How can we give away what we know in ways that support and guide others who are part of the more informal supports of a person's life?" Will their job descriptions include going to a congregation to help educate and train (Poston and Turnbull 2004)? Learning to be askers and facilitators calls for community building skills, not traditional caregiving skills (Schwartz 1996). It calls for true consultation, collaboration, and partnership that extend beyond usual service system boundaries. It changes the role of a professional to include skills such as "coach" (Gaventa 2001).

## *Future Needs: Education/Training and Reframing Professional Roles*

Skills in community building or enhancing spiritual supports are not professional skills taught in many places or programs at present, either in health care, human services, or seminaries. As stated earlier, there is growing interest, research and training for health and human service providers in models of understanding and addressing spiritual needs and interests, but that is unevenly available to trainees, students, and practicing professionals. Finding new models to include spiritual issues in professional training in many disciplines rather than simply avoiding the issues is necessary.

Those education and training challenges around spirituality and faith supports are simply part of the growing need for new professional skills in an era of consumer and caregiver advocacy, community-based informal supports, limitations on public funding for professional services, quality of life interpreted as consumer outcomes, and consumer/family empowerment or self-determination (Chambers 1999; McKnight 1995; Schwartz 1996). This growing need includes learning how to utilize a variety of informal support givers in planning and practice, learning how to give knowledge to others, and learning how to empower others. It is also a paradoxical path to a new and very significant professional role, perhaps diminished in control, but much more powerful in the potential impact on the lives of individuals, families, and communities.

In the religious community, the future needs of education and training include the more successful integration of pastoral and theological issues related to disabilities and support of family caregivers in seminary education and training. That does not necessarily mean the need to develop specific, specialized courses, but rather the inclusion of issues related to disabilities and families in a variety of theological and pastoral training subjects, e.g., pastoral care, theology, scriptural studies, religious education, and more (Anderson 2003a). It can mean development of more clinical training opportunities for clergy in settings serving people with disabilities and their families. Seminaries and faith groups can also work to include training opportunities on ministries with people with disabilities in ongoing continuing education programs. The impetus for development of that training will be greatly enhanced by the advocacy of people with disabilities, their families, and/or professional caregivers who offer to create collaborative training projects.

## *Future Needs: Research*

Those challenges in theological education and religious polity point to a major area of needed research. All of the major religious traditions need to do more extensive, in-depth research into issues related to disability within their own scriptural foundations and faith traditions. All of the major faith traditions have scriptural foundations that support inclusive supports with people with disabilities and their families. All of them also have some traditions and understandings that serve as barriers, such as traditional understandings of the restrictions in Leviticus or the passages that talk about "the sins of the parents being visited upon their children." These traditions and practices should be understood in the context of the times, in ways that inform families and clergy as they work together to understand disability within the context of their faith or spirituality. There are some important examples of this kind of research, as cited earlier in this chapter, but much more work needs to be done in all of the major faith traditions and traditional theological disciplines.

That research also needs to explore more systematically the kinds of "best practices" in faith communities that support people with disabilities and their families. This is one area with vast opportunities for collaboration with researchers in human services and health care, particularly with those with skills in qualitative research and participatory action research (Gaventa 2009b). Some of the research questions could include:

- What are the factors and strategies needed to develop inclusive congregational supports?
- What do families need and expect from their clergy or congregations? What can families and advocates to do to facilitate those supports?
- What is the impact of effective spiritual supports on the health and quality of life of people with disabilities and their families?
- Stated differently, what other kinds of outcomes grow from effective collaboration with faith communities and inclusive supports, e.g., friendships, socialization, employment, etc.
- How are effective spiritual supports, whether in a congregational setting or not, related to successful strategies in positive behavioral supports for people with challenging behaviors?
- How are spiritual supports related to the increasing diversity of cultures in this country, and the development of culturally competent supports?
- What are the best models and practices for collaboration between "scientific" or "secular" services and supports within faith communities?

## Future Needs: Policy

If one defines policy as the place where values, knowledge, and attitude inform and guide practice and action, then the future needs in policy around spiritual supports for people with disabilities and their families could be described as the need for *accessible* and *inclusive* policy changes in both "public" and "private" spheres, or in other words, in both secular and religious arenas. Can traditional professional services be "scientific" enough to recognize that spirituality is indeed an area of important practice and support? Second, can religious communities and professionals can be "faithful" enough to recognize and affirm the role of scientific and secular services and supports while also claiming their own responsibility to include and support people with disabilities and their families? The stereotypes on both sides sometimes block effective collaboration, when, for example, "secular" services see clergy and religion only as "proselytizers" and clergy see public services as "godless service providers."

The challenge and need is to develop effective policies and partnerships in both arenas of service and caregiving. Those policies can guide ways of working together, respecting the importance of different roles and perspectives while maintaining appropriate boundaries. It may not be easy. The bridge that builds that collaboration should be the joint commitment to provide the kind of services, support, and ongoing care that families with disabled members need and want, moving toward the outcomes that are most important to them. That kind of commitment can welcome as many caring supports as are wanted, needed, and possible. It can lead to a collaborative "doing what it takes" practice on everyone's part, and, in the end, be a source of continued inspiration for people with disabilities, their families, and the professionals and systems who support them, whatever their role or religious persuasion.

## References

Abrams, J. (2000). *Judaism and disability: Portrayals in ancient text from the Tanach through the Bavli.* Washington, DC: Gallaudet University Press.

Anderson, R. C. (2003a). Infusing the graduate theological curriculum with education about disability: Addressing the human experience of disability in the theological context. *Theological Education, 39*(1), 1–24. http://www.religionanddisability.org/user/ATS%20article,%20Theological%20Education,%2039(1).pdf.

Anderson, R. (2003b). *Graduate theological education and the human experience of disability.* Binghamton: Haworth.

Benton, J., & Owen, M. (1995). *Opening doors to people with disabilities.* Washington, DC: National Catholic Office for Persons with Disabilities.

Black, K. (1996). *A healing homiletic: Preaching and disability.* Nashville: Abingdon.

Block, J. (2002). *Copious hosting: A theology of access for people with disabilities.* New York: Continuum.

Bolduc, K. (1999). *His name is Joel: Searching for God in a son's disability?* Louisville: Bridge Resources.

Bolduc, K. (2001). *A place called acceptance. Ministry with families of children with disabilities.* Louisville: Bridge Resources.

Carter, E. (2007). *Including people with disabilities in faith communities: A guide for service providers, families, and congregations*. Baltimore: Paul Brookes.

Chambers, R. (1999). *Whose reality counts? Putting the first last*. London: Intermediate Training Technology.

Downey, M. E. (1986). *A blessed weakness: The spirit of Jean Vanier and L'Arche*. San Francisco: Harper and Row. In E. M. Boggs Center, *Dimensions of faith and congregational ministries with persons with developmental disabilities and their families*, Sect. V, 49–63. http://rwjms.umdnj.edu/boggscenter/products/pdf/Dimensions%20final%20August%202005.pdf.

Eiesland, N. (1994). *The disabled God: Toward a liberatory theology of disability*. Nashville: Abingdon.

Fitchett, G. (1993). *Assessing spiritual needs: A guide for caregivers*. Minneapolis: Augsburg/Fortress.

Gaventa, W. (1986). Religious ministries and services with adults with developmental disabilities. In J. Summers (Ed.), *The right to grow up: An introduction to adults with developmental disabilities* (pp. 191–226). Baltimore: Brookes.

Gaventa, W. (1990). Respite care: The opportunity for state-church partnership. *Exceptional Parent, 20*(4), 22–26.

Gaventa, W. (1997). Pastoral care with people with disabilities and their families: An adaptable module for introductory courses. In M. Bishop (Ed.), *Thematic conversations regarding disability within the framework of courses of worship, scripture, and pastoral care*. Dayton: National Council of Churches Committee on Disabilities.

Gaventa, W. (2001). Creating and energizing caring communities. In D. Doka & J. Davidson (Eds.), *Caregiving and loss: Family needs, professional responses* (pp. 57–77). Washington, DC: The Hospice Foundation of America.

Gaventa, W. (2002). Defining and assessing spirituality and spiritual supports: A rationale for inclusion in theory and practice. In W. Gaventa & D. Coulter (Eds.), *Spirituality and intellectual disability: International perspectives on the effect of culture and religion on healing body, mind, and soul* (pp. 29–48). Binghamton: Haworth.

Gaventa, W. (2006). Signs of the times: theological themes in the changing forms of ministries and spiritual supports with people with disabilities. *Disability Studies Quarterly, 26*, 4.

Gaventa, W. (2008a). Spiritual and religious supports. What difference do they make? *Exceptional Parent Magazine, 38*(30), 66–68.

Gaventa, W. (2008b). Including religious voices on disability. Which ones? *Exceptional Parent Magazine, 38*(5), 52–55.

Gaventa, W. (2009a). (Ed.). *On the road to congregational inclusion: Dimensions of faith and congregational ministries with persons with developmental disabilities and their families*. New Brunswick: The Elizabeth M. Boggs Center, Robert Wood Johnson Medical School, UMDNJ. http://rwjms.umdnj.edu/boggscenter/products.

Gaventa, W. (2009b). A place for all of me and all of us. Rekindling the spirit in-services and supports. *Mental Retardation, 43*(1), 48–54.

Gaventa, W., & Berk, W. (2001). *Brain injury: When the call comes: A congregational resource*. New Brunswick: The Elizabeth M. Boggs Center, Brain Injury Association of New Jersey, and New Brunswick Theological Seminary.

Gaylord, V. (Ed.). (2002). *Impact: Feature issue on faith communities and persons with developmental disabilities*. St. Paul: University of Minnesota.

Gleeson, T. (2002). Incorporating spiritual supports into residential services: The PSCH model. In V. Gaylord (Ed.), Impact: Feature issue on faith communities and persons with developmental disabilities (pp. 30–31). St. Paul: University of Minnesota.

Haworth, A., Hill, A., & Glidden, L. (1996). Measuring the religiousness of parents of children with developmental disabilities. *Mental Retardation, 34*(5), 271–279.

Heifitz, L. (1987). Integrating religious and secular perspectives in the design and delivery of disability services. *American Journal of Mental Retardation, 25*, 127–131.

Hornstein, B. (1997). How the religious community can support the transition to adulthood: A parent's perspective. *Mental Retardation, 35*(6), 485–487.

Hubach, S., & Tada, J. (2007). *Same lake, different boat: Coming alongside people touched by disability*. Phillipsburg: P&R Publishing.

Koenig, H. (2001). Handbook on religion and health. New York: Oxford University Press.

Landes, S. (2002). Atlanta's interfaith disabilities network. In V. Gaylord (Ed.), *Impact: Feature issue on faith communities and persons with developmental disabilities* (pp. 28–29). St. Paul: University of Minnesota.

Larson, D., & Larson, S. (1994). *The forgotten factor in physical and mental health: What does the research show?* Rockville: National Institute of Healthcare Research.

Matthews, D., Larson, D, & Barry, C. (1993). *The faith factor: An annotated bibliography of clinical research on spiritual subjects*. Rockville: National Institute of Healthcare Research.

Mcknight. J. (1995). *The careless society: Community and its counterfeits*. New York: Basic Books.

Mcknight, J. (1996). *Everyone has a gift*. Toronto: Inclusion (Video presentation).

Miltiades, H. B., & Pruchno, R. (2002). The effect of religious coping on caregiving appraisals of mothers of adults with developmental disabilities. *Gerontologist, 42,* 82–91.

Olson, M., Dollahite, D., & White, M. (2002). Involved fathering of children with special needs: Relationships and religion and resources. *Journal of Religion, Disability, and Health, 6,* 47–63.

Poston, D., & Turnbull, A. (2004). Role of spirituality and religion in family quality of life for families of children with disabilities. *Education and Training in Developmental Disabilities, 39,* 95–108.

Puchalski, C., & Romer, A. (2000). Taking a spiritual history allows clinicians to understand patients more fully. *Journal of Palliative Medicine, 3,* 129–137.

Preheim-Bartel, D., & Neufeld, A. (2011). *Supportive care in the congregation*. Goshen: Mennonite Mutual Aid.

Reinders, H. (2008). *Receiving the gift of friendship: profound disability, theological anthropology and ethics*. Grand Rapids: Eerdmans.

Reynolds, T. (2008). *Vulnerable communion: a theology of disability and hospitality*. Grand Rapids: Brazos.

Rogers-Dulan, J. (1998). Religious connectedness among urban African American families who have a child with disabilities. *Mental Retardation, 36,* 91–103.

Schwartz, D. (1996). *Who cares? Rediscovering community*. Denver: Westview.

Shogren, K., & Rye, M. (2005). Religion and individuals with intellectual disabilities: an exploratory study of self reported perspectives. *Journal of Religion, Disability, and Health, 9*(1), 29–53.

Skinner, D. G., Correa, V., Skinner, M., & Bailey, D. B., Jr. (2001). Role of religion in the lives of Latino families of young children with developmental delays. *American Journal on Mental Retardation, 106,* 297–313.

Swinton, J. (2001). *A space to listen: Meeting the spiritual needs of people with learning disabilities*. London: Foundation for Learning Disabilities. Summary retrieved from http://www.learningdisabilities.org.uk/page.cfm?pagecode=PUUP0306. May be ordered at http://www.learningdisabilities.org.uk/page.cfm?pagecode=PUBOSP#space.

Thornburgh, G. (1994). *That all may worship: An interfaith handbook to assist congregations in welcoming people with disabilities*. Washington, DC: National Organization on Disability.

Walsh, M. B., Walsh, A., & Gaventa, W. (2008). *Autism and faith: a journey into community*. New Brunswick: The Elizabeth M. Boggs Center on Developmental Disabilities.

Webb-Mitchell, B. (1994). *Unexpected guests at the banquet: Welcoming people with disability into the church*. New York: Crossroad.

Yong, A. (2007). *Theology and down syndrome: reimagining disability in late* modernity. Waco: Baylor University Press.

# Chapter 9
# Family Caregivers and Health Care Providers: Developing Partnerships for a Continuum of Care and Support

Timothy R. Elliott and Michael Parker

> I received the news of my son's injury and life sustaining surgery late in the evening of the 4th of July. I had no real idea of what the implications of a spinal cord injury were for my son and family. Over the next several months I learned the hard way what the tasks of caregiving were. No one provided me with a coherent look at the full range of caregiving tasks ahead, let alone up-to-date, practical information I needed about how to meet these challenges. All caregivers need hope… hope perhaps from an informed theological perspective that provides a sense of purpose in the face of the injury, hope perhaps from a therapist that sees return of function not just adaptation as a feasible treatment goal, or perhaps hope in the form of someone willing to simply listen… to get into the deep water with us. These are examples of the real "cups of cold water" that bonded us to professionals with whom we worked. (Anonymous father 2004).

Contrary to popular opinion, most American families do not abandon family members with chronic disease and disability to paid professionals and paraprofessionals. Family caregivers "… constitute the largest group of care providers" in the United States (Parish et al. 2003, p. 174), and as they provide the majority of long-term care in this country, the market value of their activity far exceeds that spent on formal health care and nursing home care (Vitaliano et al. 2004, p. 13). The number of family caregivers will continue to increase as our society changes with an aging populace and an escalating rate of chronic, debilitating health conditions (Carter 2008). As the number of caregivers in society increases and the health of care recipients is dependent upon the ability of the family caregivers to operate competently as de facto health care providers, the health and well-being of family caregivers is a public health priority (Talley and Crews 2007). Yet, most health care service delivery systems and practitioners fail to acknowledge and affirm the central role families play in extending health care services.

---

T. R. Elliott (✉)
Department of Educational Psychology, Texas A&M University, 4225 TAMU,
College Station, TX 77845, USA
e-mail: telliott@tamu.edu

M. Parker
School of Social Work, University of Alabama, Box 870314,
Tuscaloosa, AL 35487-0314, USA
e-mail: mwparker@sw.ua.edu

The purpose of this chapter is to discuss how health care providers can collaborate productively with family caregivers as partners providing care and assistance to persons living with debilitating health conditions. We briefly describe the current Zeitgeist associated with the growing phenomenon of caregiving among family caregivers of individuals with disabling conditions, and we discuss current practices in caregiver preparation and support. We propose the development of collaborative partnerships with caregivers in the community and discuss important aspects of assessment and service provision, with particular emphasis on the use of long-distance technologies. We argue for the identification of important caregiver tasks and competencies as a critical step toward the development of this partnership model, and offer some closing comments about the issues that have thwarted progress in this area.

## Contemporary Zeitgeist of Caregiving

Despite medical advances, caring for a person with a severe disability is increasingly challenging to America's families and systems of care because of the growth of our aging population (which increases the probability of multiple caregiving roles), medical advances that have added years to the lives of people with serious chronic illnesses and disability (Lollar and Crews 2003), reductions in nuclear family size (resulting in fewer available caregivers), increased female labor force participation (compelling caregivers to face competing work demands), diminishing access to medical assets and reductions in insurance coverage, the growing number of seriously wounded veterans returning from the Iraq and Afghanistan conflicts (Eibner 2008), increasing isolation of primary caregivers, and other changes in family structure and stability. In the case of an accidental injury in which their child incurs a permanent disability, a family will face immediate choices about where to seek the best care. After the initial health care crisis has passed, the family will then face long-term health, educational and social needs for their child and these issues may erupt in periodic crises that can stretch out for years. Such crises can thrust families into a bureaucratic maze of making successive care arrangements in a badly fragmented, long-term care system. Rather than implementing carefully constructed plans based upon the best information, in consultation with the care recipient and trusted professionals, most families find themselves overwhelmed and unprepared when facing the provision of care to a loved one who is severely impaired by a chronic disease, illness, or a disabling condition.

Across all caregiving scenarios, there is wide consensus that as a group, caregivers experience considerable burden, depression, and disruption of their well-being and social activities (Schulz 2000) and they are at risk for physical health problems (Vitaliano et al. 2003) and premature mortality (Schulz and Beach 1999). Family caring is also costly to a caregiver's earning potential and to the employers of caregivers. A recent study found that over 73% of caregivers were employed at some point in their caregiving career, and approximately 66% reported a need to adjust their work schedules to accommodate their caregiving responsibilities (National Alliance for Caregiving 2009). Family caregivers who are employed often reduce their time at work, decline in productivity or experience lost career opportunities as they provide care at home (Bond et al. 1998; Wagner and Neal 1994). The Metropolitan Life Insurance Company study indicated that caregivers experienced decreased lifetime earnings of US$ 659,130 (Metropolitan Life Insurance Company 2004). More women with children work fulltime in the United States than in any other nation in the world (Parker et al. 2003a; Wisensale 2002). As the full impact of this demographic and cultural change is experienced, the life course theme of family caregiving will be shared by a growing number of working women and men during midlife. However, competing commitments to vocation and to nuclear and extended family make women who care for family members particularly vulnerable to stress and career disruption (Moen et al. 2000; Parker et al. 2003a).

Despite these known common stressors and outcomes, substantial individual differences are apparent in how individuals respond to the caregiving role. There is evidence that many caregivers experience a sense of personal growth and meaning in their role (King et al. 2000; Kramer 1997). Some caregivers possess effective coping abilities and elaborate social networks that help them navigate the caregiving career; others rely on personal and spiritual resources, or grow personally as they honor their life-long commitment to their relationship with a family member with whom they share intimate knowledge and experience. For all caregivers, however, the career is a dynamic process as needs, issues, supports, and challenges change and fluctuate over time. Considerable variability in caregiver well-being, depression, and burden occurs between individuals who assume a caregiver role, and variability also can be observed within an individual caregiver career (Shewchuk et al. 1998).

## Caregiver Preparation and Support: Current Practices

The extant literature now sufficiently informs us of the caregiver experience and provides evidence of the considerable variation that exists among caregivers, and clearly documents the consequences incurred when caregivers are unable to adequately perform their duties as health care "extenders." Yet, to date, health care delivery systems—in both the private and public sectors—have not enacted any consistent, comprehensive continuum of services to family caregivers. Although the Affordable Care Act of 2010 reccognizes the role of family caregivers and provides incentives for developing innovative and cost-effective home and community-based services for them (Reinhard et al. 2011), States vary considerably in their response to this initiative (and some have curtailed support for "Caregiver interventions" as a cost-cutting measure (Levine et al. 2010)).

Important changes in policy and support for family caregivers have recently occured in the Veterans Health Care system (http://www.caregiver.va.gov/) and in the Department of Defense health system (particularly for family caregivers of personnel with acquired brain injuries; http://www.dvbic.org/Families—Friends/Family-Caregiver-Curriculum.aspx). The high rate of injury among many veterans of the Iraq and Afghanistan conflicts constitutes one of the largest, documented pools of veterans with severe and chronic disabilities in the history of the United States.

In many respects, most health care delivery systems utilize family caregivers as untrained and unpaid de facto health care providers who are expected to comply and cooperate with therapeutic directives proffered in a "top-down" fashion by treating clinicians. These clinicians, in turn, base their recommendations on an experience and knowledge base typically circumscribed by their particular expertise with a specific disability (e.g., spinal cord injury, traumatic brain injury), a limited sampling of issues and strengths of any given family, and the realities of available services approved by the host facility and reimbursed by a family's third-party payer.

Not surprisingly, then, the available research concerning interventions for family caregivers of persons with disabilities is intellectually Balkanized into disjointed literatures that are associated with specific disabilities (spinal cord injury, brain injury, developmental disabilities, etc.) and the ensuing interventions are dictated by the specific nature and concomitants of each disabling condition with little regard to the shared problems caregivers will have negotiating the psychosocial and health care issues they will encounter daily. The overriding emphasis on medical management of the disability—consistent with the "top-down" approach from systems that are driven by the provision of acute care services—has resulted in a dearth of meaningful studies that examine the effectiveness of interventions for family caregivers of persons with disabilities. Furthermore, the focus on medical management—although congruent with the mission of the rehabilitation team and the expertise of team members—inadvertently minimizes the experience and perspective of the family caregiver, who is compelled to learn sophisticated information and techniques, and to defer to clinical expertise under extremely stressful circumstances. Unfortunately, most rehabilitation programs ignore the implications of the available evidence concerning the caregiver experience, and with the acknowledged lack of intervention research in this area, rely on clinical lore and their expert opinion to share current practices.

For example, family members who assume a caregiving role for a loved one with an acquired spinal cord injury (SCI) encounter many clinical assumptions about the type of information and preparation they should receive. Typically, the caregiver is required to be at the rehabilitation facility to observe and learn hands-on nursing care and exercises in physical therapy. The new caregiver is usually expected to perform specific skills (toileting, bathing, transfers from bed to chair, etc.) in a relatively brief amount of time. Occasionally, rehabilitation programs offer educational sessions to instruct designated caregivers how to handle medical and other therapeutic regimens, and to teach information specific to the condition and its concomitants, and how to manage possible scenarios the caregiver will likely encounter in the community.

Generally, clinicians are not reimbursed by third-party payers for the time they spend instructing or observing family caregivers (despite the obvious urgency and expertise required for the care recipient to remain healthy once discharged into the community). In this process, caregivers who appear overly optimistic about the care recipient's prospects, or who support care recipient goals for rehabilitation that conflict with team goals, or who voice a strong difference of opinion with staff are usually described by clinicians as being "in denial" (Elliott and Kurylo 2000; Novack and Richards 1991). If caregivers are distressed and worried, they are often reassured by staff that their reactions are normal and their situation will improve over time.

Following their discharge from an inpatient rehabilitation program, families return to their respective communities with variable and inconsistent available support. Families with considerable financial resources and access to care may be able to afford (or, in some cases, qualify) for home-health services that can provide some assistance and additional therapies. Many families, however, do not qualify or cannot afford these services, and many live in rural or inner city areas where these services have been curtailed or they are no longer available. For most families, the continuum of care is relegated to scheduled outpatient appointments for physical therapies (which is contingent upon location, availability, and reimbursement sources) and annual medical evaluations, or for episodic treatment of secondary complications or emergent, acute care needs. In these standard practices, the focus of care is on the care recipient, with opportunities for the caregiver to benefit indirectly from brief interactions with health care personnel providing service to the care recipient.

## *Developing Partnerships for a Continuum of Care and Support*

Instead of the unscientific and general ineffectiveness of current practice in working with caregivers, we propose a more formal, collaborative model of support that abandons the paternalism of traditional health care services and cultivates active partnerships with family caregivers in the community. There are several advantages to this approach. It is consistent with emerging evidence supporting the use of home- and community-based services for persons living with disabilities, and it recognizes that these persons—and their family members—have a greater impact over time on their health and well-being than the services provided by any single health care professional. It acknowledges that family caregivers have ongoing yet fluctuating needs for training, support, and assistance, but they are nonetheless experts on the "... realities of their daily lives" (Mechanic 1998, p. 284). Thus, their perspectives and their input concerning the problems they face and possible solutions is valued and actively solicited.

Collaborative partnerships can be particularly effective in meeting the unique and immediate concerns of the individual caregiver (Brodaty et al. 2003). However, in order for these partnerships to be effective, it is essential that health care providers understand that some caregivers may be predisposed to experience difficulty in their role at any point in time in the caregiving career, and others may have resources at hand that enable them to benefit from less intensive, supportive programs they may access on their own recognizance. To maximize the potential effectiveness of these collaborative partnerships and to provide strategic tailored services to meet the needs of each caregiver, an informed assessment should identify characteristics of family caregivers who may be particularly vulnerable to the rigors of the caregiver role and who might require a more intense array of services. Clinical assessment should take into account the issues specific to the health condition of the care recipient, the specific challenges the family caregiver faces, and specific strengths that the family caregiver brings to the situation. A thorough assessment will rely not on clinical

**Table 9.1** Risk factors of vulnerable caregivers

| Demographic characteristics | Personal characteristics | Interpersonal characteristics |
|---|---|---|
| Lower level of education | Depressed, high levels of distress | Poor marital quality |
| Older age | Substance abuse | Problematic relationship with recipient prior to caregiver role |
| Poor health | Poor coping skills, ineffective problem-solving abilities | Interpersonal conflict, hostility |
| Unemployment | | Socially isolated, low social support |

assumptions and lore, but rather on the needs and characteristics that are unique to the individual family caregiver. Therefore, an expert triage of caregiver needs, risk factors, and unique problems is essential.

Table 9.1 depicts several recognized risk factors that characterize family caregivers who are vulnerable to the deleterious consequences often associated with caregiving. These risk factors are divided into demographic, personal, and interpersonal characteristics. Some characteristics may reflect social and behavioral patterns that are known to be indicative of marginal adjustment, generally; other characteristics may stem from circumstances independent of personal choice or volition. Although we can see how these elements may interact and influence each other, for brief and efficient screening purposes it is sufficient to first consider these components separately.

*Demographic Characteristics* Individuals who have lower levels of education and are unemployed enter the caregiver role with several disadvantages. It is likely that they lack the financial and insurance benefits often associated with higher education, gainful employment, and higher income. Caregivers with lower incomes are more likely to live with a care recipient and less likely to receive paid assistance than caregivers with higher incomes (Donelan et al. 2001). Individuals lacking the resources associated with education and employment may also lack personal and career goals that often imbue a person with a sense of competence and satisfaction. They may also have fewer social contacts and a smaller social network on which to rely for additional support. Finally, individuals with less education will experience considerable difficulty understanding basic and complex information about a health condition, its concomitants, and subsequent regimens and therapies (and are thus more likely to make errors in administering medications and assisting with therapies; Donelan et al. 2002).

Caregivers who are older appear to be vulnerable in part because the heightened demands of caregiving tax their health and physical abilities and compromise their immune response systems, and in part because stress associated with caregiving may exacerbate any existing chronic health condition of the caregiver (Vitaliano et al. 2003). Among persons caring for frail elders, for example, most are age 65 and older, and persons in this age bracket have a higher incidence of heart disease, cancer, arthritis, hypertension, and diabetes. Declines in personal health are associated with older age among caregivers, and older caregivers in poor health are more likely than others to experience problems providing therapeutic assistance (Navaie-Waliser et al. 2002). Aging caregivers also face considerable risks in managing the physical demands of adult children with disabilities, and they are also more likely to have problems with social isolation and declining financial resources; in addition, they have lingering concerns about who will care for their loved one if they are unable to provide care (Braddock 1999; Elliott and Pezent 2008).

*Personal Characteristics* Individuals who report greater anxiety and depression upon entering the caregiver role are likely to experience greater depression, anxiety, and ill health over the course of a year (Shewchuk et al. 1998). In one prospective study of family members in the initial year of caregiving for a person who had incurred a severe physical disability, evidence of a depressive syndrome was significantly predictive of depression at subsequent assessments throughout the year: Caregivers who experience problems with depression are likely to have recurring problems with depression (Elliott et al. 2003). Depressed caregivers are also more likely to report increasing problems with stress and overload, and they are more likely than nondepressed caregivers to report prescription use for emotional and physical problems.

Caregivers who have a prior or ongoing problem with substance abuse are also likely to have difficulties with the demands of caregiving. To a great extent, problems with depression and substance abuse reflect deficits in coping and problem-solving skills that are beneficial in times of duress. Effective problem-solving abilities are prospectively predictive of lower depression and anxiety scores, and with fewer health complaints among caregivers of persons with severe physical and cognitive disabilities (Elliott et al. 2001; Grant et al. 2006).

There are other data to suggest that caregivers who experience problems with emotional distress and burden may have certain personality characteristics that predispose them to emotional distress in routine and stressful situations (Hooker et al. 1998). Although we do not discount the veracity and importance of this work—indeed, we recognize recurring behavioral patterns in the caregiver career—persons with greater "affectivity" can learn effective cognitive-behavioral skills that augment their coping and adjustment. Furthermore, it is important that clinicians avoid tendencies to discount caregiver accounts of their needs and problems, and work to find ways to help caregivers resolve issues they encounter. We urge caution so that a "blame the victim" mentality is avoided, and recommend an informed, ongoing assessment that recognizes each caregiver's unique characteristics and circumstances so that appropriate services may ensue.

*Interpersonal Characteristics* Family relationships can be a source of considerable stress. Caregivers may be at risk for difficulties if they have not experienced a communal relationship with a care recipient prior to the disabling condition (Williamson and Schulz 1995). Caregivers who believe they are investing in the relationship with the care recipient and receiving few benefits in return are likely to experience resentment (Thompson et al. 1995), burnout (Ybema et al. 2002), and depression (Ybema et al. 2001). Displays of conflict, hostility, and criticism can indicate adjustment problems for both the caregiver (MaloneBeach and Zarit 1995; Soskolne et al. 2000) and the care recipient (Fiscella et al. 1997; Fiske et al. 1991), and for the overall quality of the caregiver—care recipient relationship (Knussen et al. 2005). In contrast, family caregivers who display effective problem-solving abilities in their interpersonal interactions exhibit less distress and these benefits can be observed 3 years later (Rivara et al. 1996). Effective coping behavior among family members soon after the onset of a child's traumatic brain injury is a major determinant of care recipient behavioral outcomes in the first year of injury (Kinsella et al. 1999).

Social support is often associated with caregiver adjustment and changes in social support are directly related to changes in caregiver emotional and physical health (Shewchuk et al. 1998). Many caregivers experience an erosion of social support over time (Quittner et al. 1990), but there is some evidence that this erosion may be more pronounced among caregivers who may lack adaptive characteristics and resources (Park and Folkman 1997). Caregivers who rely on their social contacts as a coping strategy appear to experience greater positive affect and report fewer health complaints than caregivers who have more avoidant coping styles (Billings et al. 2000).

*Assessing Problems and Needs Unique to Each Caregiver* Most studies of caregiver adjustment following disability employ global or disability-specific measures of stress and clinical assessment often makes some assumptions about the stressful aspects of specific demands, tasks, and stressors caregivers usually experience with various disabilities. Although these global measures and clinical assumptions have some utility, they are insensitive and lack specificity in appreciating the experiences of an individual caregiver. Other methods are better suited for understanding the experience of an individual caregiver from their phenomenological perspective.

Qualitative studies find that family caregivers experience considerable difficulty with interpersonal problems in providing care to persons with acquired disabilities (e.g., traumatic brain injuries; Chwalisz and Stark-Wroblewski 1996; Willer et al. 1991) and neuromuscular disease (Long et al. 1998). Contrary to clinical assumptions, focus groups with caregivers reveal that the most difficult problems they experience in the first year of caregiving for a person with SCI are not addressed during the initial rehabilitation program. The most difficult problems these caregivers faced concerned interpersonal difficulties ("my care recipient has a hateful attitude," "lack of appreciation," "my care recipient is demanding and bossy") and managing the subjective burden of caregiving ("finding challenging activities for my care recipient," "not enough time in the day to do previous routines and new regimens," "sense of obligation"; Elliott and Shewchuk 2002). In contrast, caregivers of adult children with developmental disabilities report problems with feeling overwhelmed, isolated, and financially strapped, and these caregivers were also critical of "professionals who don't or won't listen" and worry about their old age and who would help their care recipient following their death (Elliott and Rivera 2003).

These problems and concerns have direct implications for subsequent interventions and services that may be tailored to meet these specific concerns. Interventions that tailor problem-solving training to the specific problems experienced by an individual caregiver have demonstrated greater effects in lowering caregiver depression (Elliott et al. 2008) and in improving the social functioning of caregivers and care recipients (Elliott and Berry 2009; Elliott et al. 2008) over time than education programs. There is emerging evidence that care recipients experience decreases in personal distress as their caregivers respond favorably to home-based training (Berry et al. in press).

*Providing Relevant Strategic Services in the Home and Community* Caregivers are more likely to benefit from services and interventions that are relevant to their situation, that are readily available, and that view them as partners rather than service recipients. Ideally, services should be strategically developed and offered to caregivers to address the specific and unique concerns of each individual caregiver. These services should take into account the specific challenges family caregivers face and the strengths they bring to the caregiving situation. Caregivers who have several risk factors and appear vulnerable should receive routine monitoring for home-based services and in-home counseling and support. Caregivers who are adept in managing demands and coping with stress may fare well with less intensive programs that provide information and services as needed or as requested by the caregiver.

Furthermore, caregivers often have useful opinions about solutions to their problems, and interestingly, these solutions are not cost-prohibitive: Family caregivers of persons with SCI recommended support groups, domestic assistance, "a person who could train me (what to expect, etc.)," respite care and assistance with toileting (Elliott and Shewchuk 2002). Such recommendations reflect family caregivers' knowledge about the realities of the home situation and reflect the lack of home- and community-based assistance caregivers experience following discharge.

Brief instructional lectures or demonstrations—whether in an inpatient rehabilitation unit, an outpatient clinic, or in the home—in no way prepare a person for a career in caregiving. Educational and informational needs persist over time, depending on the changing circumstances of family life and characteristics of the caregiver. Brief instructional sessions early in the caregiver career should be construed as an orientation period in which a partnership with the caregiver is established and the needs confronting the caregiver are identified. Opportunities for refresher courses, toll-free telephone contacts that can be used as "hot lines," and manuals for home use should supplement and reinforce these instructional sessions.

In the community, family caregivers face multiple demands that limit their mobility and time commitments. It is illogical to expect family caregivers to conform their schedules around the office hours observed in the outpatient clinic. It is more expedient and reasonable to develop home-based "aftercare" programs for families who return to the community after the onset of a disability and its subsequent rehabilitation. Home-based support programs can come in many forms.

Long-distance technologies offer great potential for helping family caregivers in the home. In one clinical trial, nurses provided training in problem-solving skills to caregivers of persons following stroke rehabilitation in telephone sessions for 3 months after discharge (Grant et al. 2002). Caregivers receiving this training were significantly less depressed and reported greater satisfaction with services than those assigned to the control groups. Other studies have shown similar benefits for counseling and support provided to caregivers in telephone sessions (Roberts et al. 1995) and in videoconferences transmitted with either telephone (Elliott et al. 2008) or computer interface (Glueckauf et al. 2002), and in telephone sessions and occasional face-to-face visits in the home environment (Rivera et al. 2008).

There are also data that indicate family counseling may be effectively provided in Web-based applications (to families that have a teenage child with a seizure disorder, Hufford et al. 1999; to families that have a child with a brain injury, Wade et al. 2006a, 2006b). Moreover, family counseling provided with long-distance technologies appears to be as effective as outpatient office visits in reducing problems experienced by families, and families prefer the long-distance technologies over the traditional office visit (and it should be noted, not surprisingly, that clinicians preferred the traditional office visit; Glueckauf et al. 2002). Telephone and other long-distance technologies may also be used to provide caregiver access to support groups when mobility or distance issues impede actual participation (Brown et al. 1999).

Caregivers will also have informational needs that may not require interaction with a health care provider. For many persons, the Internet may be a viable option for accessing information. According to the most recent national survey (NAC 2009), caregivers turn first to the Internet for health information (29%), followed by consultation with doctors (28%), family or friends (15%), and other health professionals (10%). Of those who use the Internet, nearly 90% search for information about the care recipient's condition or treatment, more than half seek information about services available for care recipients, and 40% look for support or advice from other caregivers. About 58% of Americans age 50–64, 75% of 30–49-year-olds, and 77% of 18–29-year-olds currently go online (Fox 2004). Recent surveys of older Americans' use of the Internet indicate that the percent of seniors who go online has jumped by 47% from 2000 to 2004. Approximately 22% of Americans age 65 or older reported having access to the Internet, translating to about 8 million older Americans who actually use the Internet.

Interventions using this medium in caregiving have a strong potential to significantly reduce caregiver burden and to enhance the quality of life of their care recipients (Parker et al. 2002, 2003b, 2006; Roff et al. 2003). We believe that interactive health communications that take full advantage of these systems will provide important services to caregivers (Martin and Parker 2003), and recent surveys suggest that caregivers and care recipients agree. Unfortunately, family caregivers may find it difficult to digest the variety of largely untested, and highly variable information and resources available in the community and on the Internet, and this process is often further convoluted because caregivers must tailor the information they find to the particular needs of their family, often without the direct guidance of trusted professionals and experts.

## Caregiver Tasks, Readiness, and Preparation: An Essential Step

Family caregiving for persons with physical, neuromuscular, and developmental disabilities has not received the level of empirical attention afforded to caregiving associated with aging and age-related conditions. This has resulted in a lack of informed policy and gaps in the research and knowledge base. The intervention research concerning family caregivers of persons with disabilities, for example, lags far behind the gerontological literature in which many interventions and clinical trials have been reported. Similarly, family caregiver competencies—known to be critical elements in caring for elders—have not been identified or examined among caregivers of persons with disabilities.

For health care systems to develop a continuum of care and support in which empirically driven comprehensive assessment and service programs meet the ongoing and unique needs of family caregivers, it is imperative that we identify the key tasks that characterize effective caregiver preparation and readiness. This information would be fundamental to effective assessment of caregiver training and informational needs, as it would inform clinical practice and dictate the nature and quality of information available to caregivers in reading materials and in appropriate Internet sites for easy access.

In the field of gerontology, for example, Parker and colleagues (Parker 2002; Parker et al. 2003b) identified a total of 50 parent care tasks representing four domains (legal, medical, familial, and spiritual) through the systematic survey of adult caregivers and geriatric experts. Parker (2002) constructed a Parent Care Readiness Assessment (the first element of the Parent Care Readiness Program) by combining these tasks with a unique set of scoring algorithms based upon the Transtheoretical Model of Change (TMC; Prochaska and DiClemente 1983) to assess caregiver readiness to provide parent care. The TMC is a public health intervention model that matches readiness to change with the nature of the intervention. A four-factor solution was suggested that fits reasonably well a conceptualization of four domains: factor 1 was most associated with Legal–Financial themes; factor 2 was associated with Family-related tasks; factor 3 was equated to the Spiritual–Emotional domain; and factor 4 reflected the Medical Task dimension.

Using this approach, experts representing different disciplines can be surveyed to identify the common caregiving tasks associated with particular conditions. For example, family caregivers of persons with traumatic brain injury (TBI), along with state of science and practice physiatrists, rehabilitation psychologists, physical and occupational therapists, and home and nursing care experts, could be surveyed to identify the common tasks of caring for persons with TBI. Once valid and reliable tasks are identified and subjected to psychometric analysis, relevant domains of caregiving tasks can be confirmed, and state of science and practice resources and prescriptions prepared to assist family caregivers in completing high-priority tasks. Scoring mechanisms based on the characteristics of at-risk caregivers can be used to insure the relevancy of the prescriptions and recommendations provided. In short, this model provides health care providers and family caregivers with an automated assessment that leads to a tailored intervention that makes full use of available technologies to improve family caregiving competence at the point of need. In keeping with the life course model depicted in Fig. 9.1, the formulation of effective professional partnerships is viewed as essential in the ongoing caregiving experience.

We view the development of a caregiving plan as a dynamic ongoing process that involves the initial assessment of the landscape of possible tasks, and the completion

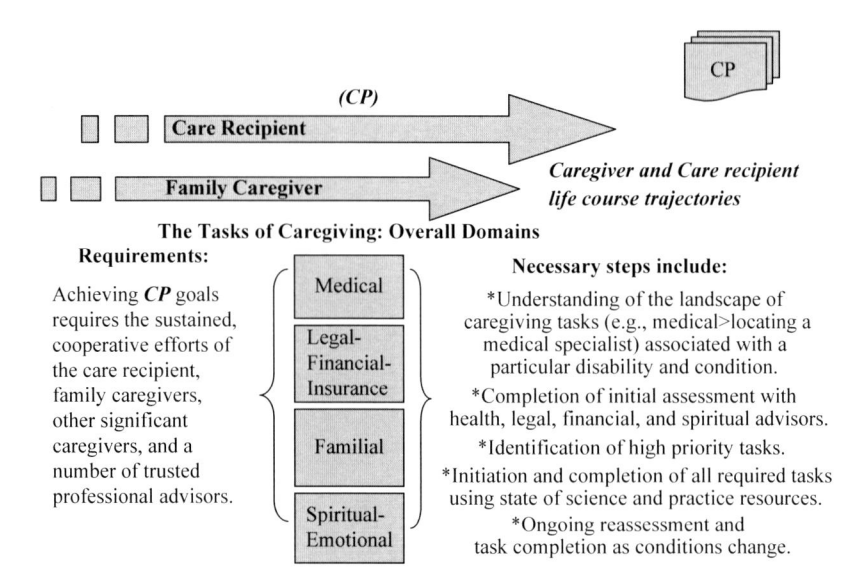

Fig. 9.1 A caregiving readiness model for developing and sustaining a comprehensive care plan

of specific tasks, followed by a reappraisal process as circumstances change. Using this approach, the caregiving plan consists of specific tasks that have been completed or are in the process of being completed. As the model illustrates, many of the tasks are complex and professionally intensive. For example, if the caregiver identifies a medical task related to the location of qualified neurologist who lives near the care recipient, the program can provide a list of qualified neurologists based on an extensive national and state resource directory that reliably captures this information and tailors geographically the informational needs for the caregiver and the family. Practitioners could use this information to locate accurate distant information for caregivers, and it may be particularly useful in assisting and directing underserved and disadvantaged caregivers who do not have access to as many resources.

Recently, the geriatric program developed using the model described in Fig. 9.1 has been formulated into a program residing on a web site (Stateofsciencecaregiving-Geriatrics.com). It consists of two primary components. The first component is a computerized self-scoring assessment instrument that will help family caregivers identify the most important tasks they need to complete to assist competently in the care of their care recipients. The second component is a series of computerized information packages (tailored prescriptions) specific to the particular caregiving needs of the end-user, as identified through the assessment the user has completed. The tailored prescriptions include URLs for top-notch Web sites as identified and recommended by some of the nation's most highly respected professionals in the field of aging as well as specific guidance about how the user can best approach each high-priority parent care task. Furthermore, the tailored prescriptions identify local resources specific to the city or county where the caregiver and/or care recipient reside. The primary target is middle-aged adults, most of whom are employed full time, who want to provide or assist in providing care for their frail elderly parents.

This procedure may be expanded in other ways. For example, future iterations may include features that allow caregivers to complete a life space assessment so providers may have an index of care recipient mobility in the home (Allman et al. 2004; Baker et al. 2003; Parker et al. 2001). This evidence-based assessment is commonly used in geriatric practice. Ultimately, a meaningful assessment of family and care recipient needs for long-term services and support (as encouraged by the Affordable Care Act; Reinhard et al. 2011) must encompass more than indicators of caregiver burden, activities of daily living and instrumental activities of daily living (Levine et al. 2010). A thorough assessment of medical tasks and managerial duties (including timing and frequency), financial challenges, care recipient behavioral problems, and co-occuring health conditions and impairments in the home are necessary to match the type and frequency of home-based services these families need (Elliott et al. 2011).

## Closing Observations

In this chapter, we have argued for a continuum of care and support that relies on active partnerships with family caregivers living in the community. We believe this approach is necessary for addressing the real-life needs of family caregivers, as it can utilize existing evidence concerning the relative needs and strengths of specific caregivers and incorporate caregiver input regarding the concerns unique to each caregiving scenario. We have also identified areas that require additional research in order for this continuum of care and support to be accomplished, and we have offered some examples from related (and relevant) areas that can inform the work we hope to see with family caregivers of persons with disabilities.

In presenting this proposal, we sidestepped three major issues that are salient to the everyday practitioner. We took a broad view of caregiving following disability, and we did confine our discussion to any single disability condition (SCI, TBI, cerebral palsy, etc.). We did not champion any single profession or discipline as the "practitioner" who would assume the lead in organizing and coordinating these programs for caregivers. In fact, we did not restrict our discussion to "rehabilitation" professions and referred to "health care providers" and "health care delivery systems." Finally, we did not address matters of funding and financial support for this continuum of care and support. No doubt many clinicians will leave our chapter wondering, "Who will pay for this?"

From our perspective, these are the very issues that keep this area and these issues Balkanized and fragmented in terms of actual practice and scientific inquiry. The emphasis on these "differences" overshadows the similarities and results in a competition for resources and control that effectively disenfranchises the family caregiver. As noted elsewhere, many health policy endeavors often have little to do with providing empirically driven cost-efficient health care and much to do with the distribution of financial and administrative resources to well-funded and active professional stakeholders (Shewchuk and Elliott 2000).

Practitioners have little influence in matters of health policy, yet all health care service delivery systems have much at stake in the efficient, rational, and ideally, scientifically informed provision of health care services. Recognizing and elevating the status of the family caregiver in the provision of health care to persons with severe disabilities is ultimately a policy issue that must be a stated priority for all stakeholders. This will require a more proactive stance that embraces a health promotion perspective, with the realization that a greater and strategic use of low-cost service providers (i.e., nondoctoral-level personnel) will be required to achieve cost-effective programs for families living with disability in our communities.

**Acknowledgments** This chapter was supported by grants to Timothy R. Elliott from the National Institute on Child Health and Human Development (1 R01 HD37661-01A3); the National Institute on Disability and Rehabilitation Research, Office of Special Education and Rehabilitative Services, U.S. Department of Education (grant numbers H133B90016 and H133A021927); and the National Center for Injury Prevention and Control and the Disabilities Prevention Program, National Center for Environmental Health (grant number R49/CCR412718-01).

The contents of this chapter are solely the responsibility of the authors and do not necessarily represent the official views of the funding agencies.

# References

Allman, R. M., Sawyer-Baker, P., Maisiak, R. M., Sims, R. V., & Roseman, J. M. (2004). Racial similarities and differences in predictors of mobility change over eighteen months. *Journal of General Internal Medicine, 19,* 1118–1126.

Baker, P. S., Bodner, E. V., & Allman, R. M. (2003). Measuring life-space mobility in community-dwelling older adults. *Journal of American Geriatric Society, 51,* 1610–1614.

Berry, J. W., Elliott, T., Grant, J., Edwards, G., & Fine, P. R. (in press). Does problem solving training for family caregivers benefit care recipients with severe disabilities? A latent growth model of the Project CLUES randomized clinical trial. *Rehabilitation Psychology*.

Billings, D. W., Folkman, S., Acree, M., & Moskowitz, J. (2000). Coping and physical health during caregiving: The roles of positive and negative affect. *Journal of Personality and Social Psychology, 79,* 131–142.

Bond, J. T., Galinsky, E., & Swanberg, J. E. (1998). *The 1997 national study of caregiving workforce.* New York: Family and Work Institute.

Braddock, D. (1999). Aging and developmental disabilities: Demographic and policy issues affecting American families. *Mental Retardation, 37,* 155–161.

Brodaty, H., Green, A., & Koschera, A. (2003). Meta-analysis of psychoeducational interventions for caregivers of persons with dementia. *Journal of the American Geriatrics Society, 51,* 657–664.

Brown, R., Pain, K., Berwald, C., Hirschi, P., Delehanty, R., & Miller, H. (1999). Distance education and caregiver support groups: Comparison of traditional and telephone groups. *Journal of Head Trauma Rehabilitation, 14,* 257–268.

Carter, R. (2008). Addressing the caregiver crises. *Preventing Chronic Disease, 5*(1), 1–2.

Chwalisz, K., & Stark-Wroblewski, K. (1996). The subjective experiences of spouse caregivers of persons with brain injuries: A qualitative analysis. *Applied Neuropsychology, 3,* 28–40.

Donelan, K., Falik, M., & DesRoches, C. (2001). Caregiving: Challenges and implications for women's health. *Women's Health Issues, 11,* 185–200.

Donelan, K., Hill, C. A., Hoffman, C., Scoles, K., Hoffman, P. H., Levine, C., & Gould, D. (2002). Challenged to care: informal caregivers in a changing health system. *Health Affairs, 21,* 222–231.

Eibner, C. (2008). *Invisible wounds of war: Quantifying the societal costs of psychological and cognitive injuries.* Testimony presented before the Joint Economic Committee on June 12, 2008. Santa Monica, CA: Rand Corporation.

Elliott, T., & Berry, J. W. (2009). Brief problem-solving training for family caregivers of persons with recent-onset spinal cord injury: A randomized controlled trial. *Journal of Clinical Psychology, 69,* 406–422.

Elliott, T., & Kurylo, M. (2000). Hope over disability: Lessons from one young woman's triumph. In C. R. Snyder (Ed.), *The handbook of hope: Theory, measures, and applications* (pp. 373–386). New York: Academic Press.

Elliott, T., & Pezent, G. (2008). Family caregivers of older persons in rehabilitation. *NeuroRehabilitation, 23,* 439–446.

Elliott, T., & Rivera, P. (2003). The experience of families and their carers in healthcare. In S. Llewelyn & P. Kennedy (Eds.), *Handbook of Clinical Health Psychology* (pp. 61–77). Oxford: Wiley & Sons.

Elliott, T., & Shewchuk, R. (2002). Using the nominal group technique to identify the problems experienced by persons who live with severe physical disability. *Journal of Clinical Psychology in Medical Settings, 9,* 65–76.

Elliott, T., Shewchuk, R., & Richards, J. S. (2001). Family caregiver problem solving abilities and adjustment during the initial year of the caregiving role. *Journal of Counseling Psychology, 48,* 223–232.

Elliott, T., Shewchuk, R., Richards, J. S., & Chen, Y. (2003, April). *Predicting changes in depression status in family caregivers of persons with recent spinal cord injuries.* Paper presented at the conference conducted by the Centers for Disease Control entitled *Safety in numbers: Working together from research into practice,* Atlanta.

Elliott, T., Brossart, D., Berry, J. W. & Fine, P. R. (2008). Problem-solving training via videoconferencing for family caregivers of persons with spinal cord injuries: A randomized clinical trial. *Behaviour Research and Therapy, 46,* 1220–1229.

Elliott, T., Phillips, C., Patnaik, A., Naiser, E., Fournier, C., Miller, T., Hawes, C., & Dyer, J. (2011). Medicaid personal care services and caregivers' reports of children's health: The dynamics of a relationship. *Health Services Research, 46,* 1803–1821.

Fiscella, K., Franks, P. & Shields, C. G. (1997). Perceived family criticism and primary care utilization: Psychosocial and biomedical pathways. *Family Process, 36,* 25–41.

Fiske, V., Coyne, J., & Smith, D. A. (1991). Couples coping with myocardial infarction: An empirical reconsideration of the role of overprotectiveness. *Journal of Family Psychology, 5,* 4–20.

Fox, S. (2004). *Older Americans and the Internet.* Internet & American Life Project, Washington, DC 20036. http://www.pewinternet.org. Accessed 24 April 2012.

Glueckauf, R. L., Fritz, S., Ecklund-Johnson, E., Liss, H., Dages, P., & Carney, P. (2002). Videoconferencing-based family counseling for rural teenagers with epilepsy: Phase 1 findings. *Rehabilitation Psychology, 47,* 49–72.

Grant, J., Elliott, T., Weaver, M. Bartolucci, A., & Giger, J. (2002). A telephone intervention with family caregivers of stroke survivors after hospital discharge. *Stroke, 33,* 2060–2065.

Grant, J., Elliott, T., Weaver, M., Glandon, G., & Giger, J. (2006). Social problem-solving abilities, social support, and adjustment of family caregivers of stroke survivors. *Archives of Physical Medicine and Rehabilitation, 87,* 343–350.

Hooker, K., Monahan, D., Bowman, S., Frazier, L., & Shifren, K. (1998). Personality counts for a lot: Predictors of mental and physical health of spouse caregivers in two disease groups. *Journals of Gerontology, 53B,* P73–P85.

Hufford, B. J., Glueckauf, R. L., & Webb, P. M. (1999). Home-base, interactive videoconferencing for adolescents with epilepsy and their families. *Rehabilitation Psychology, 44,* 176–193.

King, L. A., Scollon, C., Ramsey, C., & Williams, T. (2000). Stories of life transition: subjective well-being and ego development in parents of children with Down's syndrome. *Journal of Research in Personality, 34,* 509–536.

Kinsella, G., Ong, B., Murtagh, D., Prior, M., & Sawyer, M. (1999). The role of the family for behavioral outcome in children and adolescents following traumatic brain injury. *Journal of Consulting and Clinical Psychology, 67,* 116–123.

Knussen, C., Tolson, D., Swan, I., Stott, D., & Brogan, C. (2005). Stress proliferation in caregivers: The relationships between caregiving stressors and deterioration in family relationships. *Psychology & Health, 20,* 207–221.

Kramer, B. (1997). Gain in the caregiving experience: Where are we? What next? *The Gerontologist, 33,* 240–249.

Levine, C., Halper, D., Peist, A., & Gould, D. A. (2010). Bridging trouble waters: Family caregivers, Transitions, and long-term care. *Health Affairs 29,* 116–124.

Lollar, D. E., & Crews, J. (2003). Redefining the role of public health in disability. *Annual Review of Public Health, 24,* 195–208.

Long, M. P., Glueckauf, R. L., & Rasmussen, J. (1998). Developing family counseling interventions for adults with episodic neurological disabilities: Presenting problems, persons involved, and problem severity. *Rehabilitation Psychology, 43,* 101–117.

MaloneBeach, E., & Zarit, S. (1995). Dimensions of social support and social conflicts as predictors of caregiver depression. *International Psychogeriatrics, 7,* 25–38.

Martin, J., & Parker, M. W. (2003). Understanding the importance of elder care preparations in the context of 21st century military service. *Geriatric Care Management, 13,* 3–7.

Mechanic D. (1998). Public trust and initiatives for new health care partnerships. *Milbank Quarterly, 76,* 281–302.

Metropolitan Life Insurance Company. (2004). *Miles away: The MetLife study of long-distance caregiving*. Westport: MetLife Mature Market Institute.

Moen, P., Robison, J., & Fields, V. (2000). Women's work and caregiving roles: A life course approach. In E. P. Stoller & R. C. Gibson (Eds.), *Worlds of difference: Inequality in the aging experience* (3rd ed.). Thousand Oaks: Pine Forge Press.

National Alliance for Caregiving (2009). *Caregiving in the U.S.* http://www.caregiving.org/data/Caregiving_in_the_US_2009_full_report.pdf. Accessed 23 April 2012.

Navaie-Waliser, M., Feldman, P. H., Gould, D., Levine, C., Kuerbis, A., & Donelan, K. (2002). When the caregiver needs care: The plight of vulnerable caregivers. *American Journal of Public Health, 92,* 409–413.

Novack, T. A., & Richards, J. S. (1991). Coping with denial among family members. *Archives of Physical Medicine and Rehabilitation, 72,* 521.

Parish, S. L., Pomeranz-Essley, A., & Braddock, D. (2003). Family support in the United States: Financing trends and emerging initiatives. *Mental Retardation, 41*(3), 174–187.

Park, C. L. & Folkman, S. (1997). Stability and change in psychosocial resources during caregiving and bereavement in partners of men with AIDS. *Journal of Personality, 65,* 421–447.

Parker, M. (2002). *Parent care: Preparation and practical considerations for military families CD.* Tuscaloosa: University of Alabama.

Parker, M., Baker, P. S., & Allman, R. M. (2001). A life-space approach to functional assessment of mobility in the elderly. *Journal of Gerontological Social Work, 35*(4), 35–55.

Parker, M. W., Call, V. R., Dunkle, R., & Vaitkus, M. (2002). "Out of sight" but not "out of mind": Parent care contact and worry among military officers who live long distances from parents. *Military Psychology, 14,* 257–277.

Parker, M. W., Call, V. R., Toseland, R., Vaitkus, M., & Roff, L. (2003a). Employed women and their aging family convoys: A life course model of parent care assessment and intervention. *Journal of Gerontological Social Work, 40*(1), 101–122.

Parker, M. W., Roff, L., Toseland, R., & Klemmack, D. (2003b, March). *The Hartford military parent care project: A psycho-social educational intervention with long distance parent care providers.* Poster presented at First National Gerontological Social Work Conference, held in conjunction with Council of Social Work Education Annual Conference, Atlanta, GA.

Parker, M. W., Church, W., & Toseland, R. W. (2006). Caregiving at a distance. In B. Berkman & S. D'Ambruoso (Eds.), *Handbook on social work in health and aging* (pp. 391–406). New York: Oxford University Press,

Prochaska, J. O., & DiClemente, C. C. (1983). Stages and processes of self-change of smoking: toward an integrative model of change. *Journal of Consulting and Clinical Psychology, 51,* 390–395.

Quittner, A. L., Glueckauf, R., & Jackson, D. (1990). Chronic parenting stress: Moderating versus mediating effects of social support. *Journal of Personality and Social Psychology, 59,* 1266–1278.

Reinhard, S. C., Krassner, E., & Houser, A. (2011). How the Affordable Care Act can help move states toward a high-performing system of long-term services and supports. *Health Affairs, 30,* 447–453.

Rivara, J., Jaffe, K., Polissar, N., Fay, G., Liao, S., & Martin, K. (1996). Predictors of family functioning and change 3 years after traumatic brain injury in children. *Archives of Physical Medicine and Rehabilitation, 77,* 754–764.

Rivera, P., Elliott, T., Berry, J., & Grant, J. (2008). Problem-solving training for family caregivers of persons with traumatic brain injuries: A randomized controlled trial. *Archives of Physical Medicine and Rehabilitation, 89,* 931–941.

Roberts, J., Brown, G. B., Streiner, D., Gafni, A., Pallister, R., Hoxby, H., et al. (1995). Problem-solving counselling or phone-call support for outpatients with chronic illness: Effective for whom? *Canadian Journal of Nursing Research, 27*(3), 111–137.

Roff, L., Toseland, R., Martin, J., Fine, C., & Parker, M. W. (2003). Family-social tasks in long distance caregiving with military families. *Geriatric Care Management, 13,* 23–29.

Schulz, R. (2000). *Handbook on dementia caregiving, evidence-based interventions for family caregivers.* New York: Springer.

Schulz, R., & Beach, S. R. (1999). Caregiving as a risk factor for mortality: The caregiver health effects study. *Journal of the American Medical Association, 282,* 2215–2219.

Shewchuk, R., & Elliott, T. (2000). Family caregiving in chronic disease and disability: Implications for rehabilitation psychology. In R. G. Frank & T. Elliott (Eds.), *Handbook of rehabilitation psychology* (pp. 553–563). Washington: American Psychological Association Press.

Shewchuk, R., Richards, J. S., & Elliott, T. (1998). Dynamic processes in health outcomes among caregivers of patients with spinal cord injuries. *Health Psychology, 17,* 125–129.

Soskolne, V., Acree, M., & Folkman, S. (2000). Social support and mood in gay caregivers of men with AIDS. *AIDS & Behavior, 4,* 221–232.

Talley, R. C., & Crews, J. E. (2007). Framing the public health of caregiving. *American Journal of Public Health, 97,* 224–228.

Thompson, S. C., Medvene, L., & Freedman, D. (1995). Caregiving in the close relationships of cardiac patients: Exchange, power, and attributional perspectives on caregiver resentment. *Personal Relationships, 2,* 125–142.

Vitaliano, P. P., Zhang, J., & Scanlan, J. (2003). Is caregiving hazardous to one's physical health? A meta-analysis. *Psychological Bulletin, 129,* 946–972.

Vitaliano, P. P., Young, H., & Zhang, J. (2004). Is caregiving a risk factor for illness? *Current Directions in Psychological Science, 13,* 13–16.

Wade, S. L., Carey, J., & Wolfe, C. R. (2006a). An online family intervention to reduce parental distress following pediatric brain injury. *Journal of Consulting and Clinical Psychology, 74,* 445–454.

Wade, S. L., Carey, J., & Wolfe, C. R. (2006b). The efficacy of an online cognitive-behavioral family intervention in improving child behavior and social competence in pediatric brain injury. *Rehabilitation Psychology, 51,* 179–189.

Wagner, D., & Neal, M. (1994). Caregiving and work: Consequences, correlates and work responsibilities. *Educational Gerontology, 20,* 645–663.

Willer, B. S., Allen, K., Liss, M., & Zicht, M. (1991). Problems and coping strategies of individuals with traumatic brain injury and their spouses. *Archives of Physical Medicine and Rehabilitation, 72,* 460–464.

Williamson, G. M., & Schulz, R. (1995). Caring for a family member with cancer: Past communal behavior and affective reactions. *Journal of Applied Social Psychology, 25,* 93–116.

Wisensale, S. (2002). The inescapable balancing act: Work, family, and caregiving. *Gerontologist, 42,* 421–424.

Ybema, J., Kuijer, R., Bruunk, B., DeJong, G, & Sanderman, R. (2001). Depression and perceptions of inequity among couples facing cancer. *Personality and Social Psychology Bulletin, 27,* 3–13.

Ybema, J., Kuijer, R., Hagedoorn, M., & Bruunk, B. (2002). Caregiver burnout among intimate partners of patients with a severe illness: An equity perspective. *Personal Relationships, 9,* 73–88.

# Chapter 10
# Legal Issues Related to Caregiving for an Individual with Disabilities

Frank G. Bowe

United States policy acknowledges, but does not support, caregiving for individuals with disabilities. That is the conclusion I reached after researching the legal status of caregiving with people having disabilities. Our nation's policy is a patchwork quilt of laws that were drafted during very different periods of time, intended primarily to provide benefits for individuals with disabilities themselves. Caregivers generally were an afterthought. As a result, the federal government collects little information about caregivers, provides very little financial support for caregivers, imposes unnecessary barriers to caregivers, and needlessly complicates the work of caregivers.

Much information relevant to caregiving is available on the web. Particularly useful are the National Dissemination Center for Children with Disabilities (P.O. Box 1492, Washington, DC 20013; www.nichcy.org) and the Self-Help Group Sourcebook Online (http://mentalhelp.net/selfhelp). Where appropriate, Uniform Resource Locators (URLs) are offered in this chapter that assist interested readers to learn more.

To set the stage, a brief review is offered on the size and selected characteristics of persons with disabilities in the United States. We then examine what is known about their caregivers. Within each section, we explore implications for practice, education and training, research, and policy.

## Americans with Disabilities

The 2000 census found that approximately 50 million persons aged 5 years and over had disabilities (http://www.census.gov/prod/2003pubs/c2kbr-17.pdf), that is, about one in every five Americans. The census did not include persons residing in institutional settings; about two million such individuals have disabilities. Among

---

Frank G. Bowe is deceased.

---

Ronda C. Talley (✉)
e-mail: Ronda.Talley@wku.edu

John E. Crews
e-mail: jcrews@cdc.gov

persons aged 65 and over, 42% had physical, sensory, mental, or other disabilities. This is notable because that age cohort is about to explode, as the oldest members of the 76-million-strong "baby boom" generation reach retirement age. The proportion among working-age (16–64) individuals was much lower at 19%. Among children and youth in the 5–15 age range, just 6% had disabilities. The census bureau asked people if they had a condition that "substantially limits one or more basic physical activities such as walking" or if they were blind/visually impaired or deaf/hearing impaired, and if this/these condition(s) had lasted at least 6 months.

The number of Americans with disabilities rises for several reasons. First, medical technology today can save the lives of infants who in years past died prenatally, perinatally, or postnatally. These newborns do, in many instances, have disabilities. Second, improved diagnostic instruments and procedures today identify some disabilities that in years past escaped detection. This includes many individuals with attention deficit hyperactivity disorder (ADHD), milder forms of autism spectrum disorders, and some learning disabilities. Third, people with some disabilities are living much longer now than in years past. This author remembers discussing the projected postinjury lifespan of persons with quadriplegia (a class of spinal cord injury) with Howard A. Rusk in the mid-to-late 1970s. At that time, Dr. Rusk said, life expectancy was in the 5-year range. Today, it approaches that of persons with no disabilities. Fourth, the "pig in a python" effect of the 76-million-strong "baby boom" generation continues to be felt. The oldest members of this cohort turned 62 in 2008, and thus eligible to retire with Social Security benefits. As they, and others who follow, reach traditional retirement ages (assuming that the same proportions become disabled as was the case with past generations of persons in the 65+ age cohort, which is highly likely), they will add millions more to the ranks of Americans with disabilities.

In July 2005, the US Surgeon General, Richard Carmona, issued the first-ever *Surgeon General's Call to Action to Improve the Health and Wellness of Persons with Disabilities* (http://www.surgeongeneral.gov/library/disabilities). Prominent in the *Call to Action* was an appeal to increase knowledge of health care workers so that they may better diagnose and treat individuals with disabilities and arrange support services for them. The report cited research conducted by the Centers for Disease Control and Prevention (CDC) (see, e.g., the Crews and Talley (2012) chapter in this volume) showing that people with disabilities report their health as being worse than do persons without disabilities. The CDC analysis noted that those with disabilities are half as likely as are those with no disabilities to call their health "excellent." Conversely, they are four times as likely to describe it as fair or poor.

It is important, however, to note that many individuals with disabilities are healthy. A majority consider their health to be good or excellent, according to the National Health Interview Survey (NHIS) and the Current Population Survey (CPS), both of which are representative studies that sample about 50,000 households each year. This makes sense. People who were born deaf or blind, or with another disability, likely are healthy. Conversely, individuals with conditions such as diabetes may have poor health on a chronic or periodic basis throughout their lives.

Many Americans with disabilities function well without the need of caregivers. Millions, however, do require caregiving services. Those with intellectual disabilities (mental retardation) often need assistance with daily living, as well as financial support (www.thearc.org/faqs/respite.html). Individuals with physical disabilities frequently reside with family members, both because housing tends to be unaffordable and because it rarely is physically accessible. People with emotional conditions or autism, and many with Alzheimer's, may require support services in order to remain in community settings. In addition, persons with disabilities who are of working age are much less likely to be employed than are adults with no disabilities. For that reason, personal and family incomes tend to be well below national averages, compelling many adults to continue to reside with family members (see, e.g., Kaye 2003).

## Caregivers

We do not know how many Americans serve as caregivers for persons with disabilities. That fact is telling: no one has counted these adults. One estimate from a 1998 survey of 1,000 Americans suggests that there may be as many as 44 million caregivers in the United States and that 23% of all American adults had been "informal caregivers" during the past 12 months (Kaiser Family Foundation 2002, at www.kff.org/kaiserpolls/20020709-index.cfm). Another study, using a narrower definition of caregiving, estimated that 26 million caregivers have responsibility for one or more family members who have disabilities or other chronic health conditions (Lifespan Respite Care Act of 2006). An unknown number of nonfamily members serve as personal assistants. Their pay tends to be at or near minimum wage.

We do not know much about the health status of caregivers (i.e., whether they are themselves in need of health care, because of stress and burn-out). Most are believed to be women. An important 2004 study by the National Alliance for Caregiving and the American Association of Retired Persons (NAC-AARP 2004), *Caregiving in the U.S.* (http://www.caregiving.org/data/04finalreport.pdf) reported that nearly one out of every five (17%) of caregivers described their own health as fair or poor (Fig. 5). The Kaiser survey cited earlier noted that many caregivers acknowledged that their own health had suffered somewhat because of caregiving. I have seen this first-hand with family members, especially mothers, of children with such conditions as autism, ADHD, and a wide variety of physical and health impairments. The stress of unrelieved round-the-clock responsibilities combined with guilt feelings related to the underlying disability exacts a price. These caregivers often neglect their own health, fail to follow good nutrition principles, and as a result gain weight and even become diabetic. Researchers mining the Kaiser data have documented these occurrences nationwide (e.g., Donelan et al. 2002; Navaie-Waliser et al. 2002).

According to the National Long-Term Care Survey (2003), the services that caregivers provide cost about US$ 45 billion annually. Were their services to be compensated (family members typically serve without pay), annual expenses would rise to approximately US$ 95 billion. Another study, this one by the National Center on Women and Aging, estimated that caregivers lose, over a lifetime, some US$ 650,000 in foregone wages and retirement benefits (Women's Institute for a Secure Retirement 2004).

Caregiving may not be required on an in-person, round-the-clock basis. If so, research is needed in applying the always-on, high-speed, two-way voice/video/data technology known as broadband to caregiving. As recently demonstrated in the US House of Representatives, broadband potentially could allow a small group of support workers to provide continuous, round-the-clock, assistance to individuals with disabilities at times when in-person services are not required. That is, the technology may extend the reach of service personnel, conserve public resources, and provide remote assistance on an as-needed basis (Bowe 2005).

## National Policies on Caregiving and Persons with Disabilities

The nation's laws related to caregiving for individuals with disabilities include several offering respite care. These are poorly funded and in many cases optional rather than mandatory programs. Other important policies relate to medical care and to family leave. The national policies on accessible and affordable housing are few and grossly inadequate for one of the very few, see "Opening Doors" at the website of the Consortium for Citizens with Disabilities (http://www.c-c-d.org).

### *Personal Assistance Services*

Personal Assistance Services (PAS) are the caregiving services provided to individuals with disabilities who require these for daily living. Included are bathing, dressing, administering of medication, and related functions. The term formerly was Personal Care Assistance, for which reason the acronym "PCA" is sometimes still used. PAS is available in most states under Medicaid (see below).

Some 1.2 million individuals with disabilities receive PAS support from Medicaid home and community-based waiver programs (Kitchener and Harrington 2001) and from personal care benefit programs offered by states under the Medicaid option program (LeBlanc et al. 2001). Some obtain these services with the aid of a nearby center for independent living (CIL). There are 600+ centers in the United States. To find local centers, people go to the Independent Living Resource Utilization website at www.ilru.org, in Houston, TX.

The ILRU strongly recommends that persons with disabilities themselves do the screening, hiring, training, and supervising of PAS aides. This is a reflection of the disability-rights movement's desire to define "independent living" as, in large part, consumer control. The philosophy is one that emphasizes that while people with severe disabilities may not always be able to do things themselves, they can decide who will do them, when, and how.

Under Medicaid policy, however, PAS providers are to be selected and assigned by accredited home care or case management agencies, not by the persons who consume their services. That policy has long been opposed by disability rights advocates. A demonstration project supported by the Robert Wood Johnson Foundation and the US Department of Health and Human Services (HHS), and performed by Mathematica Policy Research Inc., of Princeton, NJ, recently showed that the advocates may be right. The survey, "Improving the Quality of Medicaid Personal Assistance Through Consumer Direction," found that reported incidents of neglect were 58% fewer when consumers directed PAS services as compared to when agencies did, that consumer satisfaction was much higher with consumer control, and that costs often were lower, as well (Foster et al. 2003).

These findings reflect the fact that the PAS providers in the study were actually employees of the individuals with disabilities, rather than of the community agencies. This meant that consumers had much greater control: they hired, supervised, and at times fired assistants. By contrast, when the services were contracted through an agency, the consumer could only complain about, but not act upon, problems with the employee. That led to very different relationships between PAS providers and consumers. This is one reason why some states differ from Medicaid. California's MediCal, for example, allows consumers themselves to hire and supervise the care workers.

Another aspect of current policy is that PAS providers may not be related to consumers (that is, members of the same immediate or extended family). This policy reflects recognition by government at the federal, state, and county levels that most current providers of PAS are family members. Were these relatives to be eligible for pay from public programs, the fear is that costs would escalate out of control. The Mathematica study suggests that this may not be true. The demonstration project allowed consumers to hire family members. Costs were not reported to be higher in that event. And consumers did on occasion fire the family members.

The Bureau of Labor Statistics projects very strong demand for PAS over the coming decades (http://stats.bls.oco/home.htm). This reflects the graying of America, the preference of many elders to remain in communities rather than go into nursing homes, and the deinstitutionalization of many individuals with disabilities pursuant to the US Supreme Court's decision in Olmstead. That decision interpreted the 1990 Americans with Disabilities Act to mean, among other things, that persons who have been placed into state facilities should be allowed to live, instead, in the community, where they should receive support services, including PAS. The Court's decision applies to individuals who are judged, by treating physicians, to be capable of living independently or semi-independently outside of institutional settings (http://www.cms.hhs.gov/olmstead/default.asp).

The implications for practice, education and training, research, and practice are numerous. With respect to practice, we need uniform standards for PAS, including personnel qualifications, consumer direction, living wages, and procedures to prevent and respond to any instances of PAS providers abusing, stealing from, or otherwise taking advantage of consumers. Training for PAS workers needs to be much more widely available than it is today. These persons are not nurses and the work they do is not properly classified as home-health care. Rather, they support individuals with severe disabilities in performing *personal* tasks so that they may then engage in work or other productive activities. Training should reflect these duties. Research is needed to expand upon the few demonstration projects currently underway, so that a foundation is established for systems change. With respect to policy, the findings in Arkansas and other states with respect to consumer direction and family members need to be incorporated into ongoing government policy, rather than limited to waivers or other demonstration projects.

## *Respite Care*

Caring for individuals who have severe disabilities can be exhausting. A child, adolescent, or adult with autism may not follow the unwritten rules of social conduct. Even waiting in line, or not taking food from other people's plates, may be beyond the ken of these persons. The stress of monitoring their behavior every hour of every day, and dealing with almost daily crises, can debilitate even the most energetic and devoted of caregivers. Similarly, the physical and medical needs of many individuals with cerebral palsy, spina bifida, and spinal cord injuries can tax the will and patience of any caregiver. The needs of many of these persons for durable medical equipment and for assistive technology devices necessitate, in most cases, ongoing battles with Medicaid over purchase of the required equipment. People with intellectual disabilities commonly need around-the-clock support. So do many people with advanced cases of Alzheimer's. Respite care, a service that offers short-term relief for caregivers, thus is often an essential service. It can provide a weekend, or even an evening, of "escape" from relentless pressure. Many persons with disabilities also appreciate respite care, recognizing how it lessens the burden on primary caregivers.

The Individuals with Disabilities Education Act (IDEA) (20 U.S.C. 1400 et seq.), the nation's landmark special-education law, authorizes respite services as "early intervention services" in Part C—infants and toddlers. States may support respite care for families having children with disabilities under the age of 3 years. However, since federal appropriations are limited, and since funds are not reserved for this purpose, the availability of respite care varies greatly from state to state. Three states with extensive programs are Texas (Texas Respite Resource Network, P.O. Box 7330, Station A, San Antonio, TX 78207-3198), Maine (Maine Respite Project, 159 Hogan Road, Bangor, ME 04401), and Georgia (Georgia Respite Network, 878 Peachtree St., NE, Room 620, Atlanta, Georgia 30901). Information is available via the "Respite Locator" website (http://www.respitelocator.org).

The Older Americans Act (42 U.S.C. 2020 et seq.) contains, in title III, a National Family Caregiver Support Program. Created in 2000, this program offers relief and support to caregivers who provide unpaid and/or informal care for persons who are elderly, including those who have disabilities. It also supports older persons who care for children under the age of 18 years. The program has never been fully funded. It does, however, finance some training resources through the National Family Caregiver Support Program Resources, including brief fact sheets on caring for individuals with developmental disabilities and on balancing duties with one's private life (both are at: http://www.aoa.gov/press/nfc_month/2004/fact_sheets).

The Public Health Service Act established the Lifespan Respite Care Program (Public Law No. 109-442) in 2006. This legislation offers grant funds to encourage states to create and maintain respite care programs serving children and adults with disabilities and other special needs.

These laws (and, in the case of the Public Health Service Act, bill) fall far short of meeting the need. With the federal deficit at an all-time record high and with many states in fiscal distress, it is not likely that existing programs will be fully funded, nor that extensive new ones will be created any time soon.

The implications for practice are self-evident. Respite care needs to be recognized for what it is: a profession that supplies much-needed services. The implications for education and training are equally obvious. The legislation assume that respite-care providers know what to do. In fact, however, most learn on-the-go. They rely on informal networks of special educators, rehabilitation counselors, and family friends for training. Research is needed to identify the nature and extent of caregivers' needs for respite care, and to tell us what are the most effective and cost-efficient models for providing respite care. As for policy, we need to greatly expand respite care making it available in all 50 states.

## Medical Care

The major sources of support in the area of medical care are Medicaid, Medicare, and private insurance. The Family and Medical Leave Act assures caregivers that they may attend to family emergencies without fear of losing employment, although they do forego pay during leave.

### *Medicaid*

Medicaid (42 U.S.C. 1396 et seq.) is the federal-state medical insurance program for people who are both poor and either have disabilities or are elderly (http://cms.hhs.gov/medicaid). Medicaid actually is 56 separate programs, because each of the 50 states and the six other entities (the District of Columbia, the four US territories, and Puerto Rico) designs its own program, including state options. Typically, Medicaid is provided when individuals with disabilities qualify for Supplemental Security Income (SSI).

The importance of Medicaid for caregiving is largely in the fact that it covers long-term care, including home-health, nursing-home, or other institutional care. Coverage of institutional care is mandatory, while community-based alternatives are allowed only under "waivers." Iowa, for example, has a "1115 demonstration waiver" called IowaCare. Approved by the federal Centers for Medicare & Medicaid Services (CMS) through mid-2010, the program moves Iowa from an institution-based to a community-based program for persons with long-term psychiatric illnesses. The institutional bias in Medicaid has frustrated families and individuals with disabilities for many years. A bill to reverse the bias—to favor community integration and the support services required to make it successful—has been introduced into every Congress for more than a decade. Now known as the Community Choice Act (formerly MiCASSA: Medicaid Community-Based Attendant Services and Supports Act), it would, if enacted, require that states offer community attendant services and supports as well as institutional care for eligible individuals in need of long-term services and supports. It will also assist states to develop and enhance comprehensive statewide systems of long-term services and supports that provide people with disabilities a choice as to where they receive these supports and services. The legislation would provide additional federal support for community support program and would serve people with greater incomes to increase employment opportunities (http://www.adapt.org/casaintr.htm).

In order to qualify for SSI, and through it for Medicaid, however, individuals and families of persons with disabilities who are under the age of 18 years must "spend down" by ridding themselves of most tangible and financial assets. Only if countable resources (such "liquid assets" as savings, stocks, bonds, etc.) do not exceed US$ 2,000 for one person or US$ 3,000 for a family will coverage be offered. In many cases, an irrevocable trust makes sense. In others, transferring assets to relatives (such as children) may be effective. A 1999 law offers an option that avoids both spend-downs and asset transfers. The Ticket to Work and Work Incentives Improvement Act allows states to present options for people to purchase Medicaid coverage. Generally, individuals with incomes below 250% of the poverty line (that is, less than 2.5 times the federal poverty level) may pay premiums for coverage. The importance of this provision is that people and families need not impoverish themselves in order to qualify for vital Medicaid services. For details, see http://www.cms.hhs.gov/twwiia/eligible.asp.

All of this suggests that Medicaid is a complex and often arcane program. It is helping people to keep up with the many rules of Medicaid is the Medicaid Aged, Blind, and Disabled Eligibility Resource Center (http://www.cms.hhs.gov/medicaideligibility/). Visitors to the site may search for state-specific regulations. A second resource is the website of the National Council on Aging (NCOA), which offers a "Benefits Checkup" page that people may use to learn about eligibility for different benefits (http://www.ncoa.org/content.cfm?sectionID=23). Also helpful are the Policy Level Guidelines issued annually by the US Department of Health and Human Services that spell out eligibility criteria for Medicaid, food stamps, and other means-tested programs (http://aspe.hhs.gov/poverty/03poverty.htm; U.S. Department of Health and Human Services 2005). Even with such resources, the regulations are so complex and the task of securing coverage so challenging that an entire industry has sprung up to advise families on Medicaid, especially about rules on spending down.

Medicaid commonly reimburses costs for assistive technology devices and services. (Medicare, by contrast, covers only durable medical equipment that is prescribed by a physician as medically necessary.) Individuals with physical disabilities and many who have communication-related conditions such as cerebral palsy require assistive technology devices for everyday living, for communication, and for employment. The devices do not obviate the need for personal caregiving services (Hoenig et al. 2003). However, they can relieve that need. A survey conducted by the National Council on Disability (NCD) in 1993 reported that individuals with disabilities who rated their quality of life without assistive technology at "3" (on a scale of 1–10) raised their ratings to "7" when they considered the added benefits of assistive technologies (National Council on Disability 1993). To state that Medicaid can reimburse families for the costs of assistive technologies is not to say that securing such reimbursements is easy. It can require months, and even years, to secure the needed products.

Despite its many problems, millions of Americans with disabilities regard Medicaid as essential. They need the assurance that this federal-state program offers. Employer-supported health care often is not available for jobs that these persons qualify to perform. Such health plans typically exclude coverage of "pre-existing conditions" (disabilities are by definition pre-existing conditions). Were the individual to lose his/her job, the health coverage could be taken away. Employers are required to offer former workers continued coverage, pursuant to the Consolidated Omnibus Budget Reconciliation Act (COBRA). However, the ex-employee must pay 100% of the premium, and many cannot afford to do so.

## *Medicare*

Persons with disabilities who receive Social Security Disability Insurance (SSDI) and those who are on Old Age and Survivors Insurance (OASDI)—what most of us refer to as "Social Security"—typically also qualify for Medicare. Medicare (42 U.S.C. 1395 et seq.) is the federal medical-insurance program for older people. Created in 1965, Medicare still retains the "end-of-life" focus upon "hospital-like" services and products (in 1965, age expectancy for persons aged 65 years or over was much shorter than it is today). Medicare will cover, for example, short- but not long-term hospitalization, and wheelchairs but not other assistive technology devices. It covers nursing-home care only for 100 days, and provides only limited home-health care. And only recently has Medicare covered prescription drugs (www.medicare.gov).

## *Private Insurance*

When people have private insurance, they often can use it to cover many expenses related to care for children and other family members. When disability occurs, private health insurance policies (usually linked to employment) characteristically will pay for whatever assistive technology devices and services are required, and sometimes modifications to the family home up to a limit (cap on coverage). Typically, coverage is capped at US$ 1 million or less. While this seems to be a lot of money, the reality is that expenses often exceed that amount within the first few years, leaving the individual and the family without adequate resources. Note, too, that many private insurance policies track Medicare: they will not approve services that Medicare would not allow. For many adults with disabilities, private health insurance is either unavailable or unaffordable. These persons may only qualify for jobs that do not offer employer-provided health care. If private insurance is supplied, pre-existing condition exclusions may render it useless at least for the first year or so of employment. Premiums may be so costly that the worker cannot afford to pay them. All of this helps to explain why so many families are willing to "spend down" to qualify for Medicaid.

Long-term care insurance is available. However, it is often very costly. Someone who is 65 years of age could pay US$ 4,000 annually for such coverage with no assurance of ever needing it. In addition, eligibility usually is restricted, primarily to disqualify anyone already diagnosed with a condition that is likely to require long-term care.

## *Family and Medical Leave Act*

The Family and Medical Leave Act of 1993 (29 U.S.C. 2654) entitles most workers to unpaid leaves of absence for up to 3 months to care for a family member. Companies and not-for-profits having 50 or more workers must comply with FMLA. They may not place the employee's job in jeopardy because of the leave (http://www.dol.gov/esa/whd/fmla).

## Implications

The implications of medical-care laws are several. With respect to practice, perhaps the most critical need is to help people to learn what is available and how they may qualify. The implications for education and training are pressing. State- and local-based staffs who administer Social Security, Supplemental Security Income, Medicaid, and Medicare often are not familiar with the rules governing these programs. Some employers, notably small companies, may not know their obligations under the Family and Medical Leave Act. The inevitable result of all this is that decisions are often arbitrary. To illustrate the scope of the problem, the Social Security Administration must employ more administrative law judges to hear complaints than are in the entire federal court system. Research can help us to project future needs for medical insurance and other protections, particularly as the baby boom generation moves into the retirement years.

With regard to policy, Medicare and Medicaid are both in desperate need of overhaul. Medicare needs drastic revision to reflect the fact that people aged 62 or 65 years no longer die within a few years. Rather, life expectancy may be to the mid-80s. As for Medicaid, it must be streamlined and simplified. There are just too many rules, regulations, and policies. SSI and Medicaid also should be made available to persons with disabilities regardless of employment status. It makes no sense to restrict eligibility only to persons who have demonstrated an inability to work. Finally, both health insurance programs are well-known to be at risk financially. Medicaid, for example, costs half the states more than they receive in tax revenues and federal assistance. Medicare is a federal-only program. The trustees of the Federal Hospital Insurance (HI) and the Supplementary Medical Insurance (SMI) trust funds report annually to Congress on these trust funds' short- and long-term financial health. The 2005 report estimates that Medicare will remain solvent until 2020. Policy reforms that enable both to continue, albeit with different rules on eligibility and coverage, are urgently required.

## *Housing*

The Fair Housing Amendments Act of 1988 (42 U.S.C. 3601 et seq.) offers some help to caregivers and to individuals with disabilities. It is, however, grossly inadequate to meet the need. Caregiving for persons with disabilities would be much easier were housing to be more accessible and more affordable than it is. Sadly, only 1–2% of the nation's housing stock (private homes, apartments, condominiums, etc.) is physically accessible. And even those homes and units seldom are affordable for Americans with disabilities.

A recent initiative, known as "visitable" housing, offers some hope. Spawned by the Georgia-based organization Concrete Change, it calls for residential housing to be visitable by persons using wheelchairs or other mobility aids. In practice, that means a house would have an entry point flush with the ground (perhaps via a ramp), first-floor doors and halls that are 32 in. or wider, and an accessible half-bath or bathroom on the ground floor. Visitable houses are not accessible homes; there is no requirement for upper floor rooms to have wide doors, for example. The group has a video describing its goals at http://www.concretechange.org. There are "visitable housing" laws in Georgia, Texas, and some other states; Florida has a "bathroom law."

The scope of the problem is staggering. Private homes are exempt from accessibility rules. For that reason, when a family member sustains a severe medical condition, especially one that results in a physical disability, the family residence is virtually never physically accessible. Tens of thousands of dollars are required to renovate the house to make it accessible. While the family could, in theory, move, the reality is that there are very few accessible homes to which they could move. The 1988 Fair Housing Amendments Act covers only new (post-1991) multifamily (four or more units) housing. In many parts of the country, few if any, apartment, condominium, or other multiunit buildings have been constructed since 1991.

Affordability is another critical concern. A recent study, *Priced Out in* 2002, reported that in 2002 for the first time ever the average monthly rent exceeded the average SSI monthly check (O'Hara and Cooper 2003). Someone with a disability who relies on SSI would have no funds remaining after paying rent to cover food, clothing, and other life necessities. The study also reported that at least 640,000 adults with severe disabilities are forced, for financial reasons, to live at home with aging parents.

Public housing ("projects") is affordable. However, only a small fraction of the units in the typical public housing projects are accessible. Federal law requires that only 5% of apartments in newly built projects be physically accessible (www.hud.gov/offices/fheo/disabilities/accessibilityR.cfm). The major federal program for constructing accessible public housing, section 811 of the Fair Housing Act (42 U.S.C. 11381 et seq.), is tragically underfunded. In the face of demand from millions of Americans with disabilities, just 3,000 accessible units are built each year. Group homes are an important option for many people with disabilities. However, there are sizeable numbers of such homes only in five states, and even in those five states, the supply falls far short of meeting the demand (www.usdoj.gov/crt/housing/final8_1.htm).

The implications for practice, education and training, research, and policy are numerous. With regard to practice, we urgently need to catalog the existing stock of accessible housing. Millions of American families are desperately searching for such units. Yet, aside from a few small registries (e.g., the Massachusetts registry at www.massaccesshousingregistry.org and the Connecticut one at www.housingregistry.com) the necessary resources are scarce. Special educators, rehabilitation counselors, public advocates, and other social-service professionals need to be trained to identify the few sources of financial assistance available to persons with disabilities and caregivers who seek accessible and affordable housing options. Research is needed to document the scope of the accessible- and affordable-housing crisis (the occasional "Priced Out" series is one of only a handful of such studies). Finally, the nation needs to confront the fact that the aging of the baby boom generation necessitates the creation of new policies, notably the imposition of rules, disagreeable as they may be to some, calling for accessibility in virtually all new private residences.

## Problems, Gaps, and Implications

The facts discussed above reveal deep-seated problems, wide gaps in coverage, and other issues that have important implications for practice, education and training, research, and policy.

### *Practice*

Practice in caregiving should feature consumer control, with the individual making the key decisions about what is done, when, how, and by whom. For persons who are not able to make those decisions, consumer control specifies that a consumer's representative, chosen by the individual with a disability, will make them. This is well-established (e.g., Foster et al. 2003) and a key feature of the MiCASSA bills.

MiCASSA would require states to develop quality assurance programs, including grievance and appeal procedures for consumers and mechanisms for reporting abuse and neglect. States that failed to comply would be federally sanctioned.

## *Education/Training*

Training for consumers should be voluntary, as specified in the MiCASSA bills, and should include selection of attendants, their supervision, and, as necessary, termination of their services. Training for caregivers should be offered in a wide variety of modalities, including distance education, and should extend beyond health care to incorporate other aspects of necessary support services, including how to assist someone to learn and retain self-help skills, to dress and bathe, to prepare for and engage in paid work, to travel around the community, to shop, and to perform personal financial transactions.

## *Research*

We need to continue the kind of research that was done by Mathematica (Foster et al. 2003) so that the most effective and efficient service models developed by the states under Medicaid waivers and other projects and programs are brought together and made widely available to policy makers and service providers alike. We need much more information about the characteristics, health care needs, and training of caregivers throughout the nation. If research were to substantiate the promise of broadband to support remote caregiving services when in-person assistance is not required, the cost-effectiveness of this option needs to be established. And we need research that identifies the national, state, county, and local status of accessible housing stock. Creating a national consensus around accessibility in residential housing will require a much more complete picture than we now have about how many one- and two-family homes are accessible, how many apartments and condominiums are either accessible or readily modified to become accessible.

## *Policy*

As for policy, of the laws reviewed in this chapter, the most important likely is Medicaid. It is worth reiterating that Medicaid is actually 56 different programs. Some state Medicaid programs offer work incentives, such as the Medicaid Buy-In program, that allow employed persons with disabilities to purchase Medicaid coverage in the event that employer-provided health care is not available. Other states, however, do not. Very few states have examined the potential for conflicts between their buy-in programs and the Medicare Modernization Act's Part D prescription drug program. A Kaiser Commission on Medicaid report suggests that buy-in participants may encounter trouble securing needed drugs and may end up paying much more for them (http://www.aphsa.org/disabilities).

PAS services are currently state-option services under Medicaid. The state-to-state variability of Medicaid serves as a disincentive for families to move (if, for example, they find an accessible home in another state). Were the family to relocate, it may well discover that critical services are not available in the new state. In addition, the family would be at the bottom of the waiting list for many key Medicaid-related services. Placement into group homes is an example. Even in New York and Michigan, which have the most extensive group-home programs, waiting lists for such placements are in excess of 7 years.

The fact that people who retire at or about age 65–70 years now have life expectancies into the 80s needs to be reflected in Medicare policies. It no longer makes sense, as it did in 1965 when the program began, for Medicare to limit key services to short periods of time and to cover only durable medical equipment. PAS is another area in which policy needs to catch up with demand. The current patchwork of waivers and demonstration projects does not suffice to meet the need. Rather, PAS should become as standard a component of services as is universal pre-K, full-day kindergarten, and other changes in national policy.

## Conclusions

A nation that recognized the importance of the work performed by caregivers, including PAS workers, would provide for their training and for their availability where needed. At present, the United States offers little education for these persons and supports their services only in selected States. A nation that valued caregiving, whether provided by family members or by paid employees, would provide health insurance, retirement benefits, and financial compensation they deserve, as well as the respite care these persons need, given the often-draining nature of their work. Similarly, Medicaid and other key programs would foster, not constrain, caregiving in the home and community, rather than in impersonal institutional settings.

A country that acknowledged the obvious fact that tens of millions of its citizens need accessible and affordable housing would insist upon physical accessibility at least in new construction and would support the building of large numbers of affordable housing units. The United States at present does neither. The time has come for change.

In these and other ways, as this paper shows, our nation lacks a coherent policy on caregiving. Instead, we are tapping into a hodgepodge of laws and programs that were designed for other purposes, hoping that they somehow will meet the need. Research cited in this chapter dashes that hope. We can no longer deny the realities that research has brought to our attention. The lack of a national policy on caregiving affects about one American in every five (because 20–23% of adults are caregivers in any given 1-year period). The foregone wages, retirement benefits, and other sacrifices people make in order to provide caregiving services now add up, over a lifetime, to more than half a million dollars per caregiver. Caregivers are, in many cases, placing their own health at risk because they are not provided with the support that they themselves need, including respite services.

What would a sound caregiving policy look like? It would, first of all, recognize a public responsibility, and not insist that all caregiving is "private" and "voluntary." For starters, we need to quantify the problem, in all its dimensions. How many people are caregivers? How many are trained for the work, which often rises to the level of skilled care? What is their health status? Then we need to review all caregiving-related laws, regulations, and policies, so as to specify exactly where existing rules constrain caregiving. An example: Consumer control over PAS is known to work. Why not revise the rules that permit it only in demonstration projects and under waiver? Another: Why need we tie eligibility for PAS services to Medicaid and SSI? The nation should not force people with disabilities to choose between services they need for survival and quality of life, on the one hand, and pursuit of the American dream on the other.

A good policy move beyond the "my home is my castle" idea of private homeownership being exempt from architectural requirements and say, instead, that the graying of America makes it in the public interest that all residences, including single-family homes, be at least visitable and preferably accessible. It would feature Medicaid, Medicare, and private health insurance policies that support care in the home and community, rather than being biased in favor of institutional care. There would be robust systems—facilities such as group homes, a strong supply of well-trained support workers, and the like—that would seamlessly assume parental responsibilities after young people age out of special education at 18–21 years of age.

Finally, a coherent national policy on caregiving would include greatly needed and long-overdue overhauls of both Medicaid and Medicare. Medicaid already costs states more than does education and many other human services. Despite the fact that states have shown real creativity in fashioning ways to improve the 50-year-old medical insurance program, federal law still requires them to seek waivers for each innovation. As for Medicare, its orientation to end-of-life services and institutional care is badly out of date. Reforming it will not only help persons who are retired or on Social Security Disability Insurance but also—because many private health policies track Medicare—privately insured individuals and families as well.

# References

Bowe, F. (2005, June 16). *Two-way technologies: A history of the struggle to communicate*. Paper presented at a demonstration for the U.S. House of Representatives. http://people.hofstra.edu/faculty/frank_g_bowe/two-way_technologies.html. Accessed 25 April 2012.

Crews, J. E., & Talley, R. C. (2012). Introduction: Multiple dimensions of caregiving and disability. In R. C. Talley (Series Ed.) and R. C. Talley & J. E. Crews (Vol. Eds.), *Multiple dimensions of caregiving and disability*. New York: Springer (Editor's Note: This volume).

Donelan, K., Hill, C. A., Hoffman, C., Scoles, K., Feldman, P. H., Levine, C., & Gould, D. (2002). Challenged to care: Informal caregivers in a changing health system. *Health Affairs, 21*, 222–231.

Foster, L., Brown, R., Phillips, B., Schore, J., & Carlson, B. L. (2003). *Improving the quality of Medicaid personal assistance through consumer direction*. Princeton: Mathematica Policy Research. http://content.healthaffairs.org/cgi/reprint/hlthaff.w3.162v1?hits=10&FIRSTINDEX=0&AUTHOR1=Foster&FULLTEXT=Medicaid&SEARCHID=1&gca=healthaff%3Bhlthaff.w3.162v1&allch=citmgr&. Accessed 25 April 2012.

Hoenig, H., Taylor, D. H., & Sloan. F. A. (2003). Does assistive technology substitute for personal assistance among the disabled elderly? *American Journal of Public Health, 93,* 330–337.

Kaye, H. S. (2003). *Improved employment opportunities for people with disabilities.* (Disability Statistics Report 17). Washington, DC: U.S. Department of Education, National Institute of Disability and Rehabilitation Research.

Kitchener, M., & Harrington, C. (2001). *Medicaid 1915(c) home and community based waivers: Program data, 1992–1999.* San Francisco: University of California.

LeBlanc, A., Tonner, C., & Harrington, C. (2001, Summer). State Medicaid programs offering personal care services. *Health Care Financing Review, 22*(4), 155–173.

Lifespan Respite Care Act of 2006. S. 1283 and HR 3248. http://thomas.loc.gov (109th Congress). Accessed 25 April 2012.

National Alliance for Caregiving & American Association of Retired Persons. (2004). *Caregiving in the U.S.* Washington, DC: Author. http://www.caregiving.org/data/04finalreport.pdf. Accessed 25 April 2012.

National Council on Disability. (1993). *Study on the financing of assistive technology devices and services for individuals with disabilities.* Washington, DC: Author.

National Long-Term Care Survey. (2003). *What is the NLTCS?* http://cds.duke.edu/nltcs/index.htm. Accessed 25 April 2012.

Navaie-Waliser, M., Spriggs, A., & Feldman, P. H. (2002). Informal caregiving: Differential experiences by gender. *Medical Care, 40,* 1249–1259.

O'Hara, A., & Cooper, E. (2003). *Priced out in 2002.* Boston: Technical Assistance Collaborative. www.tacinc.org. Accessed 25 April 2012.

U.S. Department of Health and Human Services. (2005). *The Surgeon General's call to action to improve the health and wellness of persons with disabilities.* Washington, DC: Department of Health and Human Services, Office of the Surgeon General.

Women's Institute for a Secure Retirement. (2004). *Financial steps for caregivers: What you need to know about money and retirement: A WISER guide.* Washington, DC: National Association of Area Agencies on Aging. http://www.aoa.gov/prof/aoaprog/caregiver/WISER.pdf.

# Chapter 11
# Long-Term Care Planning for Individuals with Developmental Disabilities

**Deborah Viola and Peter S. Arno**

More than 5 million children and young adults with developmental disabilities are cared for by their parents (National Association of Councils on Developmental Disabilities 2011). With respect to long-term care planning, they are not a priority of researchers, advocates, legislators, and funders. At least a quarter of the people with developmental disabilities are cared for by their parents and caregivers who are 60 years or older (New York State Family Caregiver Council 2009; Statewide Caregiving and Respite Coalition of New York 2011). Working parents provide at least 10 hours per week attending to their children's health care needs, and, as a result, their own wages and health suffer (U.S. Department of Health and Human Services (HHS) 2008). Our traditional model of long-term care is narrow and short-sighted. The Class Act, which was part of health care reform and has since been withdrawn, would have provided some financial assistance for long-term care to those who worked and contributed to the plan. Yet, less than a third of those with intellectual disabilities actually work (U.S. Equal Employment Opportunity Commission 2009). Perhaps, not surprisingly, the United States ranks near the bottom among Organization for Economic Cooperation and Development (OECD) countries in the proportion of GDP spent on services that support families of children with disabilities (Organization for Economic Cooperation and Development 2007).

The term *developmental disability* includes those individuals with intellectual and physical disabilities who essentially cannot care for themselves. According to the Administration on Developmental Disabilities (ADD):

> Developmental disabilities are severe life-long disabilities attributable to mental and/or physical impairments, which manifest themselves before the age of 22 years and are likely to continue indefinitely. They result in substantial limitations in three or more of the following areas:

---

D. Viola (✉) · P. S. Arno
Department of Health Policy and Management, School of Health Sciences
and Practice, New York Medical College, Valhalla, NY 10595, USA
e-mail: deborah_viola@nymc.edu

P. S. Arno
e-mail: peter_arno@nymc.edu

- Self-care
- Comprehension and language
- Skills (receptive and expressive language)
- Learning
- Mobility
- Self-direction
- Capacity for independent living
- Economic self-sufficiency
- Ability to function independently without coordinated services (continuous need for individually planned and coordinated services)

Persons with developmental disabilities use individually planned and coordinated services and supports of their choice (e.g., housing, employment, education, civil and human rights protection, health care) to live in and to participate in activities in the community (HHS, Administration for Children and Families 2010a).

It is important to emphasize the complexities involved. Intellectual and developmental disabilities often coexist, especially for those diagnosed with cerebral palsy or autism.

People with developmental disabilities experience disparities in access and utilization of services and supports across their lifespan. Addressing these disparities requires a dynamic, integrated, highly engaged approach across the health, education, and social welfare domains, which accounts for the complexities involved in caring for this population.

In this chapter, we propose a conceptual framework for long-term care planning that improves this integration and reflects the benefits of a collective impact approach. Such an approach creates a model that includes consumers, family caregivers, and social support programs integrated into one larger, adaptable, and accountable system to bring about reform. We begin with a discussion of the three domains and how they currently function to support those with developmental disabilities. We then discuss the limitations and strengths inherent within each domain that could constrain or facilitate integration of support and services. We conclude with a summary of critical initiatives required to assure that collective impact, through the proposed long-term care planning framework, can be achieved. While the proposed framework is built upon an evaluation and partial synthesis of what exists, it will also support and clarify the complex network that individuals and families must navigate over a life time.

Reducing the limitations of developmental disabilities for individuals and their families is essential if we are to improve the health, productivity, and general welfare of this vulnerable population. It is time to elevate these issues among policymakers and the public as we anticipate the millions of children with developmental disabilities who will become adult and older adults.

## Medical Domain

Individuals with disabilities often experience health care disparities and as a group are considered a vulnerable population. Their health care problems are often exacerbated because of poverty and unemployment. In addition, many of these individuals cannot sufficiently communicate or discuss their needs, and medical providers are inadequately trained to deal with the challenges of an individual's disability and associated special health care needs. Despite the existence of health insurance (private or public), those with disabilities are less likely to use preventive care services or to find doctors who understand their disability (Kaiser Family Foundation 2003). In 2005, the Surgeon General issued a report, *Surgeon General's Call to Action to Improve the Health and Wellness of Persons with Disabilities* (HHS, Office of the Surgeon General 2005). The report's second goal addresses the need for "health care providers to have the knowledge and tools to screen, diagnose and treat the whole person with a disability with dignity." For those who experience developmental and intellectual disabilities from a very young age, this call takes on even greater urgency. The current medical training model is neither patient-centered, nor does it consider a lifespan perspective, especially following the transition from childhood into early adulthood. Given the impact of disparities on the use of health care and therapeutic services upon existing special education services, the need for care coordination among this population is critical. This integration becomes difficult to achieve when care for people with disabilities is void of long-term relationships between providers and those with disabilities. Not only are the complexities of the health care system difficult to navigate but receiving quality care at transitional moments—school to work or aging out of the pediatric care system at age 21—when important changes are taking place in one's disability is extremely problematic. The current system cannot address the dynamic quality of disability, making it more critical for those with disabilities and their families to exert more control over their own transitions in care.

In the "Bridges to Health Model" (Lynn et al. 2007), the population is divided into 8 segments that facilitate each group's transition through the Institute of Medicine's (2001) "Quality Chasm" to assure safe, effective, efficient, patient-centered, timely, and equitable care across their life span. Individuals with developmental disabilities would be considered chronically disabled in this model, but the suffered experiences of developmental disabilities are substantially more varied and dynamic than the model allows. Disability and health are two distinct concepts: a person can have a disability and be quite healthy or in some cases people can have serious, unstable health. It is the latter that is problematic. They may be at times chronic, with normal function, or stable, with serious disability; and similar to their nondisabled counterparts, they may move from one segment to another before experiencing a "short period of decline before dying" or frailty due to aging. Their incremental health care costs have been estimated to be anywhere from two to six times higher than those without disabilities (Ganz 2007; Ouyang et al. 2008). In addition, the transition from child/youth to adulthood for those with disabilities puts these individuals at increased health care risk as a result of non-health-related factors, including leaving the education system and the availability of special education services. Thus, the bridge to care for young people with chronic disabilities may differ from the bridge required for older adults who acquire their chronic disability later in their lives; furthermore, given limited resources, the bridge may not exist for some. For example, disparities exist by race and socioeconomic status; in one study of post high school use of services by children with autism, African-American and low-income youths were far more likely to receive no services upon exiting the school system (Shattuck et al. 2011). Traditional models of caregiving for those with developmental disabilities are often interpreted from two different perspectives—the pediatric and geriatric models. The burden on families and the difficulty for those with a disability to navigate the transition suggests a need for a comprehensive care framework that combines the perspectives of both pediatric and geriatric care and encourages long-term relationships between providers and individuals with disabilities. In a model proposed by Raina et al. (2004), the authors consider the effect on psychological and physical health of families based upon the interplay between socioeconomic status, child's functional and behavioral attributes, and how these contribute to the families' balance between informal and formal care, self-perception, social support, family function, and stress management. Their conceptual framework suggests that without this integration, and considering the importance of family caregivers to those with disabilities, it is difficult to imagine building better bridges or transitions in care for those with developmental disabilities; without these adjustments it may be inconceivable to build a long-term care framework for this population.

*The Future of Disability in America* (Institute of Medicine [IOM] 2007) notes that the transition to adult status has differential consequences for children who have relied exclusively on public insurance or Supplemental Security Income, since these children must often requalify for services when they turn 18. Children who have been covered by a parent's employer-sponsored or other public insurance may find that they have become uninsured. The introduction of health care reform in the United States now protects children with private insurance through age 26; however, most federal- and state-provided services and programs have age limits of 18–21. All of this complicates the coordination and transition of health care planning for these individuals and thus often requires changes in providers, further exacerbating the lack of longitudinal care and understanding required in treating these complex disabilities.

The medical and education domains have some overlap in the provision of care and services; yet there is too little communication across domains. The social welfare domain, which is needed to support both medical care and education through the provision of critical services such as housing and employment, often operates through a disparate cluster of agencies and organizations, fostering dependency of persons with developmental disabilities on their families. Health care transitions must include a more careful consideration and involvement of the education and social welfare domains if they are to contribute towards improving long-term care for those with developmental disabilities.

## Education Domain

Most individuals with developmental disabilities are diagnosed at a young age and are often referred to as "special needs" children within the school system. Children diagnosed with special needs require special education and related services supported by a federal mandate, Individuals with Disabilities Education Act (IDEA). However, the Americans with Disabilities Act (ADA) covers both children and adults with physical or mental limitations that impact life activities; thus children with disabilities may also receive support and services in the school setting by virtue of a Section 504 plan as part of the ADA (Malsch et al. 2008). Although estimates vary, a study by the Department of Health and Human Services (2008) reports 13.9% of school-aged children have special health care needs (which include developmental disabilities); another study concluded that 9.2% of households with children have a child with sensory, physical, or mental disabilities (Wang 2005).

School-based planning is important for families and is accomplished through the Individual Education Plan (IEP; and Individual Family Service Plan for younger children). The IEP includes transition planning for graduation from high school (e.g., postsecondary, vocational, or employment) and integration within the community, from as early as age 14. Although required by law, many schools are resource-constrained, and parents are ill-prepared to press for full compliance. As many as 44% of states are not in compliance with the federal requirements of the IEP process, and 88% are not in compliance with the limited transition planning requirements already built into the IEP (Wright and Wright 2011). Despite the best efforts of various organizations such as The Arc in compensating for the lack of compliance with federal mandates, there are numerous lost opportunities as children with disabilities move from kindergarten through their high school years, even for those in the most outstanding school systems. According to the President's Committee for People with Intellectual Disabilities (PCPID 2004), transition planning statistics are alarming: 90% of adults are not employed, fewer than 15% participate in postsecondary education, and "at least 50,000 people with intellectual disabilities were on waiting lists for Medicaid waiver services for individual and family supports."

The requirements of the IEP and 504 planning documents are limited in scope regarding the information recorded and required of other health care and service providers; they are also limited with respect to integrating community-based partners and programs that could work in concert with school-based services. Based upon a physician's medical diagnosis, many therapeutic services, particularly speech, physical, and behavioral therapy, are first provided through the educational system. Once an individual exits the school system, these services are principally funded by health insurance programs, notably Medicaid. Changes in an 18-year old's qualification for public insurance or other federal and state services are usually encumbered by restrictions on the amount of income he/she can earn or the amount of support he/she can receive from family members. Moreover, Medicaid (a state-administered system) may place severe limitations on the types of services provided. Furthermore, there is little or no communication between medical providers and educators or school-based therapists. In addition, there is no database or master file, other than a caregiver's ability to assimilate and maintain all of the reports on behalf of the person with a disability, and therefore, there is no assurance of continuity of care. Oftentimes, families meet with new providers and "start from scratch." More critically, since the information is not integrated, it is impossible to determine longer term planning needs or allow for sustainable transitions into the community, similar to what develops as a youth becomes an adult in the medical domain. These demands place an inordinate burden on family caregivers who often become the information hub for the individual, requiring them to navigate the system for care and services in the community. Managing these multiple demands is often overwhelming to individuals with disabilities and their families. Without a strong social welfare infrastructure, there is little opportunity for longer-term benefits to be fully realized even if the medical and education domains were seamlessly connected through transition planning into adulthood. Enormous gaps would still exist in assuring the independence of persons with developmental disabilities to live to their full potential within their communities.

## Social Welfare Domain

Sixty-one percent of individuals with developmental disabilities live within communities and with their families (Larson 2006). The philosophical shift towards extending the "least restrictive environment" perspective of the education system has largely been a result of the 1999 Olmstead Decision. The Supreme Court "affirmed the policy by ruling in Olmstead v. L.C. that under the Americans with Disabilities Act (ADA) unjustifiable institutionalization of a person with a disability who, with proper support, can live in the community is discrimination. In its ruling, the Court said that institutionalization severely limits the person's ability to interact with family and friends, to work and to make a life for him or herself" (ADD 2000). Further guidance was rendered to Medicaid agencies to facilitate the allotment of resources to help assure the existence of community-based services for those with disabilities. In 2005, Congress passed the Money Follows the Person (MFP) program to provide states with additional resource to encourage less reliance on institutionalizing people with disabilities and reduce the financial impact on Medicaid. Even prior to the MFP, the Medicaid Home- and Community-Based Services (HCBS) waiver program (1981), was designed to encourage similar objectives, which were not always achieved and led to numerous court challenges preceding Olmstead. Despite these challenges, as of 2009 "states provided HCBS to more than six times as many persons with ID/DD... as lived in (a Medicaid facility)" (Lakin et al. 2010). To this day, it is obligatory upon communities to fully integrate these programs and policies in the provision of care and services.

The ADD funds State Councils on Developmental Disabilities to assist people with developmental disabilities in securing employment, education, housing, transportation, and access to health care. Strategic partnerships between local Chambers of Commerce can help promote employment and encourage community-based initiatives that support employment, such as improved access to transportation systems. Housing demonstration programs encourage the move from dependent, family-provided care to independent living, but require that other community supports, especially jobs programs and access to transport, are in place.

Community coherence is central to assuring that persons with disabilities have equal opportunity for education, work, transportation, housing, socialization, and quality health care. Without this, it becomes extremely difficult for individuals with disabilities to "own" his or her care, thus fostering an overreliance upon family caregivers, generally parents, who become "career" caregivers. These caregivers require community supports themselves, as well as opportunities for respite, so that caregiver burden and strain are minimized. Work-life integration for family caregivers includes community partners who provide child care, after-school programs, transportation and social services, workplace flexibility, financial resources, and volunteer and advocacy organizations. The community, defined broadly, embodies the social welfare domain; "It is the invisible framework that connects families to the people and institutions that provide care, services, and support" (Bookman 2004).

Successful communities can benefit all members, not just those with developmental disabilities, if they are able to build capacity:

> Community capacity is the interaction of human, organizational, and social capital existing within a given community that can be leveraged to solve collective problems and improve or maintain the well-being of a given community. It may operate through informal social processes and/or organized efforts by individuals, organizations, and the networks of association among them and between them and the broader systems of which the community is part. (Chaskin 1999)

In a focus group of families who care for members with developmental disabilities, "parent highways" or "information highways" seemed the most critical need for families regardless of the age of the individual with a disability. Families expressed frustration at having to play navigator because of the lack of readily available information, planning checklists, directories of services, or assurances that community providers were safe and trustworthy (Washington State Department of Social Services 2010). According to the PCID, nearly 72,000 persons with developmental disabilities were on waiting lists for residential services that would facilitate independent living in 2000, and family respite care remains "in critical short supply in most states," no doubt as a result of funding and direct service workforce shortages. This portends a potentially more serious problem: those with developmental disabilities will have no choice but to be dependent upon their caregivers, and career caregivers are burdened with long-term care planning for their care recipient as well as for themselves. Currently, there are few support systems that are integrated so that both the aging caregiver and care recipient can plan simultaneously and anticipate the end of life of the caregiver. The incentive undoubtedly exists; the Older Americans Act (HHS, Administration on Aging 2011) requires priority be given to "older individuals providing care and support to persons with mental retardation and related developmental disabilities."

It is our belief that the medical, education, and social welfare domains can be adapted to include a lifespan perspective that supports an enhanced understanding of patterns of care for people with developmental disabilities, especially following the transition from childhood into early adulthood. However, effective, efficient, patient-centered care and support will not be realized for this group unless medical professionals, educators, policy makers, community-based providers, and caregivers work together. What follows is a proposed collective impact initiative or framework that integrates the three domains into a system designed to reduce disparities in access to support and services and encourage independence in planning for long-term care for those with developmental disabilities.

## Long-Term Care Planning

How can we achieve long-term care planning for people with developmental disabilities given that the respective domains we have described are traditionally isolated by functionality, mission/goals/objectives, funding/payment schemes, and policy design? If our objective is an integrated coherent planning framework that will make a *collective impact*, it will ideally be composed of various smaller frameworks, programs, and recommendations from researchers, advocates, and government agencies who generally have worked within the scope of these isolated domains. Assuming this is a reasonable strategy, we need a process to foster this integration. A collective impact approach may facilitate this process in building a workable long-term care framework.

As described by Kania and Kramer (2011), "Collective impact initiatives involve a centralized infrastructure, a dedicated staff, and a structured process that leads to a common agenda, shared measurement, continuous communication, and mutually reinforcing activities among all participants." Participation in such an arrangement by various organizations and individuals is based upon each contributing their strengths; measurements of success for one participant supports shared success by others by virtue of reinforcement and communication. The initiative builds upon smaller successes and has the flexibility to adapt as required, e.g., to respect and respond to the dynamic and individual nature of disability. Currently, no single authority or organizing entity or system exists to help move any of the isolated solutions forward, let alone to integrate them across domains. By definition, collective impact initiatives do just that.

Given what we have described in the prior sections, it would be helpful before discussing the proposed long-term care framework for people with developmental disabilities to summarize the major barriers to integration, as well as the potential strengths, that each domain contributes to the overall initiative.

The medical domain has come under a great deal of scrutiny as a result of health care reform and its emphasis on patient-centered care and services. Many frameworks for improving health care outcomes for people with disabilities have been suggested, either as part of larger systems of care (e.g., the Bridges to Health model) or for specific subpopulations as in the Multiple Chronic Conditions Strategic Framework (MCC) from the Department of Health and Human Services (2010c). The MCC not only takes into account possible benefits from recent reform legislation, but consists of four goals that are in many ways compatible with ideas suggested by the Surgeon General and the IOM:

1. Foster health care and public system changes to improve the health of individuals with multiple chronic conditions.
2. Maximize the use of proven self-care management and other services by individuals with multiple chronic conditions.
3. Provide better tools and information to health care, public health, and social services workers who deliver care to individuals with multiple chronic conditions.
4. Facilitate research to fill knowledge gaps about, and interventions and systems to benefit, individuals with multiple chronic conditions.

These goals are reinforced and supported by goals and recommendations from the *Surgeon General's Report* as well as the IOM's *Future of Disability in America*. Specifically, the MCC framework is person-focused and fosters independence for those with disabilities. It encourages integrated community-based care models, development of health outcome targets and measurement, as well as incentives and payment reforms to encourage participation by providers. *The Future of Disability* report recommends developing a comprehensive disability monitoring system, which would standardize and strengthen disabilities research and treatment (the need for this surveillance and monitoring cannot be overemphasized). As suggested by the Bridges to Health model, national quality standards have been developed that would also benefit care planning and outcomes, including the Culturally and Linguistically Appropriate Services (CLAS) and Competency Assessment Instrument (CAI), which measures competencies needed to provide high-quality care for those with persistent mental illness. However, the medical training model itself is still diagnosis-centered, and there is little cross-disciplinary consideration given in fields of practice. For example, geriatricians and primary care physicians are given little training on how those with developmental disabilities age or are even aware of prevalence data for conditions like Alzheimer within this population. In addition, practices are still established within fields of study or residency, e.g., groups of pediatricians with no emphasis on coordination of caregivers, including those providers of clinical, therapeutic, psychosocial, formal or informal care. Transcending this limitation could be made easier by recent changes in health care reform legislation, which suggests several initiatives that would support a collective impact, including funding for Accountable Care Organizations, emphasis on patient-centered care and medical homes, and investment in electronic health records.

Unlike the medical domain, education is not ordinarily considered part of long-term care planning, since our current mindset involves planning for aging adults long after completion of schooling. For those with developmental disabilities, long-term care planning begins as early as initial diagnosis and clearly involves planning from preschool through high school. The current emphasis on K-12 individualized education planning is a limitation for those with disabilities for several reasons. There is no time built in to follow up on transition plans (if they even exist) to assure appropriate placement in the workplace or vocational or postsecondary education; there is no consideration for ongoing health care or other support services, such as speech, behavior, or physical therapy; and there is virtually no concern for the financial considerations that accompany transition from youth to early adulthood. Although there are some limited experiments with dual enrollment options, e.g., enrollment in vocational training programs while in high school, which extends the funding life associated with the IEP, there are no widespread legislative changes that could benefit the entire school-aged population of people with disabilities. The PCID report offers many insights, but one recommendation that would help eliminate this barrier and serve as an important initiative for supporting long-term care planning builds upon the dual enrollment experiments:

Develop a seamless pre K-16 system of instruction and support to remove barriers that limit the ability of federal resources—including Social Security, Medicaid, special education, vocational education, and other general education and human services resources—to be pooled with state and local funds to support students with intellectual disabilities while in high school, as they enter the workforce or postsecondary education.

Schools are limited by the level of technology they employ in IEP or 504b planning, and budget constraints no doubt make it more difficult to make use of available planning software. A very few schools conduct regular meetings or forums for exchanging information with community partners, including the local chapters of organizations such as Arc or United Cerebral Palsy, local colleges or employers that could provide programs for people with developmental disabilities, or even State Councils on Developmental Disabilities. This makes it even more critical to consider the impact of community involvement as part of the collective impact initiative.

The social welfare domain is more nebulous in definition than the other two, and it requires defining relationships between community agencies and programs. In many cases, the goals, objectives, and services overlap, and there is no mechanism to facilitate communication other than by the person with the disability, assuming he or she is capable, or through the resolve of formal and informal caregivers. Although federal law and funding promote meaningful involvement in the community, there is very little integration as we have already noted between employment, housing, and transportation, for example, to assure that those with disabilities can participate as fully as possible. Individuals with developmental disabilities are at risk of losing Social Security income and Medicaid support based on income earned or assets owned, which results in disincentives for employment. There are few income or respite services for family caregivers who often provide housing, care, and transportation out of their own time and resources, and even less planning in anticipation that the caregiver will predecease the recipient. Even if transition planning occurred during high school, it is often neglected when individuals approach midlife. At that stage of the life cycle, planning for guardianship, family caregiver transitions (e.g., usually from parent to sibling), financial stewardship (including the impact of inheritance on public support), and long-term housing and care become paramount. Issues abound for aging caregivers of those with developmental disabilities as they need to plan for their own care needs as well. There is very little capacity within communities to integrate this dual planning that needs to take place in these households. Yet some states have begun to anticipate the increasing need for "aiding older caregivers" that could serve as initiatives for reducing some of the limitations inherent in the social welfare domain. One toolkit for state and local aging agencies was developed with a grant from the Administration of Aging that involved a series of workshops conducted in 33 states (Baxley et al. 2005). These workshops focused almost exclusively on determining how community organizations could partner and collaborate with families to assure that adults with developmental disabilities had the ability to age within their families and within their communities. Their efforts were in part motivated by concerns that a "significant portion of in-home supports are provided by family caregivers, [who] will be aging beyond their capacity to provide care over the next 10–20 years," and "that approximately 50% of individuals with I/DD (intellectual/developmental disabilities) and their caregivers are unknown to either the aging or the DD service system." Furthermore, the report notes that "expectations are that the 60+ age group with I/DD will increase threefold over the next 20 years." The State Councils have also developed 77 outcome measures that "best serve the needs of their consumer population" and could inform areas of improvement within communities to better target resources. The PCID describes a funding process based upon SSI and Medicaid waiver bundling "into one seamless set of incentives for work and self-employment, safe and affordable housing, and control over transportation" that would also incent community partners in realizing a collective impact on long-term care planning for individuals with developmental disabilities.

If our common agenda for the initiative to provide a long-term care framework for people with developmental disabilities is *to reduce disparities in access to services and encourage independence in planning for long-term care for those with developmental disabilities*, then we could conceivably imagine the following scenario for an older man with a developmental disability named Daniel. Since medical training would evolve around patient-centered care, a geriatrician treating dementia would appreciate how this condition might present in a 65-year old with autism, presumably the same patient who as a younger man had been treated by primary care physicians in the same practice for many decades after seeing a pediatrician from that practice years before. Presumably, Daniel might have enjoyed several years in the workforce as an alarm technician because of his IEP transition plan that was developed when he was 14 and took him through training at a vocational school. Finally, community-based transport providers worked with the group practice to assure that people with disabilities (as well as older people) were part of a weekly scheduled route that not only delivered patients to the practice for appointments as needed, but provided transportation to the local shopping center and major employer groups within the community. Daniel's mother, who is now in need of care herself, shares in planning and community services as a result of agency partnerships between local aging agencies and those serving people with developmental disabilities. And, care over Daniel's lifespan is connected from early on through the integration of IEP school-based software and electronic health records at the practice. All of his services are part of universal health care provided through Medicaid and Medicare; he receives income support from Social Security and was able to save some money since he was not penalized for earning "too much" to disqualify from public support. His mother's will transfers her home and assets to him—and again does not disqualify him from participating in the practice or receiving necessary support services.

Although this illustrative example does little to present the complexities involved in assuring Daniel's multiple needs are met, it serves to reinforce that care is available over the person's lifespan and is delivered in a way that allows a high degree of autonomy and independence. Nowhere in this example was it necessary to have a family caregiver available to accompany Daniel as translator or record keeper, or even health historian, to assure that continuity of care takes place. Although each domain still retains its own set of outcomes and activities, they are linked by a common agenda and a broader set of shared measures related to eliminating disparities within the population of people with developmental disabilities, as illustrated in Fig. 11.1.

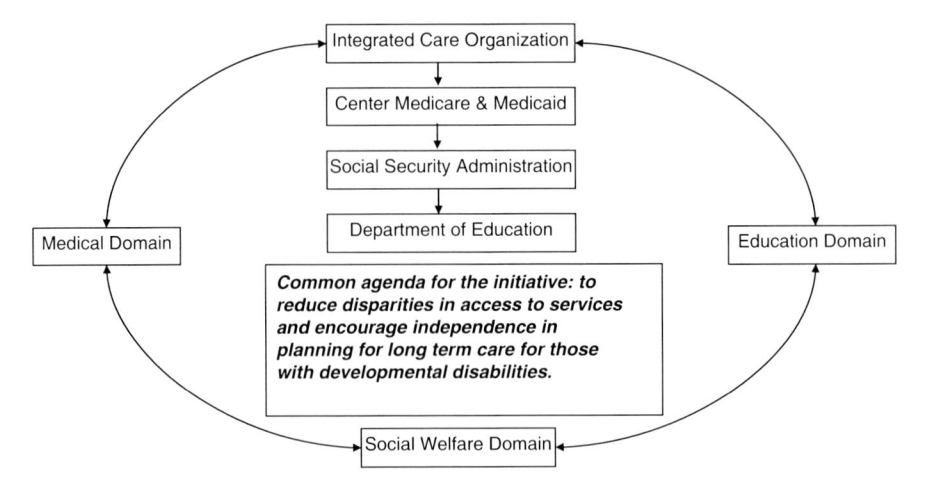

**Fig. 11.1** Long-term care framework for individuals with developmental disabilities

The resulting collective impact initiative uses an integrated care organization (ICO), similar in concept to currently legislated Accountable Care Organizations (ACOs), as its "independent backbone organization." The ICO would be a recognized legal entity networking not only health care providers, but local school boards, community organizations including major service providers and employer groups, and would have overall responsibility for shared governance and coordination of a patient's long-term care plan. The plan would be approved by the Center for Medicare Services and Medicaid, which would serve as the primary payer, essentially extending the MFP program by funneling resources and payments from the Department of Education and Social Security Administration. Legislation would be updated to reflect increased incentives to work; income caps would be raised so that individuals are not disqualified for services. Since developmental disabilities are generally diagnosed while individuals are of school age, they would be assigned to an ICO within their communities as soon as they qualify for either an IEP or 504b plan. The ICO would be held to the same standards for care as ACOs and care coordination that is patient- and caregiver-centered and would be expected to meet or exceed the *Healthy People 2020* (HHS 2010b) objectives for topic area Disability and Health (DH). The objectives and targets are listed in Table 11.1 for DH-5, improving transition planning from pediatric to adult care, and for DH-14, increasing the proportion of children and youth with disabilities who spend at least 80% of their time in regular education programs. Healthy People 2020 objectives can also be adapted to assure accountability on the part of the ICO (Table 11.2).

Collective impact initiatives are only successful if partners share a common agenda or mission, have credible measures and objectives for which they can be evaluated and held accountable, plan mutually reinforcing activities to achieve those objectives, and are organized under a structure that facilitates ongoing communication. The initiative must have a reliable funding source, so elimination of special waivers to support the isolated initiatives of the past (e.g., HCBS, dual enrollment) must be bundled into one

**Table 11.1** Healthy people 2020 summary of disability and health objectives

| Systems and policies | Barriers to health care | Environment | Activities and participation |
|---|---|---|---|
| DH-1 Identification of "people with disabilities" in data systems | DH-4 Barriers to primary care | DH-8 Barriers to health and wellness programs | DH-13 Participation in social, spiritual, recreational, community, and civic activities |
| DH-2 Surveillance and health promotion programs | DH-5 Transition planning | DH-9 Barriers to participation | DH-14 Inclusion of children and youth with disabilities in regular education programs |
| DH-3 Graduate-level courses in disability | DH-6 Medical care for epilepsy and uncontrolled seizures | DH-10 Barriers to obtaining assistive devices, service animals, and technology | DH-15 Unemployment |
| | DH-7 Use of inappropriate medications | DH-11 Visitable features | DH-16 Employment |
| | | DH-12 Congregate care | DH-17 Social and emotional support |
| | | | DH-18 Serious psychological distress |
| | | | DH-19 Nonfatal unintentional injuries requiring medical care |
| | | | DH-20 Early intervention services |

**Table 11.2** Examples of how objectives are measured

| | Target (%) | Baseline | Target setting method | Data source |
|---|---|---|---|---|
| DH-5: Increase the proportion of youth with special health care needs whose health care provider has discussed transition planning from pediatric to adult health care | 45.3 | 41.2% of youth with special health care needs had health care providers who discussed transition planning from pediatric to adult health care in 2005–2006 | 10% improvement | National Survey of Children with Special Health Care Needs, HRSA, Data Resource Center for Children and Adolescent Health |
| DH-14: Increase the proportion of children and youth with disabilities who spend at least 80% of their time in regular education programs | 73.8 | 56.8% of children and youth with disabilities spent at least 80% of their time in regular education classrooms in 2007–2008 | Modeling/projection | Individuals with Disabilities Education Act (IDEA) database, DoED, Office of Special Education |

stable funding stream similar to MFP under the direction of CMS, which includes Medicaid and Medicare payments, Social Security income, and dollars associated with IDEA- and ADA-supported resources.

We are fortunate to have many resources available to those who go through life with a developmental disability. To a large extent, we have a full complement of laws, policies, and social support programs already in place to assure that these individuals have the ability to live their lives to the fullest extent possible. What is consistently absent is an easier way to transition through one's lifespan. As a result, many families miss opportunities and fail to receive services and supports they are entitled to. By working together, we can make a collective impact on advancing the equality of individuals with disabilities through a long-term care planning framework that fosters their independence and a richer and more productive participation in their own communities.

## References

Administration on Developmental Disabilities. (2000). *The Olmstead decision fact sheet*. http://www.acf.hhs.gov/programs/add/otherpublications/olmstead.html. Accessed 24 April 2012.

Baxley, D. L., Janicki, M. P., McCallion, P., & Zendell, A. (2005). *Aiding older caregivers of persons with intellectual and developmental disabilities: A tool kit for state and local aging agencies*.

Bookman, A. (2004). *Starting in our own backyards: How working families can build community and survive the new economy*. New York: Rutledge.

Chaskin, R. J. (1999). *Defining community capacity: A framework and implications from a comprehensive community initiative*. Chicago: Chapin Hall Center for Children at the University of Chicago.

Ganz, M. L. (2007). The lifetime distribution of the incremental societal costs of autism. *Archives of Pediatric Adolescent Medicine, 161*, 343–349.

Institute of Medicine. (2001). *Crossing the quality chasm*. Washington, DC: National Academy Press.

Institute of Medicine. (2007). *The future of disability in America*. Washington, DC: National Academy Press.

Kaiser Family Foundation. (2003). *Survey of people with disabilities*.

Kania, J., & Kramer, M. (2011). Collective impact. *Stanford Social Innovation Review, 2011*, 36–41.

Lakin, K. C., Larson, S. A., Salmi, P., & Webster, A. (2010). *Residential services for persons with developmental disabilities: Statues and trends through 2009*. Minneapolis: University of Minnesota, Research and Training Center on Community Living, Institute on Community Integration.

Larson, S. A (Ed.). (2006). *Policy research brief, 17*(1). Minneapolis: University of Minnesota, Research and Training Center on Community Living, Institute on Community Integration.

Lynn, J., Straube, B. M., Bell, K. M., Jencks, S. F., & Kambic, R. T. (2007). Using population segmentation to provide better health care for all: The "Bridges to Health" model. *Milbank Quarterly, 85*(2), 185–208.

Malsch, A., Rosenzweig, J. M., & Brennan, E. M. (2008). *Disabilities and work-family challenges: Parents having children with special health care needs*. http://workfamily.sas.upenn.edu/. Accessed 24 April 2012.

National Association of Councils on Developmental Disabilities. (2011). http://www.nacdd.org/about-nacdd/what-are-developmental-disabilities.aspx. Accessed 07 May 2011.

New York State Family Caregiver Council. (2009). *Report: Supporting and strengthening caregivers in New York state.* http://www.aging.ny.gov/Caregiving/Reports/InformalCaregivers/FamilyCaregiverCouncilReport.pdf. Accessed 15 May 2011.

Organization for Economic Cooperation and Development. (2007). *Babies and bosses: Reconciling work and family life* (vol. 5). A synthesis of finding for OECD countries. Paris: OECD.

Ouyang, L., Grosse, S. D., Armour, B. S., & Waitzman, N. J. (2008). Health care expenditures of children and adults with spina bifida in a privately insured U.S. population. *Journal of Autism and Developmental Disorders, 38*(3), 546–552.

President's Committee for People with Intellectual Disabilities. (2004). *A change we have to keep.* Washington, DC: PCPID.

Raina, R., O'Donnell, M., Schwellnus, H., Rosenbaum P., King, G., Brehaut, J., et al. (2004). Caregiving process and caregiver burden: Conceptual models to guide research and practice. *BMC Pediatrics, 4,* 1.

Shattuck, P. T., Wagner, M., Narendorf, S., Sterzing, P., & Hensley, M. (2011). Post-high school service use among young adults with an autism spectrum disorder. *Archives of Pediatric Adolescent Medicine, 165*(2), 141–146.

Statewide Caregiving and Respite Coalition of New York. (2011). *Issues for aging caregivers of adults with developmental disabilities.* www.scrcny.org/mccallion.pdf. Accessed 15 May 2011.

U.S. Department of Health and Human Services. (2005). *Office of the Surgeon General. Surgeon General's call to action to improve the health and wellness of persons with disabilities.* Rockville: Author.

U.S. Department of Health and Human Services. (2008). *The national survey of children with special health care needs 2005–2006.* Rockville: Author.

U.S. Department of Health and Human Services, Administration for Children and Families. (2010a). http://www.acf.hhs.gov/opa/fact_sheets/add_factsheet.pdf. Accessed 07 May 2011.

U.S. Department of Health and Human Services. (2010b). *Healthy People 2020: The road ahead.* http://www.health.gov/healthypeople/url/. Accessed 21 May 2011.

U.S. Department of Health and Human Services. (2010c). *Multiple chronic conditions—A strategic framework: Optimum health and quality of life for individuals with multiple chronic conditions.* Washington, DC. http://www.hhs.gov/ash/initiatives/mcc/. Accessed 21 May 2011.

U.S. Department of Health and Human Services, Administration on Aging. (2011). http://www.aoa.hhs.gov/AoA_programs. Accessed 24 April 2012.

U.S. Equal Employment Opportunity Commission. (2009). *Questions & answers about persons with intellectual disabilities in the workplace and the Americans with Disabilities Act.* http://www.eeoc.gov/facts/intellectual_disabilities.html. Accessed 24 April 2012.

Wang, Q. (2005). *Disability and American families: 2000.* Washington, DC: U.S. Department of Commerce, U.S. Census Bureau.

Washington State Department of Social Services, Aging & Disability Services Administration. (2010). *Investing in a system of care: Focus group interviews with families and consumers of services for people with developmental disabilities.*

Wright, P. W. D., & Wright, P. D. (2011). *Back to school on civil rights, chart 4: Number and percentage of noncompliant states in each area according to 1994–1998 OSEP monitoring reports.* http://www.wrightslaw.com/law/reports/IDEA_Compliance_3A.html. Accessed 05 May 2011.

# Chapter 12
# Emerging Technologies for Caregivers of a Person with a Disability

Margo B. Holm and Ketki D. Raina

For caregivers of persons with disabilities, the importance of their caregiving can be reflected on a continuum that at one end supports the beginning of life and at the other end supports the end of life (see Fig. 12.1). Since the early 1980s, infants who needed a medical device to compensate for a vital organ or body function and were thus technology dependent, have been sent home from the hospital with their parent caregivers because of cost reductions and better developmental outcomes for the children (Cross et al. 1998). One of the most critical factors that determined whether technology-dependent children had extended hospital stays or were able to be cared for at home was the ability and commitment of the parent caregivers to manage the technology (Cross et al. 1998; Odom and Chandler 1990; Perkins 1993). Likewise, when support is needed at the end of life, caregivers of a family member in the final stages of life secondary to a disorder or condition such as amyotrophic lateral sclerosis, Huntington's disease, or cancer often must master technologies to administer oxygen, nourishment, and pain-relieving medications (Aranda and Hayman-White 2001; *Caring for people with Huntington's disease* 2005; Gibson and Schroder 2001; *Twilight brigade: Compassion in action* 2008). In between the two ends of the caregiving continuum, caregivers use technology to support persons with disabilities so that they can carry out the activities that constitute the fabric of their everyday lives—eating, toileting, bathing, dressing, transferring and communicating, as well as participate in the social roles valued by these persons—such as parent, volunteer, teacher, lawyer, spouse, or coach. Technologies designed to support persons with disabilities also have the potential to reduce the need for personal assistance and reduce caregiver burden.

---

M. B. Holm (✉) · K. D. Raina
University of Pittsburgh, 5012 Forbes Tower, Pittsburgh, PA 15260, USA
e-mail: mbholm@pitt.edu

K. D. Raina
e-mail: kraina@pitt.edu

**Fig. 12.1** Stages of the caregiving continuum

|————————————————————————————|
Support            Enable        Facilitate        Support
Beginning of Life  Activities    Participation     End of Life

## Relationship of Caregiving, Disability, and Functioning

One conceptual model that provides a common language and framework for describing the interactions among the caregiver, person with a disability, and technology is the International Classification of Functioning, Disability and Health (ICF; WHO 2001). The ICF has universal application and represents an integration of opposing views of disability, namely the medical model (disability is within the person) and the social model (disability is created by the social environment; WHO 2001). As shown in Fig. 12.2, the ICF connotation of health is a dynamic state that includes the ability to function in the real world, not just the absence of a disease, disorder, or condition. ICF defines body structures as the anatomical parts of the body and their components, and body functions as the physiological process of body systems. The dysfunction of body structures or body functions results in impairment. Activities are defined as the tasks or actions performed in daily living, and participation is defined as involvement in real life situations. The inability to complete activities or to participate in real life environments results in activity limitations or participation restrictions. The ICF also explains and qualifies the difference between activities and participation in another way: engagement in activities indicates that a person has the inherent capacity to do so in a standard environment whereas participation indicates performance of activity tasks and actions in real life situations. In the ICF framework, functioning indicates the healthy performance of body structures, body functions, activities, and participation; whereas, disability indicates the presence of impairments, activity limitations, or participation restrictions (WHO 2001).

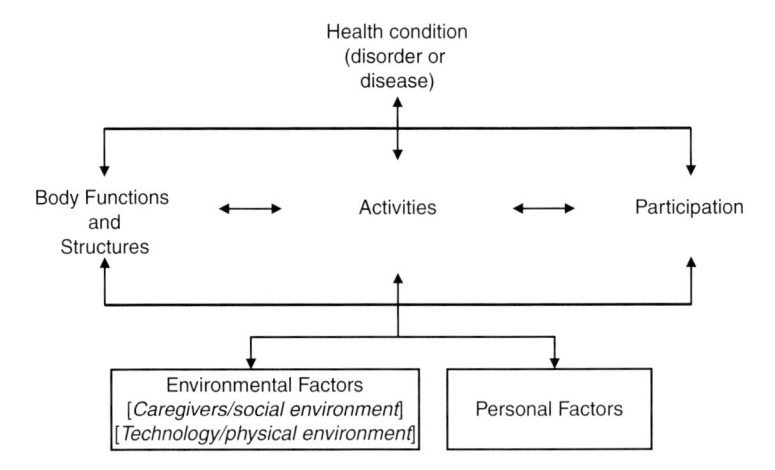

**Fig. 12.2** The International Classification of Functioning, Disability and Health (ICF) framework (WHO 2001, p. 18), adapted to show how caregivers and technology are included

The ICF framework addresses contextual factors that impact health and functioning, which are described as either environmental factors (physical, social, and attitudinal environment at the level of the person and society) or personal factors (person's background excluding health condition/state). The ICF taxonomy also recognizes products and technology and support by informal and formal caregivers as a means of enabling individuals to minimize disability and maximize functioning (WHO 2001). Because of its multidimensional perspectives of everyday functioning, the ICF provides an excellent framework for discussing emerging technologies as a support for caregivers of a person with disabilities. The use of current and emerging technologies by caregivers reflects interactions among the person with a disability, the caregiver, the technology (which at minimum should make a task or action possible), and the environmental context. In addition, the interaction should also increase ease of task performance, decrease the pain, frustration, anxiety, and fear associated with task performance, decrease the potential for injury; and improve the task safety, independence, adequacy and satisfaction of the person with a disability—and likewise... do the same for the caregiver (Bialokoz et al. 2002).

## Current and Emerging Technologies that Support Caregiving at the ICF Domain of Impairment

### *Current Practice*

A sentinel event in caregiver technology occurred in the early 1980s, when Andrew Dibner developed a personal emergency response system (Lifeline) that enabled frail elderly without professional caregivers to remain in their own homes, yet signal for medical help if necessary (Lifeline personal response and support services 2005). Early forms of the system used a telephone speaker and a wearable pendant that signaled the telephone to dial automatically for help. Whereas initially the supply of caregiving technologies was limited, currently technologies available to caregivers that are designed to resolve problems in the domain of impairment are numerous and varied. Today, "off-the-shelf" technologies are readily available for caregivers to monitor blood pressure, blood oxygen, glucose levels, heart rate, and ventilatory capacity as well as to manage incontinence, transfers, exercises, stretching, and wound care (*The caregivers marketplace* 2007; Center for Aging Services Technologies [CAST] 2005; The Wright Stuff caregiver products 2005).

### *Emerging Practice and Research*

Whereas current caregiver technologies that are designed to address problems in the impairment domain are "hands-on" devices, that is not the trend with emerging technologies. Two trends in these emerging technologies are noteworthy:

(1) technologies designed to reduce the impairment of the person with a disability, including sensor, wireless, and robotic technologies and (2) technologies for communication of information and educational content.

## Technologies Designed to Reduce the Impairment of the Person with a Disability

Emerging technologies that reduce the impairment of the person with a disability also have the potential to reduce caregiver burden. Implanted technologies such as cochlear implants have been used to reduce sensory impairments, but emerging technologies are also focusing on reducing musculoskeletal impairments, and thus the extent of personal caregiving assistance. Research in the United States, the Netherlands, and the United Kingdom has focused on bowel and bladder prostheses, and neuroprostheses for hand grasps as well as for standing and transfers in persons with spinal cord injuries (Creasey et al. 2000; Davis et al. 2001; Grill et al. 2001; Lozano 2001). Some studies have shown monetary savings with the use of neuroprostheses, as well as increased independence, function, and quality of life for the person with the disability (Creasey et al. 2000), which translated into decreased caregiver burden. Along a similar line, brain neural implant technology is being used to enable individuals who are physically "locked-in" (intact cognition, no bodily movement) secondary to stroke or spinal cord injury to control the cursor on a computer screen by thought alone (*The future of brain–computer interfacting* 2005; Sample 2005a, 2005b, March 31). Likewise, brain-computer interfaces are being used to restore speech and communication to people with amyotrophic lateral sclerosis, thus enabling social communication and the ability to make their wants and needs known to their caregivers (*The future of brain–computer interfacting* 2005).

Implanted sensors are also emerging for cardiovascular and mental function impairments. EndoSensor$^{TM}$ is a microelectromechanical system (MEMS) fabrication technology designed to measure blood pressure from within a cardiac stent. For formal and informal caregivers who must constantly monitor the blood pressure of a person who has had a stent implanted, this wireless sensor technology allows the caregiver to monitor pressure using an electronic wand that is waved over the (clothed) chest of the person with the stent (Becker 2006).

Emerging technologies to reduce impairment and enhance mental functions are more controversial than those for reducing sensory, musculoskeletal, and cardiac impairments. "Psychiatric implants," which can deliver uniform doses of psychotropic medications for 1 year to individuals with severe mental illness are seen as a breakthrough by many caregivers who must manage difficult and aberrant behaviors when medications are stopped, or as coercion of the person with the disability, since the choice of whether or not to take a medication is taken away (Talan 2005; Vedantam 2002). A similar controversy exists for the emerging "neurotechnology" of neurocognitive enhancers, which can be used to enhance mental functions of those with impaired memory, and therefore reduce caregiver burden (Farah et al. 2004).

Although some of the emerging technologies are being used in everyday practice, most are still in the research phase and therefore not easily accessed. Those that are available have often emanated from federally funded programs such as the Rehabilitation Engineering Research Centers (RERC). At the RERC on Mobile Wireless Technologies for Persons with Disabilities at Georgia Tech, one research project is focusing on sonification (use of sound waves) as a substitute for vision, to provide persons with visual impairments a "picture" of the immediate environment to enhance the safety and ease of their mobility (*Rehabilitation engineers' emphasis on helping people with disabilities will improve wireless technology for everyone* 2002). Another team at Georgia Tech is developing a wearable captioning device that wirelessly receives input from public address systems, transmits it to a personal digital assistant, and displays captioning to a micro display attached to glasses. The captions appear to float several feet in front of the user. For those with hearing impairment, this also has the potential to reduce reliance on others to interpret audio announcements that the general public receives (Sanders 2005).

Finally, emerging technology sensors can be used to help caregivers ascertain changes in body functions of those in their care. These technologies include electronic "noses" that detect the odors of growing bacteria on or around the person with a disability, toilets that have sensors to detect glucose concentrations in urine, and "watches" that have sensors capable of detecting hypoglycemia in persons with diabetes (Durham 2001). Research is also being conducted on the utility of environmental sensors in "smart houses" to enable distance caregivers to detect catastrophic events or changes in the health status of the person with a disability by sensing lack of motion or extended levels of silence in the environment (CAST 2005; Gurley et al. 1996; Whitehouse et al. 2002).

*Technologies for Communication of Information and Educational Content* Emerging technologies for distance caregiving, both by professional and informal caregivers, have focused primarily on caregiver education for monitoring the health status of those in their care (*Caring for people with Huntington's disease* 2005). One example of a health monitoring system is the Electronic HouseCall (EHC; Cyber Care, Inc.), which enables informal caregivers to set up and apply monitoring technology (blood oxygen, blood pressure, coagulation, ECG, glucose, etc.) and then send vital signs to a professional over a telephone line (*Cyber-Care's Electronic HouseCall System tested in transglobal medical data transfer over Internet2* 2001; see Fig. 12.3). EHC, as well as similar systems, include a camera for a more personal interaction as well for visual feedback to the professional on affect, shortness of breath, and pallor of the person with a disability (Balas and Iakovidis 1999; Lovell et al. 2001; T.I.E. 2005; Whitten 2002). For family caregivers of stroke survivors who help to implement rehabilitation exercise programs at home, feedback will be possible soon from haptic interfaces such as the DataGlove and Rutgers Ankle Interface (Burdea 2001). These technologies use virtual reality and send signals of hand and ankle movements during exercise to a computer screen for immediate feedback to the caregiver and stroke survivor, and simultaneously transmit the information to a database that will be accessed by the rehabilitation professional.

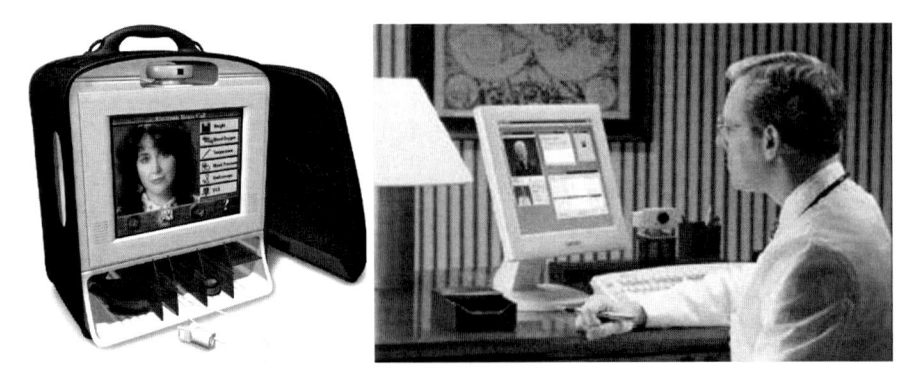

Fig. 12.3 Electronic HouseCall (CyberCare, Inc.) scenario, courtesy of Dr. John Peifer

## Technologies in Support of Caregiving at the ICF Domains of Activities/Participation

### Current Practice

At the ICF domains of activities/participation are those tasks and actions that are at the foundation of everyday life: mobility, self-care, taking care of a household, and tasks related to education, work, and employment. A myriad of low technologies (low cost; simple mechanical devices such as long-handled bath sponge, tub bench, transfer board, and commode) and high technologies (high cost; electronic devices such as mechanical lifts, incontinence alarms, and wander alerts) are currently available to caregivers (ABLEDATA 2008; *The Boulevard* 2005; *The caregivers marketplace* 2007; *Caring for people with Huntington's disease* 2005; *Twilight brigade: Compassion in action* 2008), however, the ability to access and use these technologies depends on financial resources and the ability to match the caregiver and person with a disability, the task, and the technology (Holm and Rogers 1991; Romano 1998; Scherer 1991, 2000; Scherer and Galvin 1997) so that the technology can be used effectively.

### Emerging Practice and Research

Emerging technologies focused on supporting caregivers at the ICF domains of activities/participation are being designed to: (1) reduce the activity limitations of the person with a disability, reduce caregiver burden, or eliminate the need for personal assistance through the use of sensor, wireless, and robotic technologies; and (2) communicate information and educational content.

*Emerging Technologies to Reduce Activity Limitations and Participation Restrictions*
Emerging technologies that reduce activity limitations and participation restrictions of the person with a disability can also reduce the need for personal assistance

**Fig. 12.4** iBOT allows the individual to rise vertically to eye level and balance on two wheels

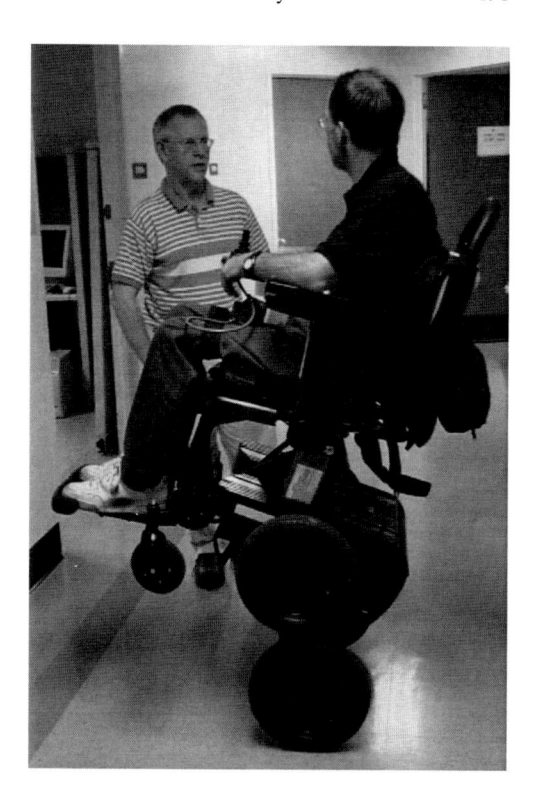

and reduce caregiver burden (Hammel et al. 2002). For functional mobility activities/participation, for example, emerging technologies include manual wheelchairs with power assists (Arva et al. 2000; Independence iBOT 2005) and the iBOT mobility system (Independence iBOT). Wheelchairs with power assists have the advantage for the caregiver of being lighter and more portable than a power wheelchair, and the advantage for the user of a push rim power boost that reduces physiologic demands (Arva et al. 2000; Herz-Unterstützungssysteme 2003; Independence iBOT 2005). The iBOT is designed to enable the user to rise vertically to eye level and balance on two wheels as well as rise to various activity surface heights. It also has the ability to climb stairs, thus eliminating stairs as an architectural barrier that limits where the user can engage in everyday activities (Independence iBOT; see Fig. 12.4).

Robotics researchers have also designed mobility devices for persons with disabilities that decrease the need for personal assistance/caregiving. For example, at JPL, Fiorini and colleagues have developed a sensor-guided wheelchair (Fiorini and Shiller 1998). The chair can navigate through crowds using a sonar system and a laser. This allows the user to move in the direction desired, at a comfortable speed, without having to make repetitive and exhaustive maneuvers. The GuideCane (Ulrich and Borenstein 2001) is another example of mobile robotic technology. It is designed to assist persons who are blind or visually impaired to move safely and quickly around obstacles and hazards. It uses ultrasonic sensors to provide feedback to the user through the device handle and this guides the user to move in a suitable direction.

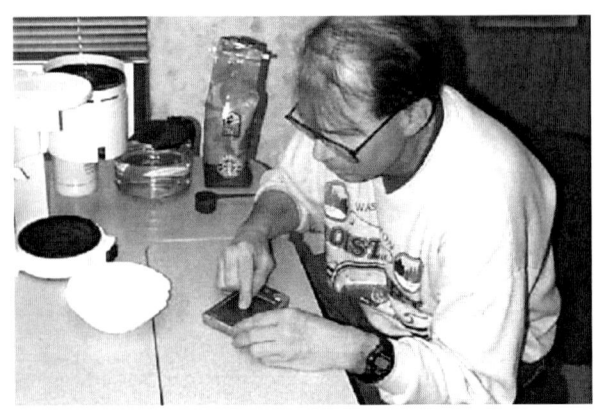

**Fig. 12.5** Carl uses the Visual Assistant to make coffee each morning

The field of cognitive orthotics is another area of emerging technology designed to facilitate activities and participation of the person with a disability and reduce caregiver burden. At the most basic level are text pager systems such as NeuroPage (Hersh and Treadgold 1994) and MedPrompt (MedPrompt: Solutions for better aging 2005), which allow the caregiver to page the user and transmit a reminder for a scheduled activity (e.g., take blue pill now). These systems are best used for redundant tasks and are best used as a cueing system for task initiation.

The power and versatility of the Pocket PC has yielded an emerging technology that can be used as a cueing device, and when cueing is needed for more complex activities/participation, Pocket PCs can be loaded with proprietary software to meet the challenge. For example, software is available that allows the caregiver, job coach, or employer to program schedules and task steps using text cues (Levinson 1995, 1997) graphic images or pictures (*AbleLink technologies: Changing lives with cognitive support technologies* 2008; see Fig. 12.5), or combinations of text, images, and voice messages (*AbleLink technologies: Changing lives with cognitive support technologies* 2008; *Caring for people with Huntington's disease* 2005; CAST 2005; Memory Aided Prompting System [MAPS] 2003). While each of the previous cognitive orthotics requires input of a specific schedule or sequence of events by the caregiver, employer, or coach, the newest cognitive orthotic technologies are designed to be anticipatory and intuitive. For example, a Pocket PC is programmed using an approach known as Planning by Rewriting (PbR; Ambite and Knoblock 2001) or another similar approach, whereby the system is interactive with the user. Thus, if an appointment is missed, the cognitive orthotic rearranges the user's schedule by choosing an optimal scenario from the choices that have been programmed into the orthotic, and then lets the user know what to do, or where to go (Levinson 1995, 1997; *PEAT: The planning and execution assistant and training system* 2005). However, developing cognitive orthotics for persons with disabilities for the purpose of reducing caregiver burden is not an easy task, as the developers of the Independent LifeStyle Assistant (I.L.S.A) discovered (Haigh and Kiff 2004). I.L.S.A. had to be retired.

**Fig. 12.6** A robotic map of part of "Pearl's" nursing facility, which Pearl learned and uses to guide residents

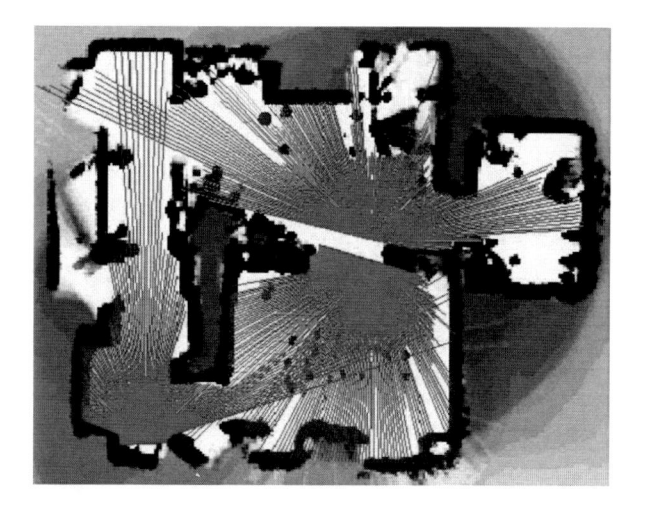

In the 1980s, Engelhardt testified before Congress (High technology and its benefits for an aging population 1984) and later published about robots as important tools for caregivers (Englehardt 1989; Englehardt and Goughler 1997). She anticipated that robots would serve numerous caregiving roles, including daily living expert assistance systems, personal servants, guardians and protectors, lifetime career assistants, and transporters (Englehardt and Goughler 1997). Just as anticipated by Englehardt, the Nursebot team (http://www-2.cs.cmu.edu/~nursebot/) has developed a personal service robot named Flo (Baltus et al. 2000), a plan-based personalized cognitive orthotic named Pearl (McCarthy and Pollack 2002; Pollack 2002; Pollack et al. 2002; Thrun et al. 1998), and also a robotic walker (Morris et al. 2002). Flo was designed as a reminding system and also had interactive capabilities such as answering questions about the weather and current television programs. Flo is also capable of finding faces and tracking them, and while appearing interested in the person speaking to it, Flo is really directing its camera and microphones toward the person. Flo's designers did this on purpose to make Flo more "socially acceptable" and to ascertain if "face tracking" would improve the degree to which persons would accept a robot as a personal assistant (Baltus et al. 2000; Ho et al. 2005; Morris et al. 2004; Wu and Miller 2005).

Pearl is also a mobile robot (Montemerlo et al. 2002) who was programmed using the PbR approach, combined with Autominder, another cognitive orthotic system that learns a person's everyday activities, updates them, and then provides reminders. Pearl learns about each new environment through a process known as "robotic mapping" (Thrun et al. 1998) whereby a human leads a robot through an environment and identifies landmarks that will be important to the robot as a caregiver/personal assistant (see Fig. 12.6). The mobile robot learns, refines, and generates a map that it then uses as a navigational guide as it carries out its responsibilities (see Fig. 12.7). A similar technology that also uses robotic mapping to navigate is a robotic walker (Morris et al. 2002). Whereas Pearl serves as a guide for residents who must walk or wheel on their own as they follow, the robotic walker not only guides, it provides

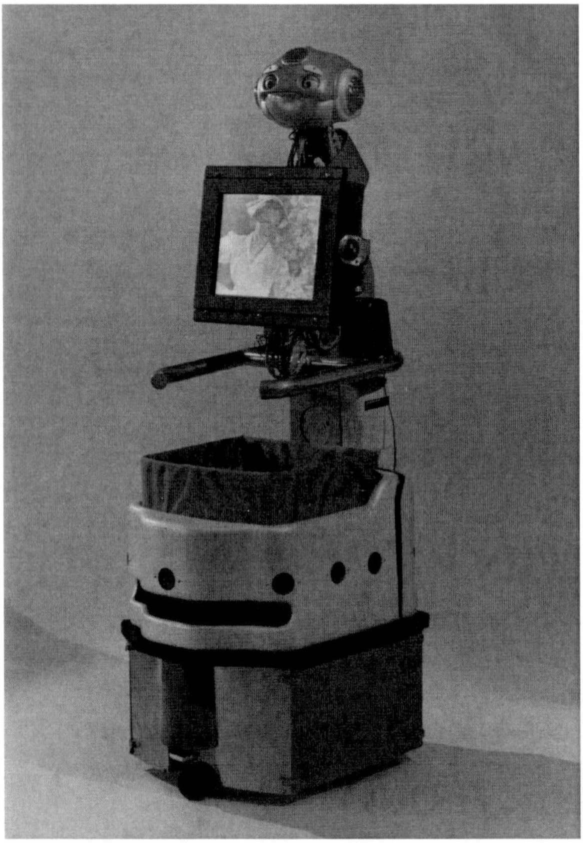

**Fig. 12.7** Pearl, a mobile robot

a source of support for the resident (see Fig. 12.8). Caregivers at the nursing facility have been very positive about Pearl and the robotic walker, because the robots relieve them of routine tasks so that they can care for others who need skilled assistance (Morris et al. 2002).

Caregiving activities occur within environments, and in addition to "smart" robots, another emerging technology is known as a "smart" or intelligent environment (*The Aware Home Research Institute* 2008; CAST 2005; Durham 2001; EliteCare 2008; Mollenkopf and Wahl 2002; Murdoch et al. 2002; Thomas 2002; van Berlo 2002). However, there is a trade-off that must be balanced between intelligent environments/distance caregiving technologies and the privacy of the person with a disability, which Lundberg and Reed have described as the "autonomy-risk equilibrium" (EliteCare 2008). Although distance caregivers are comforted by the knowledge that they can fulfill their caregiving to the person with a disability by monitoring them in their everyday environments, the trade-off is a lack of privacy for the person with a disability, especially if that person is an adult (Mynatt and Rogers 2001). Current technologies that support distance caregiving, such as temperature sensors, water

**Fig. 12.8** Robotic walker

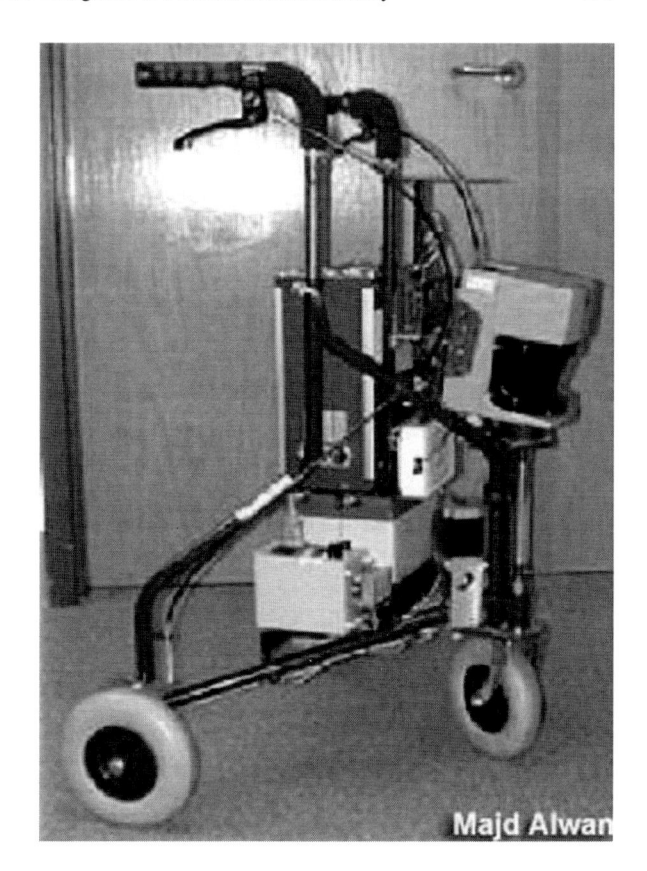

sensors, motion sensors, and wireless cameras, are inexpensive and easy to use (Aging in place///remote monitoring solution 2008; *Caring for people with Huntington's disease* 2005). For example, a wireless camera can be used by a mother with a disability, from her work computer, to monitor attendant care being provided each morning to her teenage son who also has a disability (*Caring for people with Huntington's disease* 2005). Likewise, a son in Seattle can monitor his father, recently diagnosed with dementia, in each room of his father's apartment in Pittsburgh (*Aging in place///remote monitoring solution* 2008; Murdoch et al. 2002). However, with 24-hour monitoring by the cameras, privacy is relinquished to enable autonomy and reduce risk.

Although some intelligent environments use cameras, research is focusing on technologies that are unobtrusive, intuitive, and do not interfere with either the human or built environments (EliteCare 2008). The Aware Home Research Institute at Georgia Tech is an in vivo laboratory for designing and studying sensor technologies and smart environments (Dey et al. 1999, 2001; Mynatt and Rogers 2001; Sanders 2000). Ongoing projects using camera technology include Digital Family Portrait (enables distance caregivers to track the actions of family members by date), and What Was I Cooking? (When people forget where they are in a sequence of steps, a visual display can back up to the last several actions, so that the user knows where to continue on in the sequence).

Gesture Pendant, which does not use cameras, is another Aware Home project that is exploring the ability of the user to operate home appliances with only a gesture (*The Aware Home Research Institute* 2008). Sensor technologies being developed for testing in the Aware Home also include radio frequency identification (RFID) tags that use sensors in floor mats throughout the Home, and respond to RFID tags in a user's shoes. These sensors enable unobtrusive person tracking that allows for the privacy that cameras do not—however, they only provide information about who is where in the Aware Home, not what the person is doing (*The Aware Home Research Institute* 2008).

One of Intel's Proactive Health research projects uses "motes," which are tiny off-the-shelf motion sensors that detect activity. They can be attached to everyday objects such as dishes, chairs, doors, and appliance parts that can be tracked wirelessly into a host personal computer to communicate information to a caregiver. Such monitoring by technology can allow the caregiver of an individual with cognitive impairment to take a nap, knowing that an alert will be transmitted if the knobs on the stove are moved, or the back door is opened (Dishman 2004). The Center for Aging Services Technologies tracks emerging technologies and research projects, including some previously mentioned, that are relevant to older adults and caregivers of older adults (CAST 2005).

Oatfield Estates in Milwaukie, Oregon, is an extended family residence$^{TM}$ that currently uses intelligent environment technologies for creating an autonomy-risk equilibrium (CARE$^{TM}$) for its residents. Each bungalow in the estate is wired with sensors and pervasive computing to interpret their signals. A computerized automated care system (ACS) receives and sends signals and logs all data. Residents and caregivers wear badges that enable the computers to monitor where they are located at all times, who is interacting with whom, as well as the overall physical activity levels of the residents. The badges also double as "call for help" buttons, which signal the computers, and identify to caregivers, which resident needs help, and where the resident is located. When a resident pushes a badge to call for help, pulls an emergency cord, or uses a computer touch screen (see Fig. 12.9), the ACS records when the call was placed, where it was placed from, which caregiver responds to the call, how soon the caregiver responded, and how long the caregiver spent with the resident. Thus, in addition to enabling responsiveness to resident requests, and including safety alert features (see Fig. 12.10), the ACS also gathers administrative data as a means of improving quality of care (EliteCare 2008). Other sensor technology includes load springs on the legs of residents' beds that not only weigh the residents, but also monitors if the residents are in bed, and the quality of their sleep. In addition, when a resident gets up at night, the bathroom light automatically comes on, and in the future, for residents with dementia, the computer will also remind them that they got up to go to the bathroom (Donahue 2001). For those residents that have cognitive impairments such as dementia, there are no restrictions on their movements: however, when their presence is "sensed" in the open kitchen area and no caregiver is

**Fig. 12.9** View of an Oatfield Estates computer touch screen after a resident touches the symbol on the lower right corner to request help from a caregiver

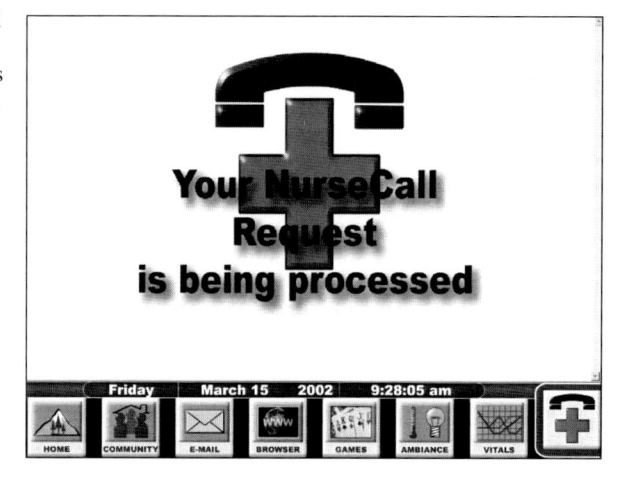

present, the ACS automatically makes all appliances inoperable. Furthermore, when residents' doors to their private rooms are closed, the sensor technology only allows the resident whose badge matches the door—or a caregiver—to gain access to the room. This feature both enhances each resident's privacy and prevents wanderers from going into the wrong rooms. For distance caregivers, if the resident agrees to a release of information, the son or daughter can sign onto the Elite Care web site

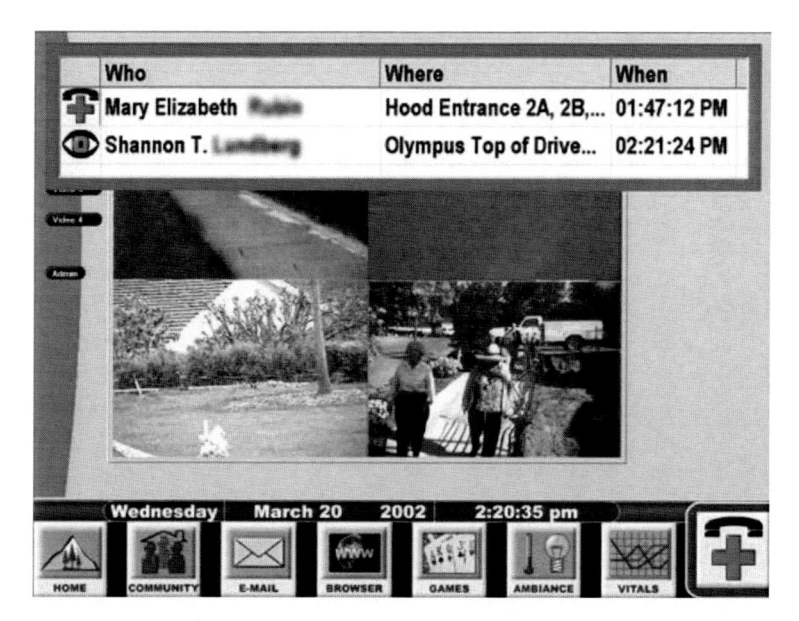

**Fig. 12.10** When residents with cognitive impairments approach the edge of the Oatfield Estates campus, their badges signal the automated care system, and a WebCam captures their image and alerts caregivers in case redirection is necessary

using a password, and find out where the resident is at the moment, as well as access trends for the week or month, including specific activities in which the resident participated.

The emerging intelligent technologies offer great promise for the autonomy of persons with disabilities and the reduction in caregiver burden. Because software algorithms can anticipate and "think" faster than human caregivers, researchers have proposed that future caregiving might include a caregiver supervising software-based "knowbots" who, in turn, would anticipate problems and manage many aspects of daily life. This emerging technology is known as proactive computing (Tennenhouse 2000). Intelligent technologies, however, raise ethical issues associated with their use (Durham 2001; Mynatt and Rogers 2001; van Berlo 2002). Reflecting on ethical issues associated with smart home technologies in the Netherlands, van Berlo (2002) commented that three issues must be considered: (1) the views of all people involved in using the technology, and the consequences of not using the technology; (2) application of the four principles of ethics, namely respect for autonomy, beneficence (what is best for the user and the caregiver), nonmalfeasance (do no harm), and justice; and (3) weighing the appropriateness of a smart technology solution to the particular case in question (p. 86).

*Technologies for Communication of Information and Educational Content* Current education and training of caregivers on the use of basic technologies to support everyday activities is usually obtained from a home care professional (Aranda and Hayman-White 2001; Gibson and Schroder 2001; Kirk 1998; Massimo 2001), from the person with a disability (Tilly et al. 2000; Walker 2001), from other informal caregivers (Perdomo et al. 2002; Rubert et al. 2002), and from educational materials available from public libraries, caregiver support groups, and Web sites that focus on caregiver resources (*AbleLink technologies: Changing lives with cognitive support technologies* 2008; *The caregivers marketplace* 2007; *Caring for people with Huntington's disease* 2005; Family Caregiver Alliance 2005; National Alliance for Caregiving 2005; National Family Caregivers Association 2005; Rosalynn Carter Institute for Caregiving publications 2006; Twilight brigade: Compassion in action 2008).

Education and training of caregivers in emerging technologies to support everyday activities has often incorporated tele-health. Tele-health is one technology that has enabled both monitoring of the health and well-being of the person with a disability as well as caregiver education and training. Tele-health technology for caregivers has included Plain Old Telephone System (POTS) technology, videophones with text, videophones with images (Buckley et al. 2001), WebCam technology (*Aging in place///remote monitoring solution* 2008; *Caring for people with Huntington's disease* 2005), computer-based systems, and combinations of the above (Elliott et al. 1999, 2001; Finkelstein et al. 2001; Sabharwal et al. 2001; Scheideman-Miller 2001; Schulz et al. 2002; Shewchuck et al. 1998; Smith 1995; T.I.E. 2005; Whitehouse et al. 2002; Whitten 2002). Tele-rehab is also gaining acceptance for the provision of occupational therapy, physical therapy, speech therapy, and vocational counseling for both the caregiver and the person with a disability. One of the advantages has been improved compliance with therapy programs (DeBevois 2006).

Although informal caregiving is not usually associated with support of life, ventilator life support systems (*Caring for people with Huntington's disease* 2005) and emerging biohybrid technologies such as a ventricular assist device (VAD; *Caring for people with Huntington's disease* 2005; Holman et al. 2001) can now be managed by informal caregivers who are adequately trained, thus enabling the person with a VAD to carry out daily activities at home. In general, caregivers found most tele-health interventions to be supportive, helpful, and easy to use, leading to greater confidence in implementing caregiving tasks, greater knowledge of caregiving resources, fewer technical errors, less isolation, and less depression (Elliott et al. 1999, 2001; Magnusson et al. 2002; Schulz et al. 2002; Shewchuck et al. 1998). The primary concern expressed by caregivers was the lack of personal contact with professionals. Caregivers also noted that in some instances, they did not have time to spend participating in a tele-health caregiver support group while other caregivers talked about problems that were not pertinent to their own situation (Schulz et al. 2002). Professionals also found the tele-health technology to be adequate and efficient (Buckley et al. 2001; Chambers and Connor 2002; Finkelstein et al. 2001).

## Policy

Policies related to the provision of technologies that support caregivers of persons with disabilities who have problems in the domain of impairment are sparse. Furthermore, those policies that do exist require a creative interpretation of the law for it to apply to caregivers (Romano 1998). For example, a powered mobility wheelchair can be justified for a person with physical and cognitive limitations, but reimbursement for the power override switch for the caregiver will be denied. Most existing policies are focused on the person with a disability not the caregiver. However, the person with the disability and the caregiver are a team in most instances; only their roles differ (Feinberg et al. 2000; Walker 2001). Caregiving for problems in the impairment domain is often related to an acute medical event wherein caregiving technologies may be funded for short-term use only. Depending on the funding source, funding can vary from full coverage to no coverage, and even with funding, families often have to contend with threats of service withdrawal (Cross et al. 1998; Kirk 1998). The Technology-Related Assistance for Individuals with Disabilities Act of 1988 (P.L. 100-407), its amendments (P.L. 103-218), and its reauthorization in 1998 (P.L. 105-394) include definitions of both assistive technology devices and services, but it applies to assistive technology devices where a "medical or legal argument can be made that the device will improve the life of the person with the disability or special need" (Romano 1998). Private insurers, school systems, and state welfare agencies have been most responsive in addressing the technology needs of the person with a disability/caregiver dyad, however, not without litigation (Romano 1998).

Just as litigation has helped to provide technology-related assistance for persons with disabilities, it has also helped to provide funding to purchase caregiving services in the form of personal assistance services legislation (Romano 1998). Even though there are financial, health care, and quality of life advantages in favor of personal assistance services for persons with disabilities who meet the criteria for attendant services, in Pennsylvania alone, in 1997 there were over 5,000 qualified persons still on the waiting list to receive those services (Doty 1998, Summer/Autumn; Prince et al. 1995; Romano 1998; Tilly et al. 2000).

On 1 January 1998, the Medicaid Community Attendant Services Act (MiCASA HR2020) was enacted, which included funding for persons with disabilities to move from a nursing home into the community and to receive education and training in the supervision of personal attendants. In 1998, there were 226 approved home- and community-based waivers under Section 1915 (c) of the Social Security Act that allowed persons who would otherwise be nursing-home-eligible to receive caregiver services in their homes (Katz 1998). Recently, a Robert Wood Johnson Foundation report concluded that the demand for caregiving is increasing and the supply of caregivers is decreasing, especially with the increase of older adults in the US population, many of whom have chronic disabling conditions (Robert Wood Johnson Foundation 2007).

In the late 1990s, the Robert Wood Johnson Foundation, in conjunction with the Health and Human Services 1115 demonstration waiver authority, implemented the "Cash and Counseling" waivers program. The program was designed to improve the efficiency of purchasing wheelchair-durable medical equipment—and then permit the resultant savings to be used by the person with a disability to buy technologies not covered by Medicare. The cash and counseling demonstration was so successful in the 15 states that it was implemented, that these states are evaluating strategies to make it a permanent option (Mahoney et al. 2006). In addition, through new provisions in the 2005 Deficit Reduction Act and 2006 Reauthorization of the Older Americans Act, the federal government has made it easier for states to introduce a Cash and Counseling option for Medicaid consumers (Robert Wood Johnson Foundation 2007).

In 2000, the National Family Caregiver Support Program (NFCSP; Public Law 106-501) was enacted in recognition that families, not just social services, are the mainstay caregivers for older adults. NFCSP includes "ElderTech" services to complement the care provided by family caregivers (Campbell 2001). On 1 February 2001, President Bush announced his new Freedom Initiative, which "will help Americans with disabilities by increasing access to assistive technologies, expanding educational opportunities, increasing the ability of Americans with disabilities to integrate into the workforce, and promoting increased access into daily community life" (Bush 2001). Title II of the Freedom Initiative also included a mandate to develop a national classification system for assistive technology devices. A classification system would help caregivers to understand the level of complexity of the technology they need to master, and persons with disabilities would understand the education and training needed by their caregivers for each classification of technology (WHO 2001).

The 110th US Congress had 27 bills before the House of Representatives and 17 bills before the Senate with a major focus on caregiving (National Alliance for Caregiving 2012). These bills focused on providing tax relief to caregivers of persons with chronic illnesses, expanding Medicare coverage and eliminating restrictions for the access of assistive technology, end-of-life issues, enhancements for medical and family leave, expanding support for caregivers by promoting educational outreach, coordination of care and respite services, prevention of elder abuse, and veterans' issues such as traumatic brain injury. Of particular interest is a bill before the House of Representatives to amend the Social Security Act to exempt medically necessary complex rehabilitation and assistive technology products, such as mobility devices and augmentative and alternate communication devices, from the Medicare competitive acquisition program (GovTrack.us. H.R. 2231—110th Congress 2007). This bill allows persons with disabilities to access customized rehabilitation and assistive technology in an expedited manner, which has the potential to improve societal participation for both persons with disabilities and their caregivers.

In addition, the Older Americans Act with its National Family Caregiver Support Program (NFCSP) was reauthorized in 2006 (U.S. Department of Health and Human Services 2012). The Act requires that the NFCSP, in collaboration with state agencies on aging, conduct research on emerging technologies that support caregivers and the ability of older adults to age-in place.

## Conclusion

Technology can be seductive, but its allure can also be misleading if the technology does not support the caregiver in meeting the needs of the person with a disability. However, in addition to basic issues of being able to access as well as to afford caregiving technologies, other questions must also be addressed for the triad consisting of: (1) the person with a disability, (2) the caregiver, and (3) the technology. Namely, when technology is needed to support caregiving, does the caregiver: (a) want to use technology?, (b) have the skills to use the technology?, (c) understand the technology?, (d) express a negative attitude, anxiety, or fear of the technology?, (e) have the resources to maintain, repair, or replace the technology?, and finally (f) have the skills to assist/support the person with a disability if and when the technology fails? (Holm and Rogers 1991). The following specific future needs/actions are recommended:

### *Practice*

1. Identification of the classifications of technologies and caregiving services that are most effective for resolving problems encountered at each ICF domain by persons with disabilities.
2. Delineation and development of competencies needed by caregivers for each classification of technology they need to use to support a person with disability.

3. Consideration of the ethical issues surrounding the use of emerging technologies for caregiving, including privacy rights and the replacement of person to person interactions with person to machine interactions.

## *Research*

1. Effectiveness and efficacy studies of current and emerging technologies to support caregivers of persons with disabilities, by characteristics of the person with the disability, characteristics of the caregiver, and classification of technology and each ICF domain.
2. Models for matching technologies to the changing needs of persons with disabilities as well as the changing needs of their caregivers.
3. Continuation of sensor technology exploration and proactive computing that can enable persons with disabilities and reduce caregiver burden.
4. Expansion of tele-health technology research that focuses on both the person with a disability as well as the caregiver.

## *Education and Training*

1. Inclusion of content, in curricula addressing human development and human services, on current and emerging technologies that enable caregivers to support persons with disabilities.
2. Delineation of caregiver training methods, by class of technology, that are known to be effective, based on characteristics of caregivers, including learning preferences.
3. Development of problem-solving interactive modules that enable family caregivers to resolve problems with complex technology devices when they fail.

## *Policy*

1. Tax incentives for companies that develop and manufacture small-volume technologies used primarily by persons with disabilities and their caregivers, and pass that savings onto the end users of the technologies.
2. Policy analysis of the implementation of President Bush's Freedom Initiative—namely, how many persons with disabilities are *direct* beneficiaries versus state governments, local governments, researchers, and business owners.
3. Federal and state funding initiatives to support research that focuses on development of affordable and accessible new technologies to support caregivers of persons with disabilities.

# References

ABLEDATA. (2008). http://www.abledata.com. Accessed 13 Aug 2008.
*AbleLink technologies: Changing lives with cognitive support technologies*™. (2008). http://www.ablelinktech.com/_handhelds/. Accessed 13 Aug 2008.
*Aging in place///remote monitoring solution.* (2008). http://www.xanboo.com/aboutus/what/whatis_aging_main.htm. Accessed 13 Aug 2008.
Ambite, J., & Knoblock, C. (2001). Planning by rewriting. *Journal of Artificial Intelligence Research, 15,* 207–261.
Aranda, S., & Hayman-White, K. (2001). Home caregivers of the person with advanced cancer: An Australian perspective. *Cancer Nursing, 24,* 300–307.
Arva, J., Fitzgerald, S., Cooper, R., Corfman, R., Spaethc, D., & Monninger, M. (2000). *Physiologic comparison of Yamaha JWII power assisted and traditional manual wheelchair propulsion.* Paper presented at the RESNA Annual Conference, Orlando, FL.
*The Aware Home Research Institute.* (2008). http://awarehome.imtc.gatech.edu/. Accessed 13 Aug 2008.
Balas, E., & Iakovidis, I. (1999). Distance technologies for patient monitoring. *British Medical Journal, 319,* 1309.
Baltus, G., Fox, D., Gemperle, F., Goetz, J., Hirsch, T., Magaritis, D., et al. (2000). *Towards personal service robots for the elderly.* http://www.cs.cmu.edu/~thrun/papers/thrun.nursebot-early.html. Accessed 13 Aug 2008.
Becker, T. J. (2006, January 28). Heart healthy: CardioMEMS moves closer to commercializing innovative sensors for heart patients. *Research Horizons Magazine.* http://gtresearchnews.gatech.edu/newsrelease/cardiomems.htm. Accessed 13 Aug 2008.
Bialokoz, A., Turner-Smith, A., Tinker, A., Lansley, P., & Bright, K. (2002). Using ICF codes to match assistive technology to persons and property. *Gerotechnology, 2*(1), 154–155.
*The Boulevard.* (2005). http://www.blvd.com/. Accessed 13 Aug 2008.
Buckley, K., Prandoni, C., & Tran, B. (2001). *Nursing management and the acceptance/use of telehealth technologies by caregivers of stroke patients in the home setting.* Paper presented at the State of the Science Conference on Telerehabilitation, Washington, DC.
Burdea, G. (2001). *Haptic feedback interfaces for rehabilitation.* Paper presented at the State of the Science Conference on Telerehabilitation, Washington, DC.
Bush, G. (2001). *New freedom initiative.* http://www.whitehouse.gov/news/freedominitiative/freedominitiative.html. Accessed 13 Aug 2008.
Campbell, M. (2001). *The promise of technology as a caregiving resource: Supplementing eldercare with eldertech.* Paper presented at the National Family Caregiver Support Program Conference: From Enactment to Action, Washington, DC.
*The caregivers marketplace.* (2007). http://www.caregiversmarketplace.com/FrameSetup.asp. Accessed 13 Aug 2008.
*Caring for people with Huntington's disease.* (2005). http://endoflifecare.tripod.com/juvenilehuntingtonsdisease/id179.html. Accessed 13 Aug 2008.
Center for Aging Services Technologies (CAST). (2005). http://www.agingtech.org/index.aspx. Accessed 13 Aug 2008.
Chambers, M., & Connor, S. (2002). User-friendly technology to help family carers cope. *Journal of Advanced Nursing, 40,* 568–577.
Creasey, G., Kilgore, K., Brown-Triolo, D., Dahlberg, J., Peckham, H., & Keith, M. (2000). Reduction of costs of disability using neuroprostheses. *Assistive Technology, 12*(1), 67–75.
Cross, D., Leonard, B., Skay, C., & Rheinberger, M. (1998). Extended hospitalization of medically stable children dependent on technology: A focus on mutable family factors. *Issues in Comprehensive Pediatric Nursing, 21,* 63–84.
*Cyber-Care's Electronic HouseCall System tested in transglobal medical data transfer over Internet2.* (2001). http://www.hoise.com/vmw/01/articles/vmw/LV-VM-07-01-1.html. Accessed 13 Aug 2008.

Davis, J., Triolo, R., Uhlir, J., Bieri, C., Rohde, L., Lissy, D., et al. (2001). Preliminary performance of a surgically implanted neuroprosthesis for standing and transfers—where do we stand? *Journal of Rehabilitation Research and Development, 38,* 609–617.

DeBevois, K. (2006). *Telerehab: Therapy anywhere, anytime.* http://www.therapytimes.com/content=6501J64E487EA4941. Accessed 13 Aug 2008.

Dey, A., Salber, D., & Abowd, G. (1999, December 13–14). *A context-based infrastructure for smart environments.* Paper presented at the International Workshop on Managing Interactions in Smart Environments (MANSE '99), Dublin, Ireland.

Dey, A., Salber, D., & Abowd, G. (2001). A conceptual framework and a toolkit for supporting the rapid prototyping of context-aware applications. *Human-Computer Interaction (HCI) Journal, 16*(2–4), 97–166.

Dishman, E. (2004). Inventing wellness systems for aging in place. *Computer Magazine,* May, 34–41.

Donahue, B. (2001). *Byte, byte, against the dying of the light.* http://www.theatlantic.com/issues/2001/05/donahue.htm. Accessed 13 Aug 2008.

Doty, P. (1998, Summer/Autumn). The cash and counseling demonstration: An experiment in consumer-directed personal assistance services (Part 1 of 2). *American Rehabilitation, 24*(3), 27–30.

Durham, M. (2001). Editors' comments: A commentary on technology and the future of health care. *The Permanente Journal, 5*(1), 5–7.

EliteCare. (2008). *Extended family residences: An alternative to assisted living.* http://www.elite-care.com/. Accessed 13 Aug 2008.

Elliott, T., Shewchuck, R., & Richards, J. (1999). Caregiver social problem-solving abilities and family member adjustment to recent-onset physical disability. *Rehabilitation Psychology, 44*(1), 104–123.

Elliott, T., Shewchuck, R., & Richards, J. (2001). Family caregiver social problem-solving abilities and adjustment during the initial year of the caregiving role. *Journal of Counseling Psychology, 48*(2), 223–232.

Englehardt, K. (1989). Computers, artificial intelligence, robotics, and aging humans. *International Journal of Technology and Aging, 2*(1), 4.

Englehardt, K., & Goughler, D. (1997). Robotic technologies and the older adult. In A. Fisk & W. Rogers (Eds.), *Handbook of human factors and the older adult* (pp. 395–413). San Diego: Academic Press.

Family Caregiver Alliance (FCA). (2005). http://www.caregiver.org/. Accessed 13 Aug 2008.

Farah, M., Illes, J., Cook-Deegan, R., Gardner, H., Kandel, E., King, P., et al. (2004). Neurocognitive enhancement: What can we do and what should we do? *Nature Reviews: Neuroscience, 5,* 421–425.

Feinberg, L., Whitlatch, C., & Tucke, S. (2000). *Making hard choices: Respecting both voices.* San Francisco: Family Caregiver Alliance.

Finkelstein, S., Speedie, S., Demiris, G., Hoff, M., & Lundgren, J. (2001). *Telemedicine in home healthcare.* Paper presented at the State of the Science Conference on Telerehabilitation, Washington, DC.

Fiorini, P., & Shiller, Z. (1998). Motion planning in dynamic environments using velocity obstacles. *International Journal of Robotics Research, 17,* 760–772.

*The future of brain–computer interfacting.* (2005). http://www.neuralsignals.com/. Accessed 13 Aug 2008.

Gibson, M., & Schroder, C. (2001). The many faces of pain for older, dying adults. *American Journal of Hospice & Palliative Care, 18*(1), 19–25.

GovTrack.us. H.R. 2231—110th Congress. (2007). *Medicare access to complex rehabilitation and assistive technology act of 2007.* www.govtrack.us/congress/bill.xpd?bill=h110–2231. Accessed 13 Aug 2008.

Grill, W., Craggs, M., Foreman, R., Ludlow, C., & Buller, J. (2001). Emerging clinical applications of electrical stimulation: Opportunities for restoration of function. *Journal of Rehabilitation Research and Development, 38,* 641–653.

Gurley, R., Lum, N., Sande, M., Lo, B., & Katz, M. (1996). Persons found in their homes helpless or dead. *New England Journal of Medicine, 334,* 1710–1716.

Haigh, K., & Kiff, L. (2004, July 25–29). *The Independent LifeStyle Assistant (I.L.S.A.): AI lessons learned.* Paper presented at the IAAI 04, San Jose, CA.

Hammel, J., Lai, J., & Heller, T. (2002). The impact of assistive technology and environmental interventions on function and living situation status with people who are ageing with developmental disabilities. *Disability and Rehabilitation, 24*(1/2/3), 93–105.

Hersh, N., & Treadgold, L. (1994). NeuroPage: The rehabilitation of memory dysfunction by prosthetic memory and cueing. *Neurorehabilitation, 4,* 187–197.

Herz-Unterstützungssysteme. (2003). http://www.herz-lungen-maschine.de/. Accessed 13 Aug 2008.

*High technology and its benefits for an aging population.* (1984). House of Representatives, 98th Congress, 2nd Session Sess.

Ho, G., Kiff, L., Plocher, T., & Haigh, K. (2005). *A model of trust and reliance of automation technology for older adults.* http://www.cs.cmu.edu/~khaigh/papers/05-Ho_Trust.pdf. Accessed 13 Aug 2008.

Holm, M., & Rogers, J. (1991). High, low, or no assistive technology devices for older adults undergoing rehabilitation. *International Journal of Technology and Aging, 4*(2), 153–161.

*Independence iBOT.* (2005). http://www.independencenow.com/home.html. Accessed 13 Aug 2008.

Holman, W. L., Ormaza, S., Seemuth, K., Boehmer, J. P., & Richenbacher, W. E. (2001). How to run an outpatient VAD program: Overview. *ASAIO Journal, 47,* 588–589.

Katz, R. (1998). The home and community-based work group: Partners with state, consumers and others to advance the PAS agenda. *American Rehabilitation, 24*(4), 1–3. (Editor's Note: Check page numbers.) http://www.findarticles.com/p/articles/mi_m0842/is_4_24/ai_54610692. Accessed 13 Aug 2008.

Kirk, S. (1998). Families' experiences of caring at home for a technology-dependent child: A review of the literature. *Child: Care, Health and Development, 24*(2), 101–114.

Levinson, R. (1995). A general programming language for unified planning and control. *Artificial Intelligence, 76,* 319–375.

Levinson, R. (1997). Tests, measurement, and technology. The Planning and Execution Assistant and Trainer (PEAT) hand-held electronic calendar and address book that features automatic cueing to start and stop daily activities. *Journal of Head Trauma Rehabilitation, 12*(2), 85–91.

*Lifeline personal response and support services.* (2005). http://www.lifelinesys.com/. Accessed 13 Aug 2008.

Lovell, N., Magrabi, F., Celler, B., Huynh, K., & Garsden, H. (2001). Web-based acquisition, storage and retrieval of biomedical signals. *IEEE Engineering in Medicine and Biology, May/June,* 38–44.

Lozano, A. (2001). Deep brain stimulation: Challenges to integrating stimulation technology with human neurobiology, neuroplasticity, and neural repair [Editorial]. *Journal of Rehabilitation Research and Development, 38,* x–xix.

Magnusson, L., Hanson, E., Brito, L., Berthold, H., Chambers, M., & Daly, T. (2002). Supporting family carers through the use of information and communication technology—The EU project ACTION. *International Journal of Nursing Studies, 39,* 369–381.

Mahoney, K. J., Simon-Rusinowitz, L., Simone, K., & Zgoda, K. (2006). Cash and counseling: a promising option for consumer direction of home- and community-based services and supports. *Case Management Journals, 7,* 199–204.

Massimo, L. (2001). Home care services and the role of "caregivers". *Minerva Pediatrica, 53*(3), 161–169.

McCarthy, C., & Pollack, M. (2002). *A plan-based personalized cognitive orthotic*. Paper presented at the 6th International Conference on AI Planning and Scheduling, Toulouse, France.

MedPrompt: Solutions for better aging™. (2005). http://www.agenet.com/service_ASP/MedPrompt_Brochure.asp. Accessed 13 Aug 2008.

Memory Aided Prompting System (MAPS). (2003). http://l3d.cs.colorado.edu/clever/projects/maps.html. Accessed 13 Aug 2008.

Mollenkopf, H., & Wahl, H. (2002). *Future societal trends and expectations of the next-generation older users of domotics*. Paper presented at the Symposium on Domotics and Networking, Miami Beach, FL.

Montemerlo, M., Pineau, J., Roy, N., Thrun, S., & Verma, V. (2002). *Experiences with a mobile robotic guide for the elderly*. http://www-2.cs.cmu.edu/~thrun/papers/thrun.pearlAAAI02.html. Accessed 13 Aug 2008.

Morris, A., Donamukkala, R., Kapuria, A., Steinfeld, A., Matthews, J., Dunbar-Jacob, J., et al. (2002). *A robotic walker that provides guidance*. http://www-2.cs.cmu.edu/~thrun/papers/thrun.robo-walker.pdf. Accessed 13 Aug 2008.

Morris, M., Lundell, J., & Dishman, E. (2004). *Catalyzing social interaction with ubiquitous computing: A needs assessment of elders coping with cognitive decline*. Paper presented at the CHI 2004, Vienna, Austria.

Murdoch, L., Kinney, J., Kart, C., & Ziemba, T. (2002). Caregiving in place: The role of technology. *Gerotechnology, 2*(1), 154.

Mynatt, E., & Rogers, W. (2001). Developing technology to support the functional independence of older adults. *Ageing International, 27*(1), 24–41.

National Alliance for Caregiving (NAC). (2005). http://www.caregiving.org/. Accessed 13 Aug 2008.

National Alliance for Caregiving (NAC). (2012). http://www.caregiving.org/FederalLegislation.htm. Accessed 13 Aug 2008.

National Family Caregivers Association (NFCA). (2005). http://www.nfcacares.org/. Accessed 13 Aug 2008.

Odom, S., & Chandler, L. (1990). Transition to parenthood for parents of technology-assisted infants. *Early Childhood Special Education, 9*(4), 43–54.

PEAT: The planning and execution assistant and training system. (2005). http://www.brainaid.com/publications/pub.html. Accessed 13 Aug 2008.

Perdomo, D., Czaja, S., & Rubert, M. (2002). Tele-REACH: A telephone intervention for caregivers. *Gerotechnology, 2*(1), 143–144.

Perkins, M. (1993). Parent–nurse collaborations: Using the caregiver identity emergence phases to assist parents of hospitalized children with disabilities. *Journal of Pediatric Nursing, 8*(1), 2–9.

Pollack, M. (2002). *Planning technology for intelligent cognitive orthotics*. Paper presented at the 6th International Conference on AI Planning and Scheduling, Toulouse, France.

Pollack, M. E., Engberg, S., Matthews, J. T., Thrun, S., Brown, L., Colby, D., et al. (2002, August). *Pearl: A mobile robotic assistant for the elderly. Paper presented at the AAAI Workshop on Automation as Eldercare*. http://www.cs.cmu.edu/~nursebot/web/papers/umich/aaai02wkshp.pdf. Accessed 13 Aug 2008.

Prince, M. J., Manley, M. S., & Whiteneck, G. G. (1995). Self-managed versus agency-provided assistance care for individuals with high level tetraplegia. *Archives of Physical Medicine and Rehabilitation, 76*, 919–923. http://www.independentliving.org/docs3/smap95.html. Accessed 13 Aug 2008.

*Rehabilitation engineers' emphasis on helping people with disabilities will improve wireless technology for everyone*. (2002). http://gtresearchnews.gatech.edu/newsrelease/MOBILEWIRE.htm. Accessed 13 Aug 2008.

Robert Wood Johnson Foundation. (2007). *Choosing independence: A summary of the cash & counseling model of self-directed personal assistance services*. http://www.cashandcounseling.org/resources/20070614-152529/FinalRWJ_CC_16pp_green_v4.pdf. Accessed 13 Aug 2008.

Romano, J. (1998). *Legal rights of the catastrophically ill and injured: A family guide* (2nd ed.). Norristown: Author.

Rosalynn Carter Institute for Caregiving. (2006). *Publications.* http://www.rosalynncarter.org/publications/. Accessed 13 Aug 2008.

Rubert, M., Czaja, S., & Walsh, S. (2002). Tele-care: Helping caregivers cope with cancer. *Gerotechnology, 2*(1), 144.

Sabharwal, S., Mezaros, M., & Duafenbach, L. (2001). *Telerehabilitation across the continuum of care for individuals with spinal cord injury.* Paper presented at the State of the Science Conference on Telerehabilitation, Washington, DC.

Sample, I. (2005a). *Chip reads mind of paralysed man.* http://www.mindfully.org/Technology/2005/Chip-Reads-Mind31mar05.htm. Accessed 13 Aug 2008.

Sample, I. (2005b, March 31). *Meet the mind readers.* London: The Guardian (UK).

Sanders, J. M. (2000). *Sensing the subtleties of everyday life.* Atlanta: Georgia Tech Research Horizons. http://gtresearchnews.gatech.edu/reshor/rh-win00/main.html. Accessed 13 Aug 2008.

Sanders, J. (2005). *Virtual voices: Wearable captioning system to make public venues accessible to people who are deaf or hard of hearing.* http://gtresearchnews.gatech.edu/newsrelease/captioning.htm. Accessed 13 Aug 2008.

Scheideman-Miller, C. (2001). *INTEGRIS rural telemedicine project:* Telerehab TM. Paper presented at the State of the Science Conference on Telerehabilitation, Washington, DC.

Scherer, M. (1991). *Matching person and technology.* Rochester: Author.

Scherer, M. (2000). *Living in the state of stuck: How assistive technology impacts the lives of people with disabilities* (3rd ed.). Cambridge: Brookline Books.

Scherer, M., & Galvin, J. (1997). Outcomes of assistive technology: Matching the right person with the right technology, then measuring the result. *Rehabilitation Management, February/March,* 103–105.

Schulz, R., Lustig, A., Handler, S., & Martire, L. (2002). Technology-based caregiver intervention research: Current status and future directions. *Gerotechnology, 2*(1), 15–47.

Shewchuck, R., Richards, J., & Elliott, T. (1998). Dynamic processes in health outcomes among caregivers of patients with spinal cord injuries. *Health Psychology, 17*(2), 125–129.

Smith, G. (1995). The risks of using complex technology in home care. *Caring, 14*(5), 30–34.

T.I.E. (2005). *Telemedicine information exchange.* http://tie.telemed.org/programs_t2/. Accessed 13 Aug 2008.

Talan, J. (2005). *Psychiatric drug implants.* http://www.mindfreedom.org/kb/mental-health-abuse/brain-experiment/psychiatric-drug-implants. Accessed 13 Aug 2008.

Tennenhouse, D. (2000). Proactive computing. *Communications of the ACM, 43*(3), 43–50.

Thomas, P. W. (2002). *Pre-summit issues paper.* Paper presented at the Access to Assistive Technologies: Improving Health and Well Being for People with Disabilities, Orlando, FL.

Thrun, S., Fox, D., & Burgard, W. (1998). A probabilistic approach to concurrent mapping and localization for mobile robots. *Machine Learning, 31,* 29–53.

Tilly, J., Wiener, J., & Cuellar, A. (2000). *Consumer-directed home and community services programs in five countries: Policy issues for older people and government.* Washington: The Urban Institute.

*Twilight brigade: Compassion in action.* (2008). http://www.thetwilightbrigade.com/. Accessed 13 Aug 2008.

Ulrich, I., & Borenstein, J. (2001). The GuideCane—Applying mobile robot technologies to assist the visually impaired. *IEEE Transactions on Systems, Man, and Cybernetics, 31*(2), 131–136.

U.S. Department of Health and Human Services. (2012). *The administration on aging: Gateway to the older Americans act amendments of 2006.* http://www.aoa.gov/oaa2006/Main_Site/index.aspx. Accessed 13 Aug 2008.

van Berlo, A. (2002). Smart home technology: Have older people paved the way? *Gerotechnology, 2*(1), 77–87.

Vedantam, S. (16 November 2002). *New techniques raise fear of coercion.* Washington Post, p. A1.

Walker, P. (2001). *A generic orientation to doing attendant work.* http://www.independentliving.org/docs2/walker2001.pdf. Accessed 13 Aug 2008.

Whitehouse, P., Marling, C., & Harvey, R. (2002). *Can a computer be a caregiver?* Paper presented at the AAAI 2002 Fall Symposium Series, Cape Cod, MA.

Whitten, P. (2002). Telehome health for COPD & CHF patients in Michigan. *Gerotechnology, 2*(1), 143.

World Health Organization. (2001). *ICF: International classification of functioning, disability and health*. Geneva: World Health Organization.

*The Wright Stuff caregiver products*. (2005). http://www.thewright-stuff.com/. Accessed 13 Aug 2008.

Wu, P., & Miller, C. (2005). *Results from a field study: The need for an emotional relationship between the elderly and their assistive technologies*. http://www.sift.info/publications/PDF/Wu-AugCog2005.pdf. Accessed 13 Aug 2008.

# Chapter 13
# Multiple Dimensions of Caregiving and Disability: Supporting Those Who Care

**Ronda C. Talley and John E. Crews**

Family caregivers form the foundation of the American healthcare system. Collectively, the wives and husbands, mothers and fathers, sisters and brothers, grandmothers and grandfathers, as well as friends, neighbors, and many others constitute the single largest block of unpaid human capital providing care today. The giving of care, or caregiving, brings together these individuals in a commitment that some wish to assume while others accept reluctantly. Family caregivers provide normative care, care that is a normal part of the life cycle, as well as exceptional care for those who are frail or elderly, or those who are born with or acquire a disability at some point in their lives. Caregiving is an issue that touches every life. Within the last decade, it has finally been recognized in American politics (Carter 2011; The White House 2001, 2011a, b) and by the general public as the important issue it is (Family Caregiver Alliance [FCA] 2003; Feinberg 2004; Feinberg et al. 2006). Caregivers are just starting to receive the attention and support they deserve (AARP 2004, 2006; The Arc 2011; The White House 2009).

Throughout this book, cutting-edge information has been presented on the current status and future directions of one segment within the caregiving universe—the caregivers of individuals with disabilities. Sixteen national experts have explored these areas to answer the questions of "what's known and what's needed" in caregiving across 12 issue areas. They have addressed caregiving for individuals with disabilities in terms of spirituality, ethnicity, psychological, educational, legislative, and policy domains.

---

The findings and conclusions in this chapter are those of the authors and do not necessarily represent the views of the Centers for Disease Control and Prevention.

---

R. C. Talley (✉)
Western Kentucky University, 1906 College Heights Boulevard,
Bowling Green, KY 42101, USA
e-mail: ronda.talley@wku.edu

J. E. Crews
Division of Diabetes Translation, Centers for Disease Control and Prevention,
4770 Buford Highway, NE, K-10, Atlanta, GA 30341, USA
e-mail: jcrews@cdc.gov

These writings have been drafted against a backdrop of caregiving and disability issues within the nation's public health framework (Talley 2007; Talley and Crews 2007a, b). In preparing this book, we have drawn from important national initiatives: *Disability in America* (Pope and Tarlov 1991), *Enabling America* (Brandt and Pope 1997), *Healthy People 2010* (U.S. Department of Health & Human Services 2000a, b), the *Surgeon General's Call to Action to Improve the Health and Wellness of Persons with Disabilities* (U.S. Department of Health & Human Services 2005), the *Workshop on Disability in America* (Field et al. 2006) *The Future of Disability in America* (Field and Jette 2007), *Healthy People 2020* (U.S. Department of Health & Human Services 2010), and *Rising Expectations: The Developmental Disabilities Act Revisited* (National Council on Disability 2011). We have also crafted this book while considering critical federal and state laws, statutes, legislation, and litigation. Recent examples of these latter include the National Family Caregiver Support Program (Administration on Aging 2011) and the Patient Protection and Affordable Care Act (PPACA 2010) in tandem with the Health Care and Education Reconciliation Act of 2010 and the Community Living Assistance Services and Supports (CLASS) Act (2010).

Furthermore, we have emphasized the very real needs and desires of the family members who provide care for a family member with one or more disabilities. Our findings resonate with those described by Dr. Perkins (2011) in her white paper on "compound" caregivers. While Perkins addresses the care of older intellectually disabled individuals, the observation may be equally relevant when applied to individuals with other disabilities:

> Within the caregiver population, older caregivers of adults with intellectual disabilities are a unique group. They face circumstances and challenges that are quite distinct from caregivers of persons that have developed illnesses, or acquired disabilities from accidents or trauma. These challenges include the fact that their caregiving role has been a lifelong endeavor, and thus they face lifespan health issues that arise from their care recipients' often complex aging process, as well as their own aging process/illnesses. Furthermore, unlike most other caregiving roles which cease upon the death or diminish after transfer to a long term care setting of the care recipient, caregivers in these circumstances often continue caregiving until their own incapacity or death. Thus, there is an added anxiety regarding the future welfare of adult sons or daughters with intellectual disabilities when the caregiver is no longer alive or able to provide care. (p. 1).

Perkins describes these demanding, often life-long responsibly well: "The collective contribution provided by caregivers to support the health and well-being of individuals with disabilities and/or chronic health issues is substantial" (Perkins 2011). While there are positive benefits of providing care, numerous negative health effects of intensive long-term caregiving has been well documented by leading researchers, including the Centers for Disease Control and Prevention (2008), Given and Given (1998), Gross (2006), Heller and Caldwell (2006), Jacobs (2004), Levine (2004), Murphy et al. (2007), Skaff and Pearlin (1992), Schwartz (2003), and Schwartz and Gidron (2002).

Family caregivers, as essential team members with professional caregivers, such as doctors, nurses, social workers, psychologists, and other medical personnel, labor to create a matrix of services and processes that form a comprehensive and coordinated support plan for the child or adult with disabilities for whom they care (Talley 2004).

## The Future of Caregiving and Disability

Several key themes emerged throughout this book. These themes need the attention and action of the caregiving community.

### *Develop the Science*

We need to continue to develop the science of caregiving and disability by understanding the magnitude and dimensions of the problem at the national, state, and community levels, among different age groups, different racial/ethnic groups, among people who have moderate-to-little financial resources. The stronger this knowledge, the more rational our decisions can be.

### *Create Policies that Make Sense, Reform Those that Do Not*

As noted throughout this book, we need to reform and make manageable and sensible the policies that affect caregivers and people with disabilities. People generally turn a sympathetic ear to those involved in caregiving, but the policies do not follow. Policies need to be constructed in a manner that encourages caregivers and/or people with disabilities to work, to live where they want, and to be able to move from state to state without losing supports, and to have as much control as possible over their own lives.

### *Develop a Comprehensive and Coordinated Research Agenda*

Expanding the research to better understand changes over time and the roles of both mothers and fathers is needed. In addition, we need to know more about the physical health, use of health services, and health behaviors of caregivers. Furthering the research to explicitly look at positive benefits of caregiving is further warranted in order to provide a more balanced perspective to the experience of raising a child with a disability. The research on parental stress and mental health is starting to uncover protective factors for families. Further work to understand protective factors will help researchers design more targeted interventions. In addition, research needs to look at protective factors for other parental outcomes.

## *Provide Seamless Support Free of Crippling Bureaucratic Burdens*

Finally, we need to make sense of the practice of caregiving. For many families the practice of caregiving is very hard work. It is not without joy, great pleasure, and pride, but it is often hard. Some families might need some training, but that might be minimal; some families might need social support, but that might not be essential. They probably all need help, help that is seamless, without burden and without bureaucracy.

## Concluding Comments

Caregiving and disability define a topic that must honor the experience of caregivers—parents, siblings, spouses, grandparents, and others—and it must honor the experience of people who are born with or acquire disabilities. The more we are responsive to each, the more we are responsive to both.

## References

AARP. (2004, April 6). *Providing care for another adult a second job for many, National Alliance for Caregiving/AARP Study Shows* (news release). Washington: AARP Public Policy Institute. http://www.aarp.org/research/press-center/presscurrentnews/a2004-03-30-caregiving.html. Accessed 5 May 2012.

AARP. (2006, March 16). *Who's caring for the caregivers? AARP unveils new report on trends in support for family caregivers: Consumer-directed services for caregivers take hold in states* (news release). Washington: AARP Public Policy Institute. http://www.aarp.org/research/press-center/presscurrentnews/caring_for_caregivers.html. Accessed 5 May 2012.

Administration on Aging, U.S. Department of Health and Human Services. (2011). *National Family Caregiver Support Program (OAA Title IIIE)*. http://www.aoa.gov/aoaroot/aoa_programs/hcltc/caregiver/index.aspx. Accessed 5 May 2012.

The Arc. (2011). *Still in the shadows with their future uncertain: A report on individual and family needs for disability supports (FINDS)*. http://www.thearc.org/document.doc?id=3140. Accessed 5 May 2012.

Brandt, E. N. & Pope, A. M. (1997). *Enabling America: assessing the role of rehabilitation science and engineering*. Washington, DC: National Academies Press.

Carter, R. (2011, May 26). *Written testimony of Former First Lady Rosalynn Carter before the Senate Special Committee on Aging*. http://www.cartercenter.org/news/editorials_speeches/rosalynn-carter-committee-on-aging-testimony.html?printerFriendly=true. Accessed 5 May 2012.

Centers for Disease Control & Prevention. (2008). *CDC seeks to protect the health of family caregivers*. http://www.chronicdisease.org/nacdd-initiatives/healthy-aging/meeting-records/HA_CIB_HealthofFamilyCaregivers.pdf. Accessed 5 May 2012.

*Community Living Assistance Services and Supports Act*. (2010). http://www.aoa.gov/AoARoot/CLASS/Law/docs/CLASSAct_Amendments.pdf. Accessed 5 May 2012.

Family Caregiver Alliance. (2003). *The road to recognition: International review of public policies to support family and informal caregiving: Policy brief*. http://www.caregiver.org/caregiver/jsp/content/pdfs/op_2003_the_road_to_recognition.pdf. Accessed 5 May 2012.

Feinberg, L. F. (2004). Caregiving on the public policy agenda. In C. Levine (Ed.), *Always on call: When illness turns families into caregivers* (updated & expanded). Nashville: Vanderbilt University Press.

Feinberg, L. F., Wolkwitz, K., & Goldstein, C. (2006, March). *Ahead of the curve: Emerging trends and practices in family caregiver support* (research report). Washington: AARP Public Policy Institute. http://www.aarp.org/research/longtermcare/resources/Articles/2006_09_caregiver.html. Accessed 5 May 2012.

Field, M. J., Jette, A. M. & Martin, L. (2006). Workshop on disability in America: a new look. Washington, DC: National Academies Press.

Field, M. J. & Jette, A. M. (2007). The future of disability in America. Washington, DC: National Academies Press.

Given, B. A., & Given, C. W. (1998). Health promotion for family caregivers of chronically ill elders. *Annual Review of Nursing Research, 16,* 197–217.

Gross, J. (2006, March 25). As parents age, baby boomers and business struggle to cope. *New York Times,* p. A1. http://www.nytimes.com/2006/03/25/national/25care.html?ex=1300942800&en=ab7386f2cbddb234&ei=5088&partner=rssnyt&emc=rss. Accessed 5 May 2012.

Heller, T. & Caldwell, J (2006). Supporting aging caregivers and adults with developmental disabilities win future planning. *Mental Retardation, 44 (3),* 189–202.

Jacobs, B. J. (2004). From sadness to pride: Seven common emotional experiences of caregiving. In C. Levine (Ed.), *Always on call: When illness turns families into caregivers* (updated). Nashville: Vanderbilt University Press.

Levine, C. (Ed.). (2004). *Always on call: When illness turns families into caregivers* (updated & expanded). Nashville: Vanderbilt University Press.

Murphy, N. A., Christian, B., Caplin, D. A., & Young, P. C. (2007). The health of caregivers for children with disabilities: Caregiver perspectives. *Child: Care, Health and Development, 33*(2), 180–187.

National Council on Disability. (2011). *Rising expectations: The Developmental Disabilities Act revisited.* http://www.ncd.gov/publications/2011/Feb142011. Accessed 5 May 2012.

Patient Protection and Affordable Care Act, 2010. http://www.cms.gov/Regulations-and-Guidance/Legislation/LegislativeUpdate/downloads//PPACA.pdf. Accessed 7 May 2012.

Perkins, E. A. (2011). *Compound caregivers: Overlooked and overburdened* (white paper). Tampa: University of South Florida, Florida Center for Inclusive Communities. http://flfcic.fmhi.usf.edu/docs/FCIC_CompoundCaregivers_070811.pdf. Accessed 5 May 2012.

Pope, A. M. & Tarlov, A. R. (1991). *Disability in America: toward a national agenda for prevention.* Washington, DC: National Academies Press.

Schwartz, C. (2003). Parents of children with chronic disabilities: The gratification of caregiving. *Families in Society, 84*(4), 576–584.

Schwartz, C., & Gidron, R. (2002). Parents of mentally ill adult children living at home: Rewards of caregiving. *Health & Social Work, 27*(2), 145–154.

Skaff, M. M., & Pearlin, L. I. (1992). Caregiving: Role engulfment and the loss of self. *Gerontologist, 32*(5), 656–664.

Talley, R. C. (Ed.). (2004). *Caring for yourself while helping a loved one with a disability.* RCI caregiving pamphlet series: Twelve tips for caregivers. Americus: Rosalynn Carter Institute for Caregiving. http://www.rci.gsw.edu/RCIBookStore/Manuals_and_Booklets_files/Disability.final.pdf. Accessed 5 May 2012.

Talley, R. C. (2007). *Advancing caregiving as a public health issue. The need for surveillance and intervention.* Paper presented at the annual meeting of the American Public Health Association.

Talley, R. C., & Crews, J. E. (2007a). Framing the public health of caregiving. *American Journal of Public Health, 97*(2), 224–228.

Talley, R. C., & Crews, J. E. (2007b). Talley and Crews respond. Public health caregiving: Up to the challenge. *American Journal of Public Health, 97*(11), 1931–1932.

U.S. Department of Health & Human Services. (2000a). *Healthy people 2010: Understanding and improving health* (2nd ed.). Washington: U.S. Government Printing Office

U.S. Department of Health & Human Services. (2000b). *Healthy people 2010: With understanding and improving health and objectives for improving health* (2nd ed., 2 vols.). Washington: U.S. Government Printing Office.

U.S. Department of Health & Human Services. (2005). *Surgeon General's call to action to improve the health and wellness of persons with disabilities*. Rockville: U.S. Department of Health and Human Services, Office of the Surgeon General. http://www.surgeongeneral.gov/library/disabilities/calltoaction/calltoaction.pdf. Accessed 5 May 2012.

U.S. Department of Health & Human Services. (2010). http://www.healthypeople.gov/2020/default.aspx. Accessed 7 May 2012.

The White House. (2001, February 1). *President's new freedom initiative*. http://georgewbush-whitehouse.archives.gov/infocus/newfreedom/. Accessed 5 May 2012.

The White House. (2009, January 30). *Vice President Biden announces Middle Class Task Force* (press release). http://www.whitehouse.gov/blog_post/vice_president_biden_announces_middle_class_task_force_1/. More information available at http://www.whitehouse.gov/strongmiddleclass/. Accessed 5 May 2012.

The White House. (2011a, June 22). *On anniversary of Olmstead, Obama administration recommits to assist Americans with disabilities* (press release). http://www.whitehouse.gov/the-press-office/2011/06/22/anniversary-olmstead-obama-administration-recommits-assist-americans-dis. Accessed 5 May 2012.

The White House. (2011b, November). *Presidential proclamation—National Family Caregivers Month*. Washington, DC. http://www.whitehouse.gov/the-press-office/2010/10/29/presidential-proclamation-national-family-caregivers-month. Accessed 5 May 2012.

# Index

**A**
Accountable Care Organizations (ACOs), 343, 348
Activities of daily living (ADL), 91, 116, 173, 174, 177, 179
AD patients. *see* Alzheimer's disease
African Americans, 14, 75, 197, 202, 203, 205, 207, 209, 212, 215, 216, 332
Agency, 26, 27, 33
  balanced, 27, 41
  unbalanced, 27
Alaskan Natives, 204
Alzheimer's disease, 10, 39, 92, 176, 179
American Indians, 202, 204, 205, 216
American Speech-Language and Hearing Association (ASHA), 130
Americans with Disabilities Act (ADA), 15, 134, 167, 170, 305, 334, 337
Anger, 10, 34–36, 38, 39, 57, 69, 76, 176
Anxiety, 270
Arthritis, 13, 147, 178, 185, 213, 270
Asian Americans, 197, 202, 204, 205, 210, 213, 214, 216
Asperger's disorder, 40
Attention deficit hyperactivity disorder (ADHD), 299
Autistic spectrum disorders, 141

**B**
Biopsychosocial model, 25
Bitterness, 58, 59
Bladder catheterization, 23
Breast cancer, 113

**C**
Cancer, 10, 38, 270, 361
Care recipient, relationship of, 6
Caregiver burden, 37, 41, 58, 63, 70, 72, 75–77
Caregiver burden, concept of, 11, 58
Caregiver burden, perception of, 77, 78
Caregiver burden, reduced, 78, 277, 338, 361, 364–366, 368–371, 376, 383
Caregiver depression, 44
Caregiver education, 11, 92, 93, 100, 102, 103, 105, 112, 114, 116, 123
Caregiver expectations, 76
Caregiver experiences, 76
Caregiver Health Effects Study (CHES), 180, 184
Caregiver-care recipient dyad, 7, 8
Caregiving, 3, 4, 6, 7, 29, 58, 69, 73, 74, 78, 95, 116, 175, 197, 215, 314, 378, 411
  dynamics of, 30
Caregiving demands, 14, 29, 30, 36, 135, 136, 145, 179
Center for independent living (CIL), 303
Centers for Disease Control and Prevention (CDC), 96, 166, 167, 203, 300
Cerebral palsy, 198, 281, 306, 311, 329
Cervical cancer, 204
Childhood disability, 8, 12, 14, 62, 70, 136, 138, 139, 141, 143, 145, 151, 152, 172, 175, 184, 207, 229, 414
Childhood disability, epidemiology of, 132
Children, 7–9, 11, 12, 16, 23, 30, 33, 39, 61, 62, 66–68, 70, 92, 148
CHIP programs, 148, 149
Chronic disease, 15, 43, 178, 210, 261, 263
Chronic illness, 23, 31, 33, 37, 43–45, 57, 62, 65, 70, 71, 75, 77–79, 209, 381
Chronic state of crisis, 29
Cognitive disabilities, 7, 30, 271
Cognitive impairment, 40
Cognitive impairments, 73, 198, 375, 399
Collateral caregivers, 96
Communication processes, 27, 28, 123

Comprehensive System of Personnel Development (CSPD), 106
Congenital defects, 23, 33
Consolidated Omnibus Budget Reconciliation Act (COBRA), 311
Critical caregiver tasks, identification of, 15
Culture, 76, 77
Current Population Survey (CPS), 300
Cystic fibrosis, 29

**D**
Dementia, 40, 75, 172, 176, 181, 211, 347, 373, 375
Depression, 12, 36, 58, 59, 263, 264, 270, 272
  stress associated, 182
Depressive symptomatology, 142
Developmental disabilities, 116, 140, 141, 178, 243, 273, 277, 327–334, 336, 337, 339, 340, 342–346, 349
Diabetes, 92, 203, 270, 300, 367
Diagnostic services, 95
Disability, 7, 9, 10, 24, 197
Disability, aging, 422
Disability, definition of, 166
Disability, severity of, 7, 91, 167, 176, 180, 182
Distress, 5
Domains of disability, 176
Down's syndrome, 176

**E**
Education, 12, 14, 15, 77, 90, 94, 95, 99, 101, 102, 112, 115, 117, 119, 120, 122–124, 169, 235, 250, 328, 337–339, 368
Education, types, 114
Emotional care, 4, 12
Emotional caregiver, 5, 11
Emotional problems, 58
Emotional stress, 3, 12, 142
End of life issues, 30, 381
End-of-life care, 6, 16
Epilepsy, 29, 352
Ethnicity, 75–77, 99, 196, 197, 200, 202, 209, 212, 214, 215, 219, 411

**F**
Family belief systems, 27, 28
Family caregiver, 5, 9, 11, 12, 15, 32, 42, 46, 47, 65, 76, 250, 263, 274, 277, 279, 280, 282, 329, 333, 336, 346, 411
Family caregiver, feelings of, 57, 62, 77, 78
Family caregiving, 4–6, 12, 27, 28, 38, 57, 58, 113, 143, 164, 172, 174, 179, 199, 264, 265, 277, 279

Family dynamics, 23, 24, 27, 29–32, 42, 43, 45, 208
Family dynamics, of care giving, 164
Family life cycle, 30, 72
Fatigue, 45, 57, 69, 177
Fear, 37, 39, 57, 59, 60, 66–68, 71, 73, 74, 76, 234, 305, 308, 363
Financial care, 5
FMLA, 46, 313
Frustration, 34, 36, 46, 58, 67–69, 71, 74, 76, 228, 339, 363

**H**
Health care providers, 15, 261, 262, 265, 268, 279, 281, 348
Healthcare
  professional caregivers, 10, 118
Hispanic Americans, 14, 197, 202, 203, 205, 207, 210–212, 214, 216
Hospice, 9, 37, 41
Huntington's disease, 38, 361
Hypertension, 270
Hysterical mothers, 66

**I**
ICIDH, 170
Illness, typology of, 29
Individual education plan (IEP), 247, 334, 335, 344, 347, 349
Individuals with Disabilities Education Act (IDEA), 3, 16, 106, 134, 307, 334
Informal caregiver, 5
Insomnia, 8, 12, 143
Integrated care organization (ICO), 348
Intellectual impairments, 40, 176, *see also* Domains of disability
International Classification of Diseases (ICD), 170
International Classification of Functioning, Disability and Health (ICF), 16, 138, 170–172, 175, 198, 362, 363, 368, 383
Interventions
  family-based, 41, 42, 145
  individual, 41
  medical, 66, 95, 118
  potential of, 184
  tailored, 279

**L**
Lawmakers, 46–48
Long term care planning, 327, 329, 339, 340, 343, 344, 346, 350
Longevity, 139, 168

# Index

## M
Maternal caregiving, 11
Maternal depression
  risk for, 76
Mediation care, 4
Mental disability, 5, 39, 40, 44, 113
Mental health, 4, 10, 11
Mental health problems, 142, 143, *see also* Depression
Mental impairments, 4
Mobility impairments, 198, *see also* Domains of disability
Mother-child interaction, 141

## N
National Alliance for Caregiving (NAC), 4
National Council on Disability (NCD), 311
National Family Caregiver Support Program (NFCSP), 48
National Family Caregivers Association (NFCA), 4
National Health Interview Survey (NHIS), 132, 150, 300
Negative feelings, 36, 76, 77
Nurse(s). *see* Professional caregivers

## O
Obesity, 203
Objective burden, 58
Occupational therapy, 8

## P
Pain, 177, 213, 228, 363
Pain-relieving medications, 361
Parental stress, 139, 141, 151, 414
Parent-child interactions, 140
Parenting Stress Index, 182
Parkinson's disease, 31
Paternal caregiving, 11
Patient-centered care, 340, 341, 343, 347
PCID, 339, 344, 346
Personal Assistance Services (PAS), 303–306, 319–321
Physical disability, 44, 113, 142, 144, 168, 176, 270, 301, 311, 315, 327
Physical morbidity, 132
Physical therapy, 8
Physician-patient encounters, 13
Physicians, 9, 25, 98, 169, 305, 342, 347
Policy makers, 8, 10, 23, 44, 47, 318, 330, 340
Problem-determined system, 24
Professional caregivers, 9, 11, 15, 27, 92, 102, 103, 111, 114, 116, 120, 228, 231, 233–235, 244, 363, 413

Psychiatric illnesses, long-term, 309
Psychiatric implants, 365
Psychiatric symptoms, 143, 146
Psychological morbidity, 132
Psychological problems, 58
Psychopathology, 43
Psychosomatic problems. *see* Depression

## Q
Quadriplegia, 23, 299

## R
Race, 6, 197, 200–202, 212, 214, 240, 332
Rehabilitation programs, 41
Robust programs, 8

## S
Schizophrenia, 179
SCI. *see* Spinal cord injury
Sensory impairments, 176, 198, 364, *see also* Domains of disability
Sensory losses, age related. *see* Domains of disability
Siblings, 8, 33, 61, 92, 96, 97, 100, 121, 140, 215, 415
Sickle cell disease, 39
Social education, 62
Socioeconomic status, 6, 43, 75, 77, 138, 197, 208–210, 216, 218, 332
Speech therapy, 8
Spina bifida, 306
Spinal cord injury, 169, 198, 261, 265, 266, 299, 306, 365
Spirituality, 14, 228–232, 234, 251, 411
Stress, 140
Stroke, 75, 92, 116, 198, 235, 275, 365, 367, 368
Supplemental Security Income (SSI), 148, 149
Supplementary Medical Insurance (SMI), 314
Support programs, 3, 8, 93, 94, 99, 102, 106, 111, 112, 123, 216, 329, 349

## T
Technologies, 281, 361, 364, 368, 380, 382
Technologies, bio-hybrid, 377
Technologies, emerging, 16, 363–366, 368, 369, 375, 377, 381, 383
Technologies, long-distance, 262, 275, 276
Technologies, medical, 132
Technologies, robotic, 364, 369
Therapy services, 95
Training, 11, 15, 94, 99, 100, 104, 105, 109, 114, 119, 120, 122, 123, 268, 298, 306, 316, 317, 415

Training caregivers, 116, 122
Train-the-trainer models, 110
Trauma, 23, 29, 43, 413
Traumatic brain injury (TBI), 29, 196, 198, 272, 278, 279, 281, 381
Triangulation, 42

**V**
Visual impairments, 20

**W**
Western culture, 37
World Health Organization (WHO), 113, 170, 171, 198

Printed by Books on Demand, Germany

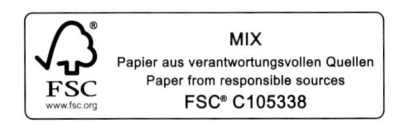